Pharmacology

A handbook for complementary healthcare professionals

Commissioning Editor: Claire Wilson
Development Editor: Kerry McGechie
Project Manager: Frances Affleck
Designer: Charlotte Murray
Illustrator: Artbits
Illustration Manager: Merlyn Harvey

Pharmacology

A handbook for complementary healthcare professionals

Elaine M Aldred

BSc (Hons), DC, Lic Ac, Dip Herb Med, Dip CHM

Chiropractor, acupuncturist, western and Chinese herbalist in private practice;
Lecturer in Pharmacology and Toxicology at the Northern College of Acupuncture;
Lecturer in Western Medicine at the Northern College of Acupuncture, UK

Forewords by

Charles Buck

Reader in Acupuncture and Chinese Medicine,
Northern College of Acupuncture, York, UK

Kenneth Vall

Principal, Anglo–European College of Chiropractic,
Bournemouth, UK

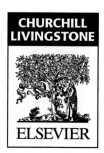

CHURCHILL
LIVINGSTONE

ELSEVIER

EDINBURGH   LONDON   NEW YORK   OXFORD   PHILADELPHIA   ST LOUIS   SYDNEY   TORONTO   2009

CHURCHILL
LIVINGSTONE
ELSEVIER

An imprint of Elsevier Limited

First published 2009

ISBN: 9780-4430-6896-0

British Library Cataloguing in Publication Data
A catalogue record for this book is available from the British Library

Library of Congress Cataloging in Publication Data
A catalog record for this book is available from the Library of Congress

Notice
Knowledge and best practice in this field are constantly changing. As new research and experience broaden our knowledge, changes in practice, treatment and drug therapy may become necessary or appropriate. Readers are advised to check the most current information provided (i) on procedures featured or (ii) by the manufacturer of each product to be administered, to verify the recommended dose or formula, the method and duration of administration, and contraindications. It is the responsibility of the practitioner, relying on their own experience and knowledge of the patient, to make diagnoses, to determine dosages and the best treatment for each individual patient, and to take all appropriate safety precautions. To the fullest extent of the law, neither the Publisher nor the Author assumes any liability for any injury and/or damage to persons or property arising out or related to any use of the material contained in this book.

The Publisher

Printed in the United States of America

Transferred to Digital Printing, 2011

The
Publisher's
policy is to use
**paper manufactured
from sustainable forests**

Foreword

When the UK's *New Scientist* magazine ran a special issue on complementary and alternative medicine (CAM), one contributor doubted whether an alternative therapist would know the difference between a leukocyte and a lump of cheese. This is a good example of the tendency for observers to display uninformed prejudices outside their field of expertise and thereby misrepresent the true state of the lead CAM professions. At that time, the medical herbalist at my clinic had a PhD in genetics, I was supervising acupuncture MSc students and my assistant acupuncturist had a PhD in biochemistry having previously worked for some years as a lecturer in a distinguished UK medical school. Clearly a gap exists between perception and reality. CAM professionals might not have to hold higher degrees in science but unless we are content to inhabit the medical fringes no practitioner can afford to be ignorant of clinical sciences. Today we are expected to be medically literate; medical ignorance is a hallmark of the vestiges of fringe medicine. Elaine's book reflects this new maturity by offering readers a compact, lucid and practical overview of pharmaceutical sciences.

Prejudices such as those mentioned above have served a useful function as they have helped dispel complacency and acted as a motivating force towards ongoing improvement in professional standards and education. This has already happened to such an extent that the notion of CAM practitioners as well-meaning but scientifically ignorant purveyors of placebo is outdated and quite inappropriate for today's serious CAM therapists. In just a few decades the training and regulation of professions such as acupuncture, osteopathy–chiropractic, nutritional therapy and herbal medicine has been transformed. Today's therapists value comprehensive medical skills comparable with established medicine in the West; the colleges expect it and the profession's regulators expect it. Science-based medical knowledge has wider ownership. The imperative to develop and maintain higher levels of skills comes from patients too; savvy consumers expect to see skills that are in line with those seen in conventional healthcare. Patients often come to consultations already well-informed about their condition and with an understanding of the pros and cons of conventional biomedical treatment. Many will lose faith if their practitioner does not appear to understand modern medicine but, at the same time, few are content to be passive and trusting recipients of care, pharmaceutical or alternative. Instead, patients want involvement, active participation and a clear understanding of their options – conventional and alternative. Patients increasingly wish to understand what they are taking and they expect their therapists, both CAM and biomedical, to understand them too. This expectation applies all the more to those of us who offer herbs or nutritionally based treatments; we need to know how the substances we and others prescribe affect our patients.

This is not to proclaim that CAM therapists have abandoned or diluted their holistic or traditional paradigms, there is no reason why we cannot operate different medical systems side by side. This recognition that there is strength in diversity and choice can also be taken as a general measure of professional maturity in medical practice. Few modern CAM practitioners would maintain the fundamentalist view that their holistic explanatory models are entirely contrary to, or intended to replace, science. Instead, they are seen as complements or alternatives. Diverse healthcare models can be appreciated as valid and real – able to grasp clinical reality in different ways. Each model has its strengths and weaknesses, its insights and its blind spots; skilled practitioners should know which model is appropriate for the clinical situation in hand. Primary care physicians usually appreciate, for instance, that pharmaceutical options are limited for early and mid-stage osteoarthritis and so often refer patients for acupuncture or other treatment; most CAM therapists would acknowledge that a patient with a 2-kg ovarian cyst is probably best referred for surgery. Now, as emerging CAM professionals gain a deeper understanding of biomedicine, increasing numbers of orthodox medical practitioners and managers are aware of evidence-based alternative models of health. In the UK the trend towards mutual understanding is reflected in more CAM awareness modules in nursing, medical and physiotherapy training schools.

In some countries such integration is already long established. Doctors and medical insurers in Germany routinely provide herbal treatment for depression and acupuncture for migraine, back pain and knee arthritis because these are proven to be cost effective. China's health service describes this relationship between modern and traditional medicine in their 'walking on two legs' healthcare policy. Over 200 million patients are treated annually in China's hospitals using traditional Chinese medicine and acupuncture. For 40 years, China has decreed that its traditional doctors must learn biomedicine and that its biomedical doctors learn the basics of traditional medicine. A conventional dermatologist there, when faced with a patient with alopecia, for example, knows that biomedicine has little to offer and is very likely to refer for Chinese herb treatment. Conversely, when a Chinese herb doctor sees elderly patients with stomach pain they will routinely refer for gastroscopy to rule out malignancy. This enlightened interchange is surely beneficial for patients but might be seen as threatening to the protectionist instincts of some sections of established medicine. A rational, humanitarian-based appraisal of patients' best options is too easily distorted by the imperatives of business and medi-politics in promoting prejudice and defending territory.

Elaine's book is emblematic of the emerging spirit of maturity in the lead CAM professions. Professional standards now rule. More and more universities in Europe, North America and Australia offer CAM degrees or validate the qualifications awarded by private CAM colleges, often up to higher degree levels. In the UK, professions such as acupuncture and herbal medicine have been models of self-regulation for many years with an eye to scrutiny from government health regulators and the public. With mature educational accreditation processes now in place, akin to those in established healthcare professions, we can better ensure that educational and course content standards are high. *Pharmacology: A handbook for complementary healthcare professionals* is part of this trend.

With today's CAM curriculum expanding to include more clinical science content, students are often surprised to discover how much they enjoy the anatomy and physiology modules in their training – they are mostly seen as relevant and engaging. Pharmacology, though, can be a tough component to teach. A large and complex subject, heavy with biochemical jargon, its relevance to CAM practice is not always immediately apparent. Students complain, 'We do not want to be allopathic medic', 'We don't prescribe drugs, why do we have to learn pharmacology'. Answer? 'Herbs, many supplements and even many foods *are* drugs, you have to understand what they do'. Furthermore, patients coming to our clinics, more often than not, are already taking prescribed drugs and clinicians need to understand how these drugs affect them. The problem is that if you are training as a CAM therapist and your biomedicine textbooks contain no mention of the substances you are intending to use therapeutically, learning can easily become a dismal struggle. Really efficient learning processes take place when we are being engaged and entertained by the material and this is more likely to happen when the material is relevant to our needs and relates to us as learners. This is why existing texts are problematic and is why this new text so neatly meets the long-standing need for a clear, succinct and relevant summary of a vast field.

As pharmacology tutor on various CAM courses at first degree and Master's levels, Elaine has been frustrated by the lack of relevant existing texts. Devising her own ways of making the subject relevant, concise and interesting, *Pharmacology: A handbook for complementary healthcare professionals* has grown out of her handouts and teaching materials, resulting in a text that understands and acknowledges the CAM student perspective. Well placed to present this material, Elaine is truly medically multilingual and multicultural, she writes as an insider both to CAM and biomedicine.

Those who contribute to the education of CAM therapists are more effective when they have the rapport that comes with having a mindset that matches that of the learner. Good teachers are often insiders to biomedicine who have defected to become insiders to CAM, with the flexibility of mind to recognise the power and value of biomedicine but able to stretch their minds beyond that into other perspectives. Colleges have sometimes employed tutors well-qualified to teach the biomedical modules but whose perspective on CAM is that of an outsider. Students quickly sense that something is wrong, the teaching focus shifts to irrelevancies, educational rapport fails and learning suffers. Elaine's contribution in offering this book is, in this sense, a hermeneutic one, informed by and inherently respectful to both science and CAM.

Elaine's eclectic outlook encompasses a spirited mix of convention, medical heresy and the territory in between. She followed her first degree in biochemistry and chemistry with a diploma in chiropractic, a diploma in Western herbal medicine and later professional acupuncture training. Coming next to study Chinese herbal medicine, she fell under my tutelage for four years at the Northern College of Acupuncture (UK), where I was principal lecturer. A knowledge vampire, Elaine took every drop she could get from the college, its tutors and from her ever-present rucksack of weighty Chinese and Western medical tomes. Later employed to teach pharmacology at the college, she identified the need for a textbook pitched to be more digestible for CAM therapists. I am not aware of any other textbook that covers this ground in this way.

Readers will find here the standard take on the relationship between pharmaceutically active substances and our biochemistry and physiology all presented in an efficient lucid format. Few words or ideas are redundant or wasted. This is made more engaging for us by the use of examples of medicinal herbs and dietary components.

So, before you begin let's clear up that leukocyte–cheese issue, I think I understand the difference. *Leuko* is Latin for 'milk' and *cyte* basically means 'blob',* so leukocyte means 'blobby stuff made out of milk' – also known as cheese!

Still not Read on ...

Charles Buck
Reader in Acupuncture and Chinese Medicine
Northern College of Acupuncture, York, UK

---

*Actually, *cyte* comes from the Greek *kytos* meaning 'hollow vessel'.

Foreword

This book, entitled *Pharmacology: A handbook for complementary healthcare professionals*, is a useful tool for all healthcare practitioners within the so-called complementary sector. The author, Elaine Aldred, represents this sector well, as she holds degrees and competencies in chiropractic, acupuncture and herbal medicine. She has written this book as a result of her frustration as a lecturer with material currently available to students in the complementary healthcare sector, and also for practitioners out in the field as a quick and relevant source of comprehensive information on pharmacology.

Being the principal of the Anglo–European College of Chiropractic, a higher education institution devoted to chiropractic education, and also a practitioner, I share Elaine's frustrations and I will be pleased to add this book to the reading list for our students. It will also become handy in my own practice as there is no doubt that we need to understand the correct approaches to the use of pharmacology in patient treatments. Specifically, understanding pharmacodynamics and kinetics, the risk–benefit profile of a drug, its drug interactions and the relevance of its use in our patient care is essential in a holistic approach to health.

The content of the book has a logical approach, starting with an explanation of the basic principles of pharmacology and gradually putting the building blocks together for a complete understanding of the use and action of pharmacology suitable for its audience.

For this audience it is essential not only that the basic principles of pharmacology are dealt with to give the student or practitioner a solid grounding but that the material also allows for a deeper and more detailed understanding.

As the aim of the book is to bridge the gap between orthodox and complementary fields in the understanding of pharmacology, it is inevitable that it focuses on vitamins and minerals relevant to pharmacology, ensuring the complementary practitioner's understanding of possible interactions of supplementation provided in conjunction with orthodox medication. The book therefore describes the major classes of drugs that affect the respiratory, cardiovascular and gastrointestinal systems, and how these relate to physiological and gastrophysiological mechanisms.

The section on plant metabolites used in herbal medicine adds great value to the book for the complementary practitioner, particularly for those who need to develop a deeper understanding of the use of herbal medicine and, of course, for students from all sectors of complementary medicine.

The section on toxicology and laboratory tests follows a fairly standard format but is nevertheless an essential ingredient in a book like this.

The introduction to the principles of evidence medicine is perhaps brief but still important. All complementary medicine is being judged by the yardstick of orthodoxy and it rarely matches up to expectations. Someone once said that if you play tennis you should not be judged by the rules of golf. I fear that complementary medicine often finds itself in this dilemma. Our treatment of patients or patient encounters are often so individualistic and specific that evidence of efficacy or efficiency is often lost in the orthodox randomized clinical trial paradigm. This does not mean that there is no evidence that what we do works, it means that we have to strive to find a new paradigm for such measurement.

Although this book is not intented to be a bedtime read, it can be read cover to cover, equally useful for student and practitioner, and I thoroughly recommend it.

Kenneth Vall
Principal
Anglo-European College of Chiropractic
Bournemouth, UK

"Even the journey of a thousand miles begins with the first step"

Old Chinese Proverb

X

Contents

xiii

Acknowledgements

I would like to thank the herbal students of the Northern College of Acupuncture for being so co-operative and diligent in their studies. Without them it would have been very difficult to understand how to present this book.

Dr Richard Adams, Dr Gina Bajek and Dr Alistair Mclachlan for their input on the orthodox medicine section.

Dr Jenni Bolton and David O'Neill of the Anglo–European College of Chiropractic Bournemouth for their advice on Chapter 42 Information gathering and the final analysis.

My family, as always, for supporting me physically and emotionally, allowing the opportunity for me to write.

Introduction

This book has probably been in the making for at least 20 years. At Chiropractic College, I was forced to wade through enormous tomes on orthodox pharmacology in order to weed out those drugs relevant to my professional needs from the more obscure ones whose use was limited to the highly supervised environment of a hospital.

As a herbalist, my frustration only grew further as I found that the chemistry associated with the therapeutic use of herbs was presented in an equally technical manner, and seemly divorced from my clinical needs. Although these kinds of book are excellent as reference tools, for overloaded students or busy practitioners there is simply too much material to be sifted through in the time they might have available. Another problem can arise from the books' authors being experts on the subject but usually not clinicians. This tends to make the material difficult to relate to everyday clinical practice.

Things finally came to a head for me when I was asked to teach pharmacology to herbal students, which made me actively address a subject that is considered by most students to be nothing more than a 'hoop-jumping' exercise in the process of becoming qualified. This made me seek a way of making pharmacology meaningful. To this end, I decided to teach pharmacology from the ground up, giving basic principles on which the students could build and relate to their clinical experiences.

Overcoming a natural resistance to the subject, however, is difficult on the grounds that pharmacology is perceived by students and practitioners as a subject only accessible to those with a scientific frame of mind. On a workable clinical level this is simply not true.

I was certainly not the most adept scientist at school and found my university course a trial. I realized later that this was because my subject was being presented from a purely academic viewpoint, with little reference to its application in the real world. I need – like many other complementary practitioners when presented with pure science – my work to be linked to the information presented if it is to be meaningful.

So, when writing this book I decided to cut the principles of pharmacology back to the bare minimum to leave a platform from which to present the subject as applicable to the complementary healthcare profession. Although this book can be used as a quick-reference book for a specific subject, if the reader takes time to methodically work through it, then pharmacology in the field of herbal medicine, nutrition and orthodox medicine not only becomes clear but also a source of enlightenment. This enlightenment should break down the final resistance to a subject that is not only fascinating but empowering to the practitioner who grasps it with both hands. Taking it on board, it is possible to see that art and science can live side by side, providing you have an open mind.

Having said this pharmacology is not an area of instant comprehension. Like playing a musical instrument, it takes time to build up proficiency. The way the book has been constructed, however, with numerous cross-references, should make the process easier.

This book has not been written as a definitive guide to every possible aspect of pharmacology, in fact it might, by those well-versed in the subject, be criticized as too simplistic. I have for example mainly used bibliographies, restricting references to instances where the material is not commonly found in the textbooks available on the subject. It is my experience that in a book of this nature too many references are off-putting.

Any omissions are generally in areas where the items are not normally encountered in clinical practice, e.g. in Chapter 22 'Terpenes', the sesterpenes – which are not normally found in plant material – have been left out, as have the more obscure orthodox drugs. I have relied on 20 years of clinical experience to cover the subjects you are mostly likely to need on a daily basis; the final chapter outlines some basic principles on how to investigate a query further.

Pharmacology can be learned by rote, so it is possible to know that flavonoids are antioxidants or that chemotherapy kills cancer cells. However, understanding the underlying principles of pharmacology enables a practitioner to use it intelligently: to see beneath a presenting condition to recognize that it might be a side effect of a drug, or to anticipate a possible interaction of a herb with a drug.

A reasonable grasp of pharmacology is rapidly becoming a necessary skill in the field of complementary medicine as the choice and use of orthodox medications becomes more complex and might possibly impact on the treatment being given.

A Few Notes on the Text

On the basis of 'a picture speaks louder than words', chemical structures will be shown where appropriate to give the reader a better understanding as to why a particular chemical might exert a particular effect or merely for comparison with a chemical of a similar property. However, some orthodox medication, for instance that used for epilepsy, is so varied that it is not possible to relate structure to function so easily.

The 'orthodox medication' sections do not cover the more specialized medications or medication that are used only with close medical supervision, e.g. hospital use, unless they are in some way relevant to clinical practice.

Throughout the book, unless a specific topic is being discussed, the generic name of the chemical will be used. This might refer to a component of a herb, nutritional supplement, food or drug.

The priority in which medication is given will not be discussed as the guidelines dictating the order in which, for example, hypertensive drugs should be administered alters depending on new research that emerges. A chapter outlining sources for such information is included at the end of the book.

As none of the readers of the book will be prescribing medication, it is enough to be aware of their respective country's guidelines, for example the National Centre for Health and Clinical Excellence (NICE) in the UK produces guidelines for doctors to follow.

There is an element of 'chicken and egg' to presenting pharmacology, in that it might be necessary to introduce complex molecules before the reader actually needs to understand them in more detail. However, for the sake of completeness and cross-referencing (always a good method of understanding a subject) they have been included briefly.

Conclusion

If you take the time to work through the book systematically you will be able to start to read drug and herbal monographs in more depth and with more application, and to interpret research papers to a reasonable degree and relate them to your clinical experience. The final chapter in the book gives information on reliable websites and also a very basic introduction to aspects of evidence-based medicine and pure laboratory research.

Understanding the principles of pharmacology will enable you to make more informed choices in the treatment of your patients and will add to your ability to successfully manage a case.

Section 1

Basic pharmacological principles

The atom: the smallest unit of pharmacology

2

To achieve a confident working knowledge of pharmacology you need a sound understanding of the structure, and therefore the function, of the basic unit of chemistry: the **atom**.

What is an Atom?

- An atom is the smallest complete unit that cannot be broken up by chemical means. It has chemical properties in its own right.
- Atoms of exactly the same composition behave in exactly the same way in chemical reactions.
- These identical atoms are called **elements** (later in the text, this term will be used interchangeably with atom).
- Different atoms or elements can combine with each other to form chemical compounds, which can be relatively small, like a water molecule, or extremely large and complex, like the DNA helix.

Atoms consist of (Figure 2.1):

- a **nucleus**

- **electrons** orbiting around the nucleus.

The Nucleus

The nucleus is made up of **protons** and **neutrons**:

- **Protons** have a positive charge.
- **Neutrons** have no charge.

For the level of pharmacology covered in this book, the presence of **neutrons** is acknowledged here for completeness but they will not be discussed any further.

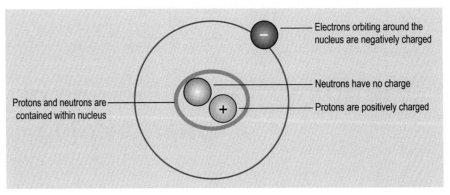

Figure 2.1 Composition of an atom. Overall charge is neutral as the negative charge of the electron orbiting around the nucleus is neutralized by the positive charge of the proton in the nucleus.

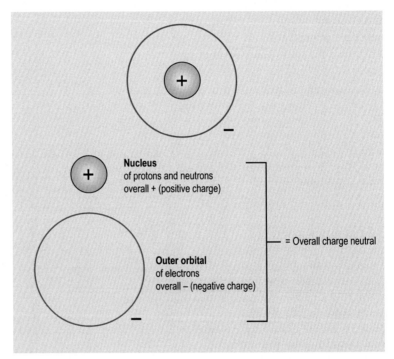

Figure 2.2 The general atomic structure without the details of the composition of the nucleus. From now on the nucleus will be represented without differentiation of protons or neutrons.

The Electrons

Like moons around a planet, **electrons** orbit around the nucleus (Figure 2.2). The space in which they move around the nucleus is therefore called an **orbital**.

How are Electrons Arranged Around the Nucleus?

Convention dictates that each orbital has a fixed number of available slots that can be filled until they reach capacity. Once an orbital becomes filled, the electrons start to fill the available slots in the next, higher orbital (the next orbital away from the nucleus). In this way, the bigger the atom, the more electrons it will have, and the more orbitals these electrons will need to fill (or occupy) around the nucleus, as can be seen in Figure 2.3.

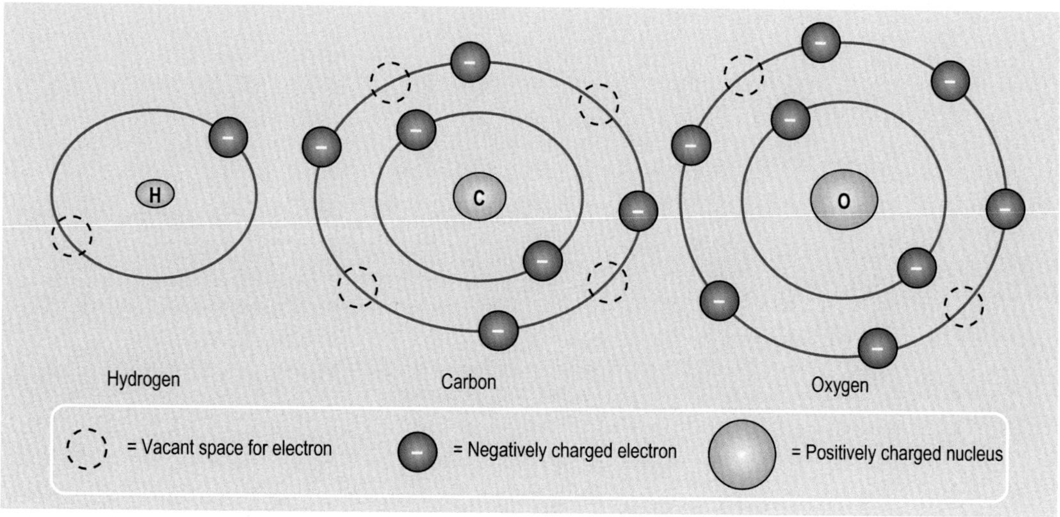

Figure 2.3 Demonstrating how atoms of different sizes have different orbitals.

It is important not to think of **electron orbitals** as being two dimensional; in fact, they can take several different three-dimensional paths around the nucleus. For simplicity's sake, however, the atomic structure is kept to a circular two-dimensional shape in diagrams, as this is accepted convention.

The Structure of an Atom

An atom always seeks stability. So, under normal conditions, the number of electrons orbiting around the nucleus exactly equals the number of protons in the nucleus:

Number of electrons = Number of protons

The Electron is the Key to Pharmacology

Usually, protons in the nucleus remain tightly bound to the nucleus. This means they have to **stay where they are** and will take part in a reaction only under extreme conditions, e.g. in the presence of bombardment by high-energy particles such as a radioactive reaction. As this is not a chemical reaction, it is not relevant to pharmacology. Electrons, however, are not so tightly bound and it does not take too much energy to encourage the electrons to take part in different chemical reactions:

- Electrons interacting with other atoms (which is what happens in **bonding**) can form more complex structures (**molecules**) (Chapter 3 'Bonds found in biological chemistry', p. 11 and Chapter 4 'Bonds continued', p. 21).
- Electrons can also shift in position to an unoccupied orbit at a higher level, rather like a ball being kicked from flat ground to a level higher up a slope. The return of the electron (the ball rolling back down the slope) to its original position releases valuable energy that can be harnessed and used by a biological organism. This is what happens in photosynthesis (Figure 2.4; Chapter 9 'Carbohydrates', p. 63).
- Electrons can also be traded like currency between specialized molecules to create energy (this happens in units in the cell called **mitochondria** which contain special molecules to do this, in a process called **oxidative phosphorylation**). This is similar to having water flowing down a hill and having small water wheels positioned at intervals to take advantage of the energy the movement of the water creates (Figure 2.5)

9

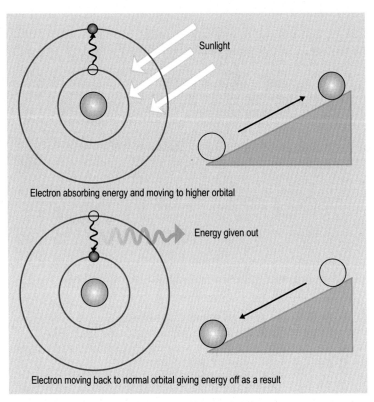

Figure 2.4 Showing the movement of an electron in photosynthesis.

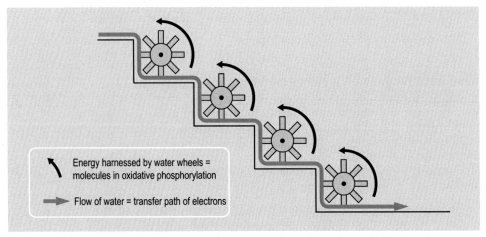

Figure 2.5 Analogy showing how electron transfer creates energy and how this can be harnessed.

- Under certain circumstances, electrons can also be made to take part in reactions that should not occur and are detrimental to the function of human tissue. These aberrant molecules are called free radicals (see Chapter 7 'Free radicals', p. 41).

From these few examples it is possible to see the important role electrons have to play in pharmacology.

Bonds found in biological chemistry

3

Each electron orbital has a specific allocation of spaces available for electrons to fill (see Figure 2.3, p. 9). In the case of the outer orbitals, it is unusual to find all the spaces empty or full and one atom will seek out another compatible atom so that they can share their respective electrons and fill their outer orbitals. This arrangement creates great stability for the associated atoms, which is why, whenever possible, bonds are formed, between individual atoms.

Taking the examples of hydrogen and carbon used in Chapter 2 (Figure 2.3), it is possible to see that hydrogen:

- has one electron in the outer orbital
- needs to combine with elements that will provide one electron to fill its outer orbital.

However, carbon:

- has two electrons in the first orbital, which is therefore full
- has four electrons in the second orbital
- needs four electrons to complete its outer orbital, making a total of eight electrons for a full orbital.

The final result of this union is that four hydrogen atoms attach themselves to one carbon atom, thus filling the outer orbitals of both the carbon and the hydrogens satisfying the needs of both elements (Figure 3.1).

It is a matter of simple arithmetic to work out where this leads: a more complex molecule – ethane – can be formed from two carbon atoms and six hydrogen atoms Figure 3.2. The process can be continued to make an even longer compound called propane (Figure 3.3).

Note: as drawing chemicals out in this way can become complicated, there is a need for a method of abbreviation. Each figure, therefore, contains examples of

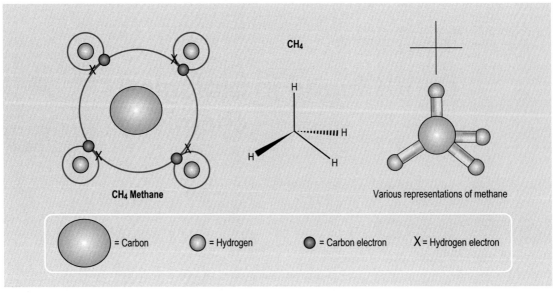

Figure 3.1 Formation of methane, with additional diagrams showing some of the more common chemical representations of this molecule.

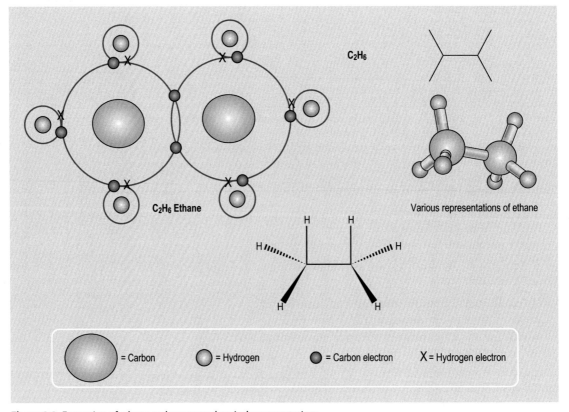

Figure 3.2 Formation of ethane and common chemical representations.

various chemical shorthands used to represent these structures. This will enable you to become used to seeing them. Naming and representation will be covered in more detail in Chapter 5 'Nomenclature: representation of chemical structures and basic terminology'.

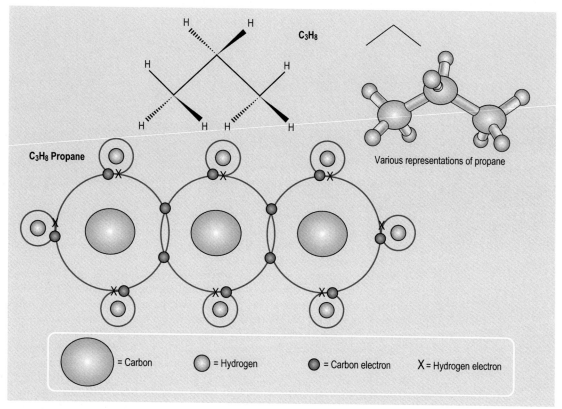

C_3H_8

C_3H_8 Propane

Various representations of propane

⬤ = Carbon   ◯ = Hydrogen   ⬤ = Carbon electron   X = Hydrogen electron

Figure 3.3 Formation of propane.

The Significance of Different Types of Bond

The way elements bond dictates the function of the particular chemical compound they create. A basic understanding of how atoms interact will help you understand the pharmacology you will encounter in your work.

Covalent Bonds

Bonds, formed by completely equal sharing of electrons, such as the previous examples, are called **covalent bonds**. This principle of bond formation can be applied to other elements, such as oxygen, nitrogen and sulphur, to create various organic compounds that can be structural or part of the metabolic processes of a plant or animal.

Covalent bonds have set bond lengths and angles, dictated by the electron orbitals of the atoms that are bonding together. Each atom has a distinctive arrangement of electrons due to the:

- electrical field produced by the orbiting electrons
- distance the outer orbital is from the nucleus
- shape of the orbital (Figure 3.4), as mostly electrons do not move in a perfectly circular orbit around the nucleus.

For a greater appreciation, blow up balloons of different shapes and arrange them as you see them in Figure 3.4. The different balloons are the accepted shapes of

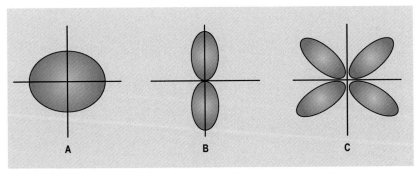

Figure 3.4 Different shapes of electron clouds.

electron orbitals and the shape of the electrostatic force created by this orbital. Notice how it is possible to bend the orbital shown in B around the axis, but that in C the movement around the axis is restricted because the sides of the balloons push against one another limiting movement.

Electron clouds are not solid but are negatively charged (like similar poles on magnets), which means that they repel one another to a particular distance and therefore into a particular shape, as in the balloon experiment. Therefore, when several of these clouds are in close proximity, which is what occurs when several atoms bond to form a molecule, the molecule acquires a specific shape.

Naturally, the above is a very simplistic explanation of what really happens, but it is important at this stage to appreciate that chemistry, and therefore pharmacology, is three dimensional, and it is very necessary to starting thinking in three dimensions to gain a proper appreciation of pharmacology, as the three-dimensional concept is very important when considering how chemicals (substrates) fit into sites that activate physiological processes.

Each substrate and site has a specific shape and in many cases only certain molecules will be allowed to fit into the site, which may be on an enzyme, the surface of a cell or at a nerve ending (see Chapter 11 'Amino acids and proteins', p. 85 and Chapter 19 'Pharmacodynamics: how drugs elicit a physiological effect', p. 137).

Importance of Covalent Bonds

Covalent bonds are the strongest bonds in nature and under normal biological conditions have to be broken with the help of enzymes. This is due to the even sharing of electrons between the bonded atoms and as with anything equally shared there is no conflict to weaken the arrangement. There are two types of covalent bond:

- non-polar: possess no charge
- polar: possess a charge.

● Non-polar covalent bonds (Figure 3.5(i), Figure 3.6)

- These are very strong bonds.
- The electrons in the adjacent atoms are shared equally, which means that there is no push/pull effect (dipole moment; see below).

Example of relevance to pharmacology: Covalent bonds are found in protein chains where two sulphurs are joined together (**disulphide bonds**) (Figure 3.7). In antibody molecules, the disulphide bond firmly holds the two parts of the antibody together, allowing the rest of the structure to hinge around it. This flexibility is an important part of the function of an antibody as it allows the antibody binding sites to adapt in binding to antigens and reach more antigen sites.

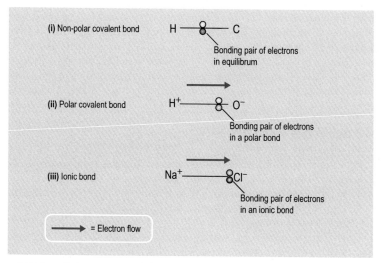

Figure 3.5 The relative positions of the bonding pair of electrons in (i) a non-polar covalent bond, (ii) a polar covalent bond and (iii) an ionic bond.

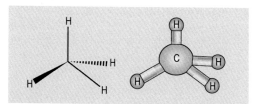

Figure 3.6 Non-polar methane. Electrons are shared evenly between the carbon and hydrogen atoms. Note how each hydrogen is not only at the same distance from the carbon but also arranged at the same angle.

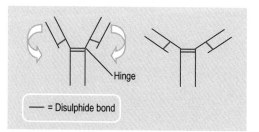

Figure 3.7 The disulphide bond in an antibody maintains rigidity while also providing flexibility.

• Polar covalent bonds (Figure 3.5(ii))

- A **polar covalent bond** is still very strong, but the electron sharing between the atoms is unequal.
- **One atom is able to pull more strongly on the electrons than the other**, so that the part of the molecule which pulls the electrons towards it is **relatively negatively charged** while the other part of the molecule which has had the electrons pulled away from it is **relatively positively charged**.

The following is an example of the pharmacological relevance of a polar covalent bond:

Water has the formula of H_2O = one oxygen atom + two hydrogen atoms

The atomic composition of oxygen compared to that of hydrogen is far more attractive to electrons than both of the hydrogen atoms and it is able to exert a much more powerful pull on the shared electrons than the hydrogen atoms. The **oxygen therefore becomes more negatively charged** as it pulls the bonding pair of electrons closer towards it.

The average electron density around the oxygen atom is 10 times the amount around the hydrogen atom. This **charge separation** creates something called a **dipole moment**, as the oxygen has a **partial negative charge** and the hydrogen a **partial** positive charge (Figure 3.8(i)). Water is actually a fascinating molecule, the pharmacological importance of which will become evident as the book progresses.

The dipole moment described above also occurs in amino acids (Figure 3.8(ii); see also Chapter 11 'Amino acids and proteins', p. 86) and becomes important in the temporary binding of chemicals to proteins, which are made up of amino acids, for example at enzyme binding sites or binding of chemicals to plasma proteins.

'Oil and Water Don't Mix'

Whether a molecule is **charged** (**polar**) or **not charged** (**non-polar**) has great relevance when it comes to pharmacology. As explained above, the electron bonding between two elements such as carbon and hydrogen is equally shared so the union is well balanced. Because of this equilibrium, methane (see Figure 3.1 and Figure 3.9) has no charge (i.e. it is **non-polar**).

However, as you have seen, oxygen **exerts a much greater electrostatic charge than hydrogen**, and so draws electrons towards itself, creating a **dipole moment** and therefore a charged molecule (see Figure 3.5(ii) and Figure 3.9). You now know that where there is a dipole moment the molecule becomes charged.

You might have heard the phrase '**oil and water do not mix**'; more than likely this is something you will have experienced when making a vinaigrette dressing. Shaking the components of the dressing together seems to mix them, but the effect is only temporary and the mixture soon separates out into two layers, with the oily part sitting on top. Mixing two different types of oil, however, is easy and there is no separation.

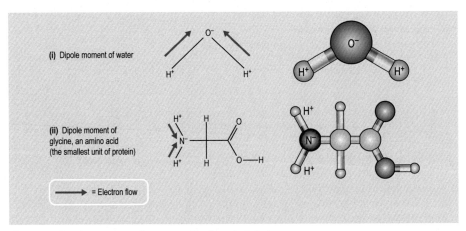

(i) Dipole moment of water

(ii) Dipole moment of glycine, an amino acid (the smallest unit of protein)

⟶ = Electron flow

Figure 3.8 Dipole moments of a water molecule and of glycine.

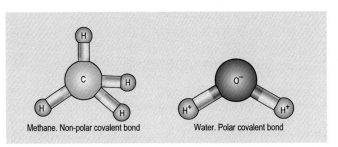

Methane. Non-polar covalent bond

Water. Polar covalent bond

Figure 3.9 The non-polar covalent bond of methane (CH_4) and the polar covalent bond of water (H_2O). (Look also at the shape of the molecule created by the bonds.)

The separation occurs because water and oil have different characteristics, water being **polar** (**charged**) and oil (the backbone of which is made up of carbons) being **non-polar** (**uncharged**).

Polar compounds tend to be **water loving** (**hydrophilic**) whereas **non-polar** compounds tend to be **water hating** (**hydrophobic**). Some natural compounds are large enough to have a bit of both qualities in their structure, which creates some very interesting pharmacological situations.

The importance of polar and non-polar compounds will soon become clear, and a basic understanding of this type of bond, and of hydrogen bonds, will make basic pharmacology much easier to understand.

Ionic Bonds (Figure 3.5(iii))

As previously discussed, all atoms like to have full outer orbitals (see Chapter 2 'The atom: the smallest unit of pharmacology', p. 7). Elements such as chlorine and sodium are very unstable on their own because:

- chlorine is short of one electron in its outer shell
- sodium has only one electron in its outer shell.

Both elements are desperately seeking a way of creating stability, in this case by chlorine acquiring another electron in its outer shell and by sodium losing its electron:

- Chlorine + 1 electron = stability
- Sodium − 1 electron = stability

When the nucleus is relatively large and only one electron is involved, the reactivity of the element is very vigorous as it achieves stability. This is why, when sodium and chlorine atoms come into contact, a great deal of energy is released (this can be seen in the safe environment of a laboratory).

The chlorine snatches the electron from the sodium atom, making its outer orbital stable, but leaving sodium with a positive charge (Figure 3.10). The sodium atom has thus become a positively charged sodium ion (Na^+). This is because the protons in the nucleus normally exactly equal the negative electrons in the outer shell (see Figure 2.1, p. 8). Sodium is now short of an electron and so, overall, gains a positive charge:

- Before ionic bonding = 11 protons + 11 electrons
- After ionic bonding = 11 protons + 10 electrons
- Therefore **overall positive charge is +1**

Using the same principle, the chlorine has an extra electron, which gives it an overall negative charge, so it is now a negatively charged chloride ion:

- Before ionic bonding = 11 protons + 11 electrons
- After ionic bonding = 11 protons + 10 electrons
- Therefore **overall negative charge −1**

As always, the reality is not as simple as this, but for the purposes of the book it is fine to make this assumption.

As ions of opposite charge are attracted to one another, like opposite poles of a magnet, they form a type of bond called an **ionic bond**. Thus a salt crystal (of the variety you use on your food) is a lattice of ionic bonds (Figure 3.11).

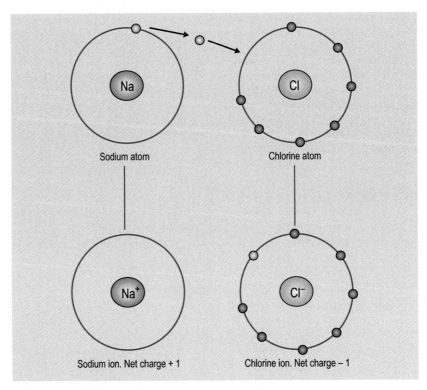

Figure 3.10 The formation of ions.

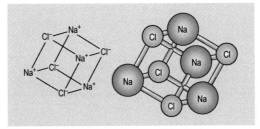

Figure 3.11 The basic lattice of a sodium chloride salt crystal and its three-dimensional model. These units link together to form visible crystals.

Hydrogen Bonds

Hydrogen bonds are very special as they are, strictly speaking, not true bonds but forces of attraction between the hydrogen atoms in one molecule and atoms of high electronegativity in other molecules. This situation is due to the uneven sharing of the bonding electron pair in a polar covalent bond (see Figure 3.5(ii)).

The strength of the hydrogen bond is only one-tenth that of a covalent bond, but when a large number of hydrogen bonds are formed between two molecules or areas of the same molecule the overall result is very strong.

The section on polar bonds above shows that the hydrogen attached to nitrogen or oxygen becomes relatively positively charged, as the nitrogen and oxygen atoms, pulling the electrons towards them, become relatively negatively charged (see Figure 3.8)

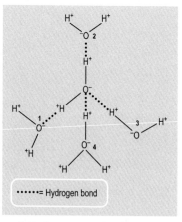

Figure 3.12 One water molecule can form four hydrogen bonds.

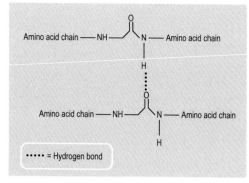

Figure 3.13 Hydrogen bonding in protein chains.

Hydrogen Bonding in Water

The relatively negatively charged oxygen atom in a water molecule is able to attract positively charged hydrogen atoms attached to other water molecules. Simple mathematics then dictates that each water molecule has the potential to form four hydrogen bonds with surrounding water molecules (Figure 3.12). This enables water to form a type of lattice even as a liquid, a phenomenon that accounts for its relatively high boiling point compared with molecules of a similar size, which are gaseous at the same temperature. It also explains why ice floats and water freezes from the top downwards.

There is a constant exchange of hydrogen between water molecules but the overall integrity stays the same providing the temperature does not get too high and agitates the molecules beyond a level where they can stick together.

A molecule that has a tightly and securely bound non-polar covalent bond cannot form a hydrogen bond.

This form of hydrogen bonding is important in biological organisms in the following ways:

- It holds separate strands of amino acids (**polypeptides**) together to create three-dimensional structures (Figure 3.13). This enables protein to have a structural function (e.g. collagen) but also enables the protein comprising the structure of enzymes to have a specific shape, creating distinctive sites for substrates to fit into.
- It ensures the two strands of the DNA double helix stay together, but at the same time is weak enough to allow the two strands to separate when duplication of the DNA occurs (see Chapter 12 'Purines and pyrimidines', p. 91).
- It helps antibodies to bind to their antigen.

Van Der Waals Attraction

All molecules, even non-polar covalently bonded ones, experience some attraction to each other. This is known as Van der Waals attraction. For the purposes of this book it is enough to be aware of this phenome non, but no more.

Bonds continued

4

Chapter 3 introduced bond formation. This chapter looks at more complex bonds, where several electrons are shared to form double or triple bonds. These bonds are relevant to the type of chemistry you will encounter in clinical practice.

21

Double Bonds

Carbon and oxygen atoms can form a double bond. Figure 4.1 gives examples of double bonds found in pharmacology. The chemical shorthand for these structures is shown alongside the detailed diagrams of electron distribution.

Why is a double bond significant?

When carbon atoms are joined by a single bond, rotation can easily occur around the bond. When there is a double bond this mobility is not possible (Figure 4.2). The structure of the double bond will not allow this rotation and rigidly fixes the shape of that molecule around the double bond. This inability to change orientation is very important in pharmacology. For example, chemically active compounds might have the same molecular formula but different chemical reactions as the components of the compounds orientated differently in space. The different actions of *cis* and *trans* fatty acids on the body are important examples of geometrical isomerism (see Chapter 6 'Isomers', p. 38 and Chapter 10 'Lipids', p. 74).

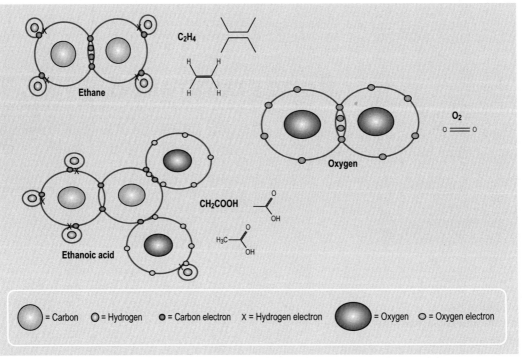

Figure 4.1 Various formations of double bond with oxygen and carbon. A carboxylate group requires a double bond between the carbon and the oxygen.

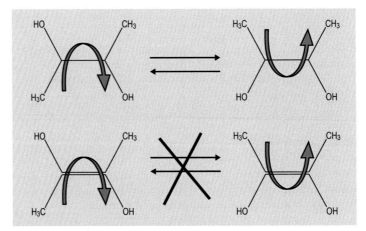

Figure 4.2 A double bond in a molecule limits rotation.

Triple Bonds

Triple bonds (Figure 4.3) occur in nature in cyanogenic glycosides (see Chapter 24 'Glycosides', p. 183) but they are not as common as single or double bonds.

Aromatic Rings

What happens when alternating double and single bonds join to form a ring? If this occurs a very interesting structure called an **aromatic ring** forms. The bonds in an aromatic ring are particularly interesting.

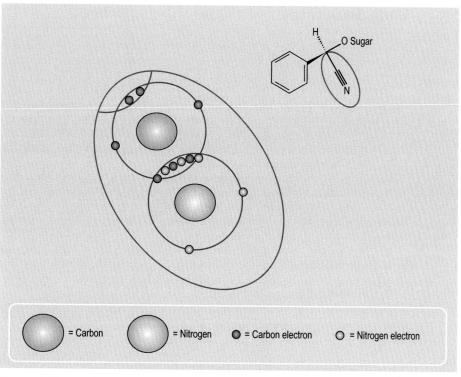

Figure 4.3 The triple bond of a cyanogenic glycoside and the arrangement of electrons.

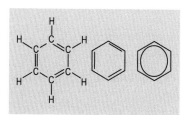

Figure 4.4 Three representations of benzene. The two versions on the left show the alternating double and single bonds; that on the right represents an overall sharing of the electrons around the ring.

The basis of the aromatic ring is benzene (Figure 4.4). In theory, benzene has three double bonds, but a molecule that is not a ring structure and has double bonds reacts very differently chemically to benzene. There are also other quibbles with bond lengths and shape, which are outside the scope of this book.

The chemical assumption that has to be made is that the electrons associated with the benzene ring are, more or less, evenly shared around the ring, so it is impossible to tell where the double and single bonds are. Thus, although the benzene ring can be thought of as a hexagon, and although the bonds are shown for the purposes of presenting a standard structure, there are, in effect, no alternating double and single bonds. In many cases, the ring is shown as the far right notation in Figure 4.4, which indicates the sharing of the electrons. This sharing gives the structure unique qualities when it comes to chemical reactions, because the hydrogen atoms around the ring can be substituted and replaced by a new functional group (see Figure 5.1, p. 30) while the benzene ring stays intact rather than breaking open and changing shape.

Long Structures

What happens when longer structures are formed? Because carbon molecules form covalent bonds with each other they can create very long, stable chains. Important examples are terpenes and amino acids.

Isoprene units, which are molecules of five carbon atoms, can join together to form carbon structures that are 10, 15 or 20 carbon atoms long (see Figure 22.1, p. 167). These comprise a very important class of molecules called terpenes (see Chapter 22), which form the aromatic components of aromatherapy oils (monoterpenes; see Figure 22.3, p. 169), steroidal-type compounds (see Figure 22.7, p. 172) and carotenes (see Figure 22.8, p. 174).

These long chains are called **polymers**, and are effectively repeating segments of smaller molecular units called **monomers**, e.g. isoprene units. Amino acids can also do this, forming **polypeptide chains** (polymers of amino acids), which – when they become long enough – cross-link to form proteins (see Chapter 11 'Amino acids and proteins').

The backbone of most organic compounds is largely made up of carbon and hydrogen atoms (hydrocarbons) with functional groups attached to the backbone (see Figure 5.1, p. 30). As with amino acids, these functional groups are responsible for the chemical characteristics of those molecules.

Important note: The same functional group will undergo the same or similar chemical reactions regardless of the size of the molecule.

The Significance of Polar and Non-Polar Bonds

As you saw in Chapter 3:

• a non-polar compound is uncharged (p. 16)
• a polar compound is charged (p. 16).

Understanding the difference between the two types of bond, and their chemical activity in different mediums, will allow you to make an educated decision about the action of a chemical from a drug, herb or food in a particular environment in the body.

The body is full of water. **Water is a very polar substance** (see Figure 3.8, p. 16) and, therefore, **if a chemical is polar it is likely to easily mix with water** (see Chapter 3 'Bonds found in biological chemistry', p. 16). **Polar chemicals are hydrophilic (water loving).**

However, cell membranes are largely made up of fats (lipids), which are **non-polar and hydrophobic (water hating)** and there are also stores of fatty tissue around the body. Therefore, any non-polar drug or herb taken into the body is, in theory, likely to move relatively easily through cell membranes, providing it is not too large, and to end up stored in fat if it is not utilized.

Polarity, however, is relative and some substances have a tendency to be more polar or non-polar, depending on the environment. A good example of this can be seen in the digestive tract, where the pH in the stomach is approximately 1 and that in the small intestine is nearer 8. pH affects the absorption of the chemicals from a drug or herb by ensuring the majority of solution of the chemical is pushed towards being **polar (water soluble)** or **non-polar (fat soluble)** (see Chapter 8 'Acids and bases', p. 55).

So, **the more non-polar or hydrophobic a substance is, the easier it will be absorbed into the body** (remember, cell membranes are largely made up of lipids). Pharmaceutical companies take this into account when they decide in which part of the digestive tract the drug needs to be absorbed. It is also worth noting as a herbalist,

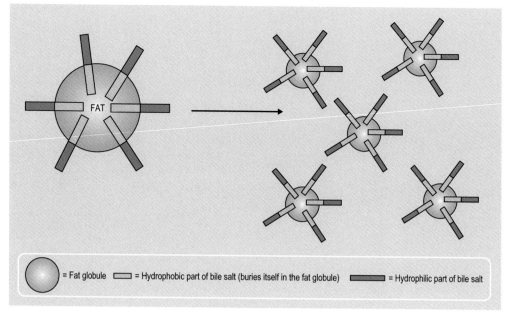

Figure 4.5 The effect of bile salts on fat in the small intestine.

because changes in pH occur with age or disease, then the absorption of their herbal prescription might be affected (see Chapter 15 'Methods of administration', p. 119). This will be discussed in more detail in Chapter 8 'Acids and bases'.

Emulsification

Emulsification is a very important process. A compound known as an **emulsant is both hydrophobic and hydrophilic (amphipathic)**. For example, when fat enters the small intestine, the hydrophobic parts of the bile salts released from the bile duct latch onto the fat, leaving the hydrophilic parts free (Figure 4.5). This encourages part of the fat globule to break off and the smaller globules become surrounded once again by the bile salts. In this way, a large amount of fat (lipid) has been made available to the lipases (the enzymes that breakdown lipids) in the small intestine (i.e. **the surface area has been increased**). The smaller size makes it easier for the lipases to access the parts of the lipids they need to react with.

Reactions You might Encounter in Literature Related to Bonding

It is not necessary to understand the details of the following reactions, but they commonly occur when organic chemicals are separated (hydrolysis) or joined up (condensation).

Hydrolysis

Hydrolysis occurs when the bond in an organic molecule is broken apart and the O–H component of water is used to form two new molecules. The OH group joins itself to one part from the organic molecule and the H atom from the water molecule joins to the other (Figure 4.6).

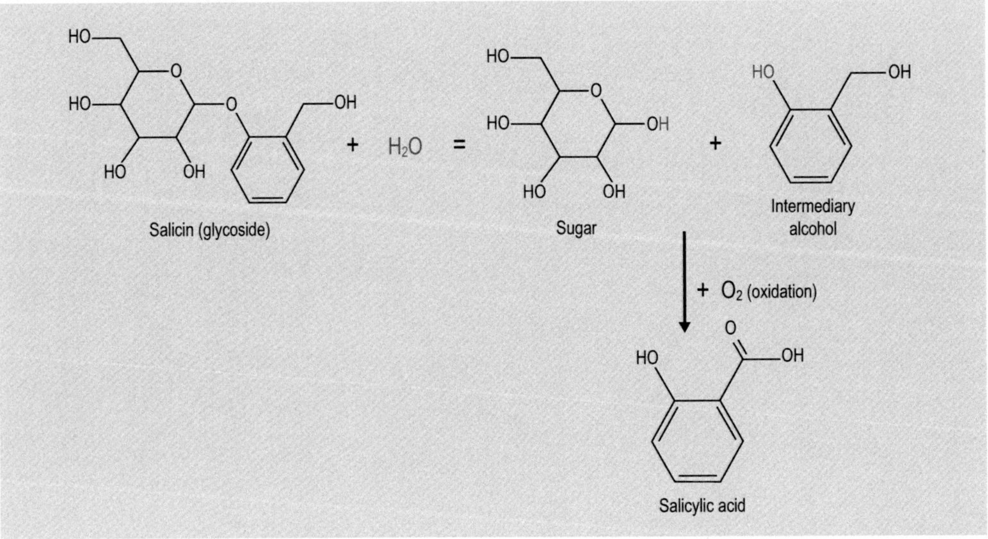

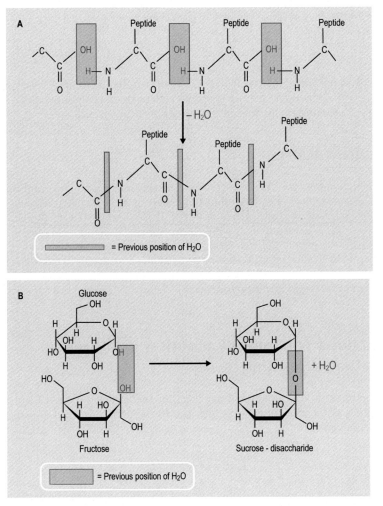

Figure 4.6 Hydrolytic cleavage of a glycoside followed by oxidation of a glycone (i.e. that part of the molecule that is not a sugar).

A

Peptide Peptide Peptide

= Previous position of H_2O

B

Glucose

Fructose Sucrose - disaccharide

= Previous position of H_2O

Figure 4.7 (A) Formation of polypeptide from amino acids. (B) The formation of a disaccharide sugar from two monosaccharides.

The cleaving of a sugar molecule from the organic component of herbs, many of which are attached to a sugar (see Chapter 17 'Metabolism', p. 132 and Chapter 24 'Glycosides', p. 181), is due to hydrolysis.

Condensation

This reaction allows individual amino acids and carbohydrates to join to form polymers (see Chapter 9 'Carbohydrates', p. 67 and Chapter 11 'Amino acids and proteins', p. 83) (Figure 4.7).

Oxidation

When oxidation occurs (see Figure 4.6), oxygen is added to a molecule. Another definition of oxidation involves movement of electrons, but for simplification it is only necessary to think in terms of addition of oxygen.

Nomenclature, representation of chemical structures and basic terminology

5

You now know how atoms join together to form larger, more complex molecules. The more complex the molecule the more difficult it becomes to draw. It is, however, possible to describe the structure of a compound no matter how big it is. So how are these diverse chemicals differentiated from one another?

The system of words used to name compounds is called **nomenclature**. The International Union of Pure and Applied Chemistry (IUPAC) has developed a standard approach to naming compounds.

You are unlikely ever to be called on to name a compound, but you might well see compounds named in scientific papers or pharmacology books. Although at first this might seem overwhelming, particularly if the compound is very complex, it is not as bad as it seems. The standardized naming system incorporates a logical numbering system, which, like shorthand, enables someone familiar with the system to visualize the precise structure of even the most complex compound.

On occasions, you might see the old-style nomenclature that was used before the IUPAC system. This is still generally understood by the scientific community, despite the IUPAC system being the favoured one. In the course of this chapter this older system will also be discussed.

The Functional Groups

Figure 5.1 demonstrates the different types of **functional groups** you are likely to see. **Each of these functional groups has a characteristic chemical reaction**.

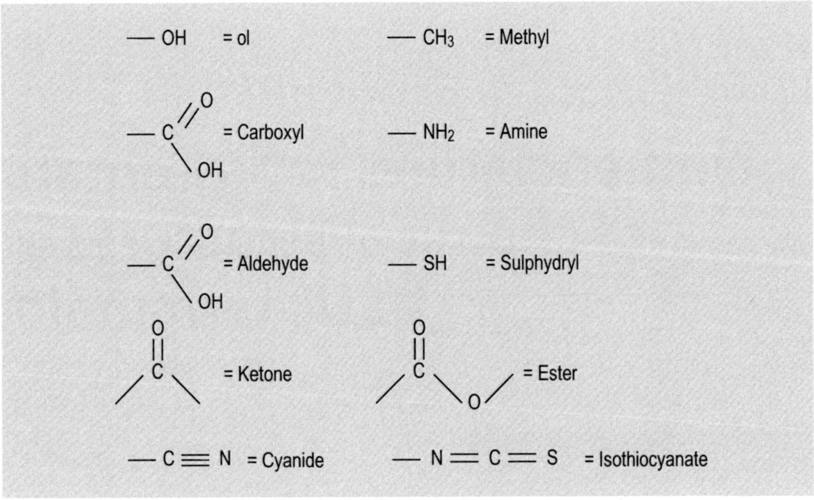

Figure 5.1 Common functional groups encountered in pharmacology.

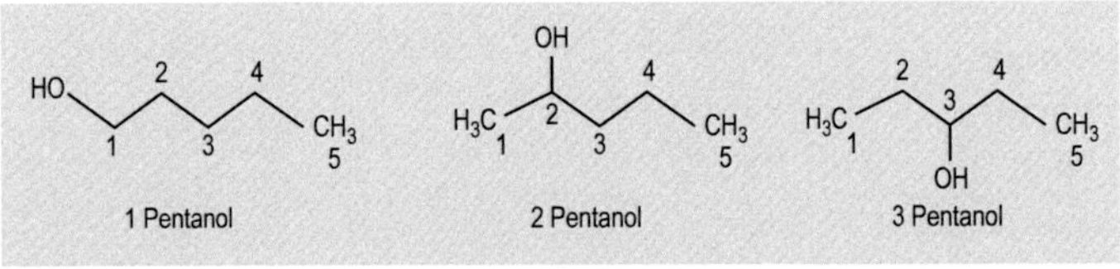

Figure 5.2 The naming of an alcohol group.

It is not necessary for you to know these in detail, but it is helpful to appreciate them with regards to a particular pharmacological activity.

Shorthand can sometimes be used for the chemical formulae of short functional groups such as:

- CH_3: the **methyl group** can be represented as **Me**.
- C_2H_5: the **ethyl** group is represented as **Et**.

There can be quite a variety of these; with a little deduction they are fairly obvious.

Many of these functional groups will be attached to a **hydrocarbon** backbone, which is composed of carbon and hydrogen atoms (see Chapter 4 'Bonds: continued', p. 24).

Naming Compounds with a Hydrocarbon Backbone

- Many of the compounds in pharmacology are based on a hydrocarbon backbone.
- When a hydrocarbon is named, the chemist will first identify the carbon backbone, which tends to be the longest continuous chain of carbon atoms, and will apply the naming procedure from this.
- The first carbon is 1, the second is 2, etc.

Figure 5.2 shows how this applies in a simple alcohol. The same principle applies to other functional groups.

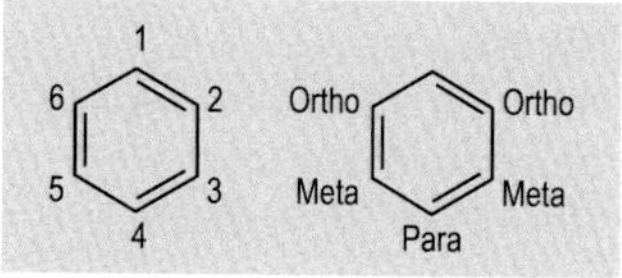

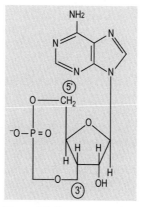

Figure 5.3 The numbering of an aromatic ring.

Figure 5.4 The structure of cyclic AMP.

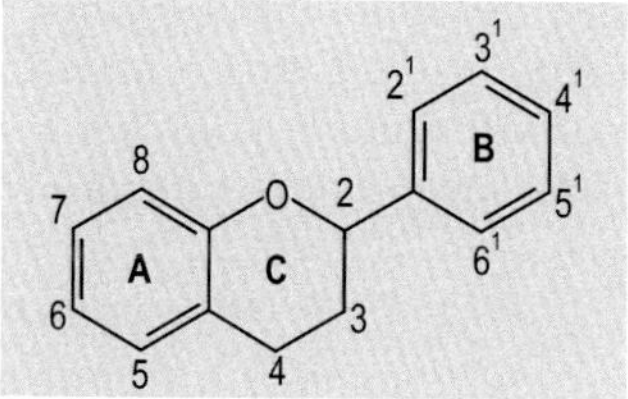

Figure 5.5 The numbering of a complex aromatic structure.

Naming Aromatic Compounds

The left-hand side of Figure 5.3 shows the new IUPAC style of nomenclature; the right-hand side shows the old style of nomenclature, which can still be seen in some literature. A benzene ring is an example of a **conjugated** compound where double bonds alternate with single bonds.

More Complex Structures of Substances Encountered in Pharmacology

Cyclic adenosine monophosphate is usually just known as cAMP (Figure 5.4), but you might also see it as 3'-5' cAMP, which is technically more precise. This notation indicates that a phosphate is linked to both the 3' and 5' hydroxyl groups of an adenosine molecule to form a cyclical structure.

When several rings are involved in the structure, as can be seen in compounds such as flavonoids, it becomes necessary to differentiate the rings (Figure 5.5).

Naming Isomers

See Chapter 6 'Isomers' (p. 35).

Naming Sugars

Sugars are a particular area where nomenclature is used extensively to cover all aspects of the sugar structure as there are so many variations. A basic introduction to this is given in Chapter 9 'Carbohydrates' (p. 66).

Naming Lipids

See Chapter 10 'Lipids' (p. 74).

Further Shorthand

When a very long chain of similar molecules is present in a chemical, a shorthand is used to simplify the presentation of the structure. Take, for example, coenzyme Q10 (Figure 5.6). The unabridged structure on the right is complicated to draw and requires careful counting to calculate the number of carbon atoms in the chain. However, in the abbreviated form on the left it is easy to appreciate the size of the molecule. This shorthand identified the recurring unit – in this case CH_2–CH=CH_2 – which occurs ten times.

R Groups

You might see R in a formula. This is usually used when compounds with the same basic structure have different chemical groups attached to them. R groups are a common feature of chemical literature, providing a quick, convenient way of expressing variable groups attached to a basic structure.

Figure 5.7 demonstrates the variations of the coumarins (see Chapter 21 'Phenols', p. 156), psoralen, bergapten and xanthotoxin, in which R is the side-chain group.

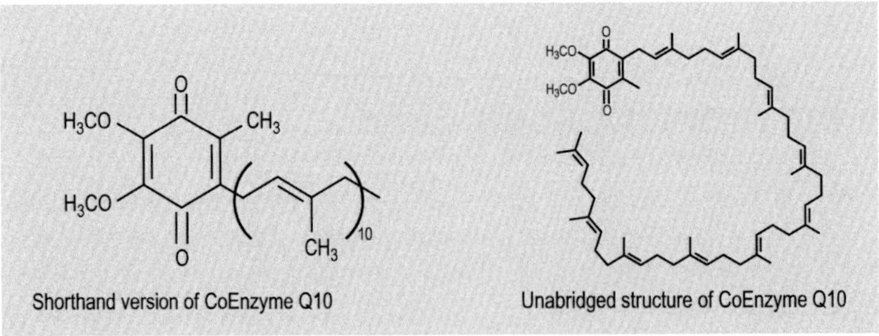

Shorthand version of CoEnzyme Q10   Unabridged structure of CoEnzyme Q10

Figure 5.6 The abbreviation of long carbon chains.

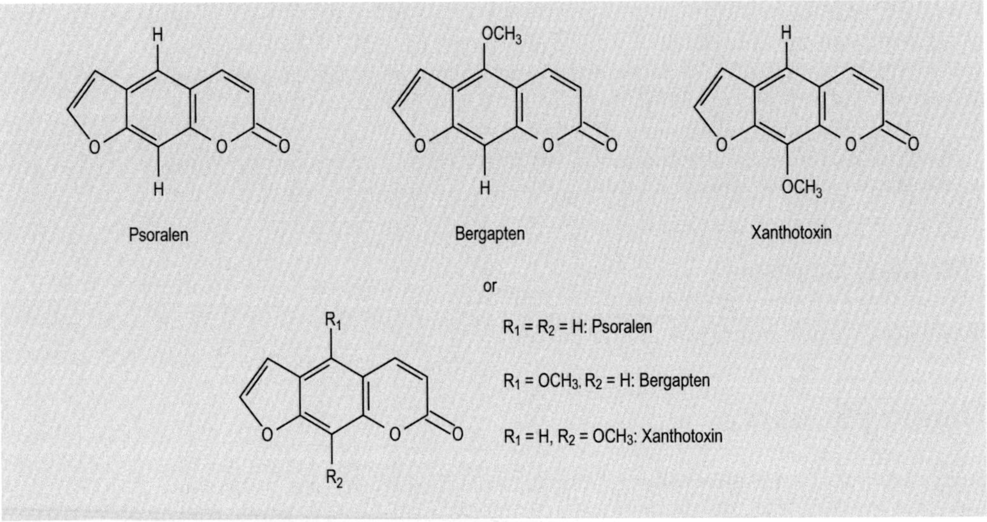

Psoralen   Bergapten   Xanthotoxin

or

R_1 = R_2 = H: Psoralen

R_1 = OCH_3, R_2 = H: Bergapten

R_1 = H, R_2 = OCH_3: Xanthotoxin

Figure 5.7 The use of R groups in pharmacology.

Two-Dimensional Representations of Three-Dimensional Shapes (Figure 5.8)

As seen in Chapter 3, chemical structure can be represented in several ways, particularly if it is necessary to represent a three-dimensional structure. There are other devices for indicating three-dimensional structures, many of which are self-evident (Figure 5.8).

Some General Terminology

- Dimeric: there are two basic units in the structure of the compound.
- Trimeric: there are more than two basic units in the structure compound.
- Moiety: a specific segment of a molecule.

Primary, Secondary, Tertiary

Although you are most likely to come across the terms 'primary', 'secondary' and 'tertiary' when working with alcohols and bases, they can be used for other compounds (however, amino acid configuration is slightly different; see Chapter 11 'Amino acids and proteins', p. 83). The definition depends on the number of hydrogen atoms attached to the carbon atom bearing the group (Figure 5.9).

Naming Orthodox Medication

Modern medication tends to be known by its brand name, which is likely to be different in each country. For example, the chemical name for the drug Prozac

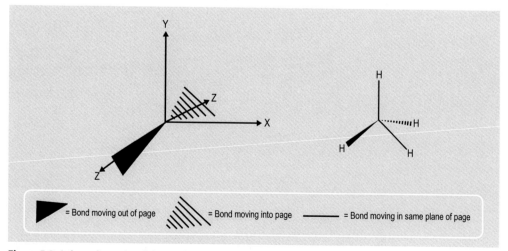

Figure 5.8 A three-dimensional chemical structure can be represented two dimensionally.

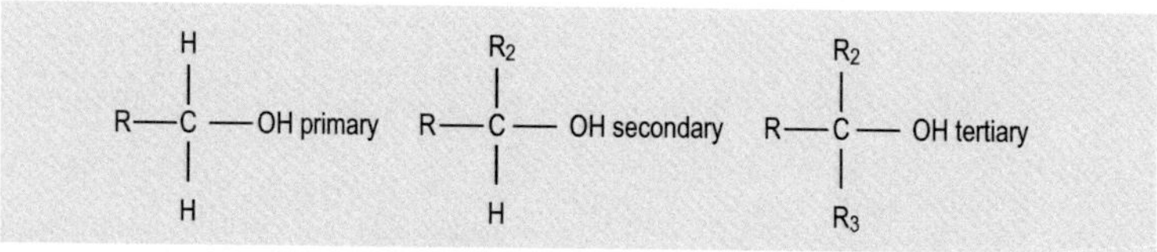

Figure 5.9 The difference between primary, secondary and tertiary alcohols.

is fluoxetine, but 'Prozac' – the brand name – is the name most commonly used. Looking at the chemical structure will leave you in no doubt as to whether you are looking at the same chemical compound.

If you are looking at medication in an international context, it is best to search by the chemical name, although several online search mechanisms will look specifically for medication (see Chapter 42 'Information gathering', p. 342).

Isomers

Chapter contents

If two compounds have the same molecular formulae (in other words, the same number and types of atoms) but the atoms are arranged differently, they are classed as **isomers**. Care has to be taken with this definition, however, as the two examples in Figure 6.1 are not isomers but the same molecule bent into a different shape because the mobility of the single bond allows it. In this example, the arrangement of atoms differs by their arrangement in space only.

Bear in mind that a single bond enables a molecule to rotate freely around it, so the apparent change in the shape in the molecule does not make it an isomer (compare this with the limited rotation around a double bond, see Figure 6.5).

There are several different types of isomer:

- Structural isomers: chain isomerism, positional isomerism.
- Stereoisomers: enantiomers, diasteroisomers, E–Z isomers.

Structural Isomers

Chain isomerism

Chain isomers (Figure 6.2(i)) occur because functional groups can branch off from the main carbon backbone. The number of carbon and hydrogen atoms remains the same but the structures are very different.

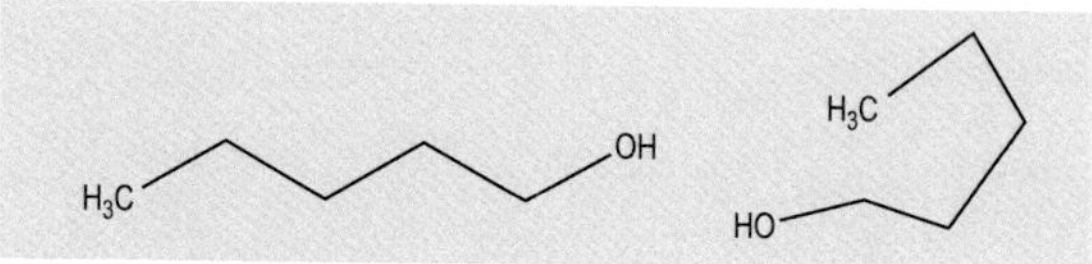

Figure 6.1 Compounds that are not isomers.

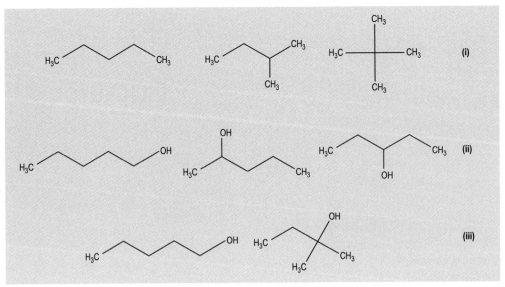

Figure 6.2 The different forms of structural isomerism. (i) Chain (ii) positional (iii) mixture of chain and positional.

Positional Isomerism

In positional isomers (Figure 6.2(ii)) the structure of the carbon backbone remains the same but the functional groups or side chains are moved around the backbone.

Combinations

It is possible to have a mixture of chain and positional isomerism (Figure 6.2(iii)). Positional isomerism can occur around an aromatic ring (see Figure 5.3, p. 31), hence the need for precise nomenclature.

Stereoisomers

It is at this point that thinking in three dimensions becomes important. Stereoisomers are isomers whose components are connected around the same point, but whose arrangement in space is different.

Entaniomers

Enantiomers are stereoisomers that are mirror images of each other and all the components of the compound radiating from one point are different. The term for this is **chiral**. The position of the compound around which this occurs is a **chiral centre** (see Figures 6.3, and 6.7). Take, for example, natural alanine, which is found in only one isomeric form: L-alanine (Figure 6.3). If alanine is produced synthetically, then both forms L and D alanine, are found. This is significant when it comes to giving a patient nutritional supplementation, as the L isomer is more likely to fit into the receptor site of an enzyme, which explains why natural products are favoured in nutritional supplementation.

• What exactly do D and L mean?

Light normally vibrates in all directions, but if put through a polarizer it will vibrate in only one direction (Figure 6.4(i)). If another polarizer is placed at exactly 90°,

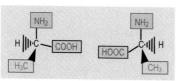

Figure 6.3 The two isomers of alanine.

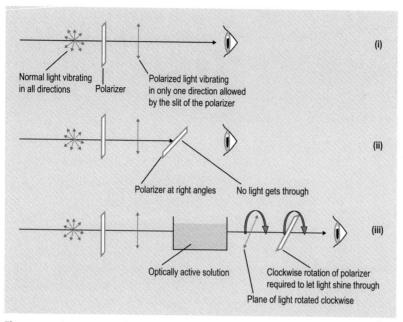

Figure 6.4 The principles of the polarization of light and how optically active solutions can affect it.

no light will get through. You can test this yourself with two pairs of good-quality sunglasses. Line them up, and then turn one through 90 degrees. The lens will appear black because no light is getting through (Figure 6.4 (ii)).

If a solution of an optically active isomer is placed in the path of monochrome (one wavelength only) polarized light, then the light will change orientation. To make it visible again, the next polarizer will have to be twisted either clockwise (*dextro*-rotation) or anticlockwise (*laevo*-rotation) to see light again (Figure 6.4 (iii)). This is where the notation dextrorotatory (D) and laevorotatory (L) comes from. The notation now being phased in is:

- Dextrorotatory: clockwise – signified by a (+).
- Laevorotatory: anticlockwise – signified by a (−).

It is possible to see both dextrorotatory and laevorotatory compounds in the same solution at the same time. This is known as a **racemic** mixture. Special equipment used in general analysis employs this characteristic. It is a fast and non-destructive way to see which optical isomer is present in a solution.

All chiral compounds will rotate light (optically active).

Disastereoisomers

- These stereoisomers do not have a mirror image.
- They are characterized by differences in their pharmacological properties.

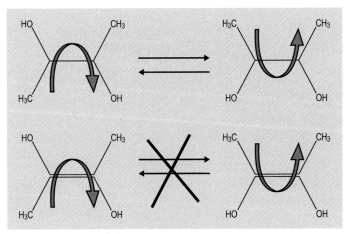

Figure 6.5 Limited rotation around a double bond.

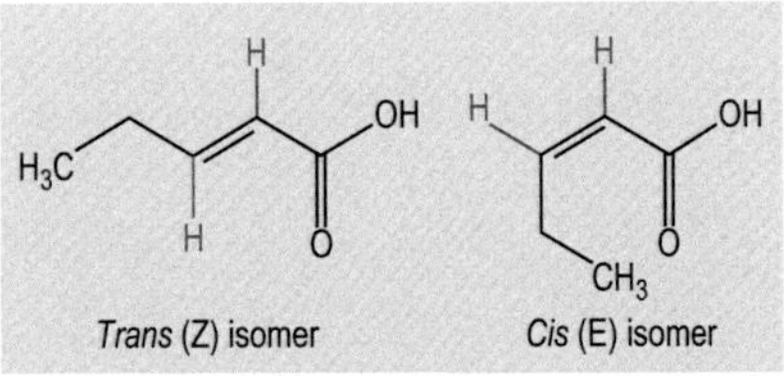

Trans (Z) isomer   *Cis* (E) isomer

Figure 6.6 Different forms of an isomer with their old and new style nomenclature.

● E–Z (*cis–trans* isomerism, geometrical isomerism)

An example of E–Z isomerism is shown in Figure 6.5 in the case of a compound with a double bond (which has already been shown to prevent rotation; see Figure 4.2, p. 22). The only way to make these compounds identical is to break the bond and rotate it, before rejoining the bond again.

This orientation around a bond can have metabolic significance with regards to the structure of a compound and a patient's health (see Chapter 10, 'Lipids', p. 76) because, as diastereoisomers, compounds possess different chemical properties.

In the literature, you will see these types of isomer referred to in two different ways (Figure 6.6). The older terminology of *cis* and *trans* is slowly being replaced by E (for *cis*) and Z (for *trans*). However, as *cis* and *trans* are well known, certainly in the area of fatty acids, as far as the general public is concerned it is useful to be conversant with both.

What Happens When a Compound has More Than One Chiral Centre?

Chemical compounds can have more than one chiral centre. Alpha tocopherol (Figure 6.7) is a good example of this. In this case, the nomenclature S or R is used to denote whether the methyl group is to the left (S) or right (L), respectively, counting from the aromatic end. The other notations of (+) or (−) can also be used for the various types of tocopherol (see Chapter 13 'Vitamins and minerals', p. 107). All natural tocopherol is RRR. Synthetic tocopherol can have SRR, SSR, SRS, SSS, RSR, RRS, RSS and RRR forms, which is why nutritionists stress the use of natural tocopherol.

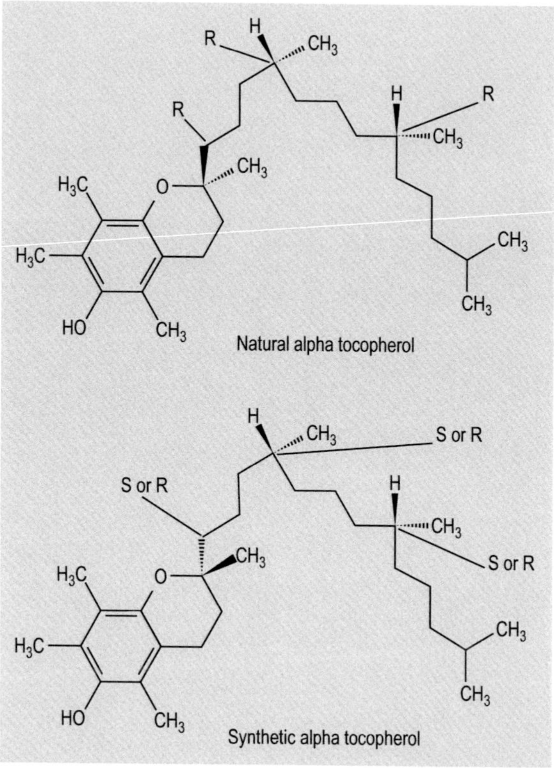

Figure 6.7 Different structures of natural and synthetic alpha tocopherol, showing chiral centres.

Alkaloids

Most alkaloids are chiral molecules, which means that their isomers can have very different chemical properties. As the extraction of alkaloids from plants for the treatment of cancer is becoming more common, pharmaceutical companies have found it vital to understand the differences between alkaloid stereoisomers, as some are more chemically active than others.

Free radicals

Chapter contents

Free radicals are talked about a great deal in the realms of nutrition but very few practitioners understand exactly what they are.

How are Free Radicals Formed?

Electrons like to exist in pairs, so when atoms are chemically separated from their **covalent bonds** (see Chapter 3 'Bonds found in biological chemistry', p. 13) they do not normally split to leave a single unpaired electron. When this *does* happen, a free radical is formed.

Free radicals are very unstable due to the single unpaired electron, so they are very keen to 'steal' an electron from the nearest stable (**non-radical**) molecule to gain stability. Free radicals can be formed by:

- The loss of a single electron from a normal molecule (non-radical).
- The gain of a single electron by a normal molecule (non-radical).

The 'attacked' molecule loses its electron and in turn becomes a free radical. This occurs quickly – in much less than a second – and the process rapidly starts a chain reaction that, once started, can cascade and ultimately result in the disruption of a cell.

What Causes Free Radicals?

- Chemicals: gases responsible for pollution, herbicides, alcohol, carcinogenic chemicals such as benzene.
- Cigarettes: fresh cigarette smoke contains high concentrations of nitric oxide, which reacts with oxygen to form nitrogen dioxide. This is a free radical and is capable of attacking unsaturated lipids at the double bonds.
- Radiation: UV light, X-rays and radioactive material. When exposed to high-intensity visible light, cells in culture are damaged, particularly the mitochondria, which are rich in the protein haem and in flavin co-containing proteins (see Chapter 13 'Vitamins and minerals', p. 93). This is what happens to skin when someone is exposed to excessive UV light.

How do Free Radicals Cause Damage?

Free radicals cause damage in four ways:

1. Damage to lipids: cell membranes and organelles (e.g. mitochondria) are largely composed of lipids. When they incur damage from free radicals their function becomes impaired.
2. Damage to proteins: free radicals attack the amino acids that are the building blocks of protein structures.
3. Damage to genetic material: free radicals attack the nucleic acids (RNA and DNA), thus affecting the function, growth and repair of cells dependent on proper protein function. This is the first step in the development of cancer.
4. Lysosome destruction: lysosomes are small, enzyme-containing lipid-membrane sacs. When the lysosome is destroyed, the enzymes are released and the cell effectively digests itself. The destructive effect of the enzymes is passed to adjacent cells and creates a widespread effect.

Normal Occurrences of Free Radicals

The body needs free radicals for certain functions:

- Phase I of the liver detoxification system (see Chapter 17 'Metabolism', p. 129) is necessary if other reactions are to take place under the appropriate control. The phase I pathway in the liver involves cytochrome P450 and produces free radicals as a necessary intermediary product. The phase II pathway – the conjugation pathway – adds chemical groups to the free radicals, terminating (**quenching**) them and returning them to normal (non-radical) molecules. If phase I is **upregulated** (made to work more efficiently) but phase II does not have the capacity to match this increased production of free radicals, the patient will become ill.
- The free radical hydrogen peroxide is required for the synthesis of the hormone thyroxine by the thyroid gland.
- Macrophages and neutrophils generate free radicals to kill off the bacteria they engulf by phagocytosis.
- Nitric oxide (a free radical) is now thought to be an important part of vasodilatation and neurotransmission.
- Oxidative phosphorylation: a series of free radical electron carriers in the mitochondria is responsible for energy production (see Figure 2.5, p. 10).

In a healthy individual, the free radicals that are formed by the body are dealt with via a variety of radical '**quenching**' systems. However, if too many free radicals form then there is a problem.

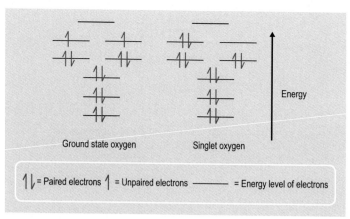

Figure 7.1 The distribution and spin direction of all the electrons of atmospheric oxygen (O_2) in its ground state and excited (singlet) state.

Reactive Oxygen Species

Oxygen is vital to life. Ultimately, it is responsible for producing energy in living organisms, although plants are also able to use carbon dioxide for this purpose. Oxygen is an interesting molecule because in its unexcited or '**ground state**' it has two unpaired electrons, in separate orbitals.

When an oxygen molecule interacts with other molecules to form a covalent bond, it needs to accept two electrons that are spinning in the opposite direction to its own electrons in the outermost orbital or they will not fit (it would be rather like trying to put two like poles of a magnet together, which results in repulsion). In the presence of energy, one of the electrons can change its direction of spin and pairs up with the other one to create **singlet oxygen** (**activated oxygen**) (Figure 7.1). This is not as stable as the **ground state oxygen** and will change back fairly quickly (less than 0.04 microseconds) but in that time it will have affected its surrounding environment.

Singlet oxygen is not a free radical but it can be formed during some free radical reactions and can trigger the formation of free radicals. Singlet oxygen can be formed by macrophages during phagocytosis and by light (in chlorophyll).

Singlet oxygen interacts with other molecules in two ways:

- It combines with them chemically.
- It transfers its excitation energy to them. The oxygen then returns to the **ground state** whereas the molecule the oxygen has interacted with becomes excited.

Thus, oxygen is activated by two different mechanisms.

- Absorbing energy: electrons orbit but, like the earth around the sun, they also spin in a particular direction. If enough energy is absorbed by the oxygen molecule then the spin of one of the orbiting electrons can be reversed (in the case of singlet oxygen the spin is reversed and the electron paired temporarily). This change activates oxygen. The oxygen will now react with organic molecules in a way it could not before it had been activated.
- Gaining an additional electron: oxygen can gain an extra electron (i.e. it is **reduced**) to form something called a **superoxide**, which in turn produces hydrogen peroxide. **Hydrogen peroxide is not a free radical** because its electrons are paired (Figures 7.2 and 7.3), but it can go on to produce problematic metabolic products. Its potential for damage is compounded by the fact that hydrogen peroxide easily passes through cell membranes and can therefore easily move out of the cell in which is was formed. This mobility means that it can spread around the body easily.

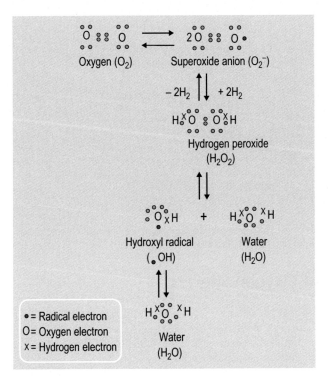

Figure 7.2 The formation of a free radical with oxygen.

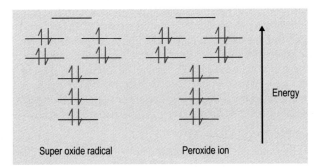

Figure 7.3 Electron configuration of the superoxide radical and peroxide ion. Note the unpaired electron of the superoxide radical and the two sets of paired electrons of the peroxide ion (which means it is not a radical).

The products of reduced oxygen are activated products but are not free radicals, only the oxygen can be said to be a free radical (because it has two unpaired electrons it is called **biradical**).

Superoxides

The most important source of the superoxide radical is the electron transport chains in the mitochondria and endoplasmic reticulum (where the cytochrome P450 is stored and works in the liver). The electrons should pass from one component of these chains to another, but the relay system is not perfect and there is thought to be some 'leakage'.

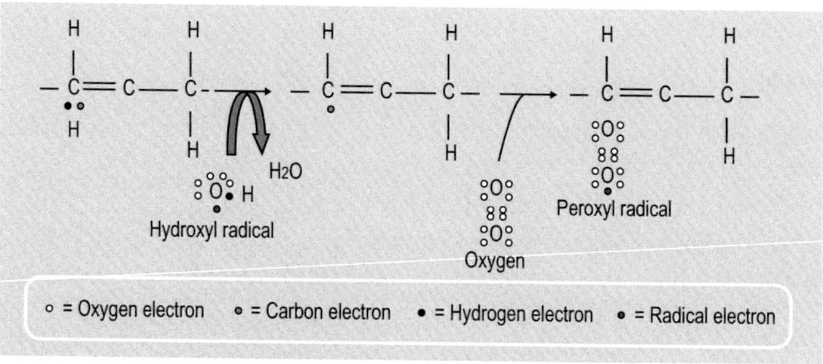

Figure 7.4 The action of free radicals on lipids.

Effects of Free Radical Damage

- Cancer: damage to the DNA causes mutations that affect the normal function of the cell, eventually leading to malignancy.
- Atherosclerosis: this is attributed to free-radical-induced oxidation of the chemicals in the body (see Chapter 27 'Problems with lipid metabolism, p. 204).
- Hepatocellular damage from excessive consumption of alcohol: not so much as a direct result from the alcohol but the products produced by the damage done by the alcohol.
- Lung conditions: free radicals present in cigarette smoke are thought to inactivate alpha 1-antitrypsin in the lung, which can lead to emphysema.
- Possible involvement in Parkinson's disease, schizophrenia and Alzheimer's disease.
- Ageing.
- Chronic inflammatory diseases.

Damage to Lipids

Oils go rancid as a result of oxidation (see Chapter 4 'Bonds continued', p. 27). In the late 1800s, it was observed that – when exposed to air – a layer of walnut oil on water would absorb three times its own volume of air in 10 days. For this reason, margarine manufactures must slow or prevent this oxidation process.

Cells walls are comprised of lipids and, as hydrogen peroxide so easily permeates these membranes, peroxidation of the fatty acid part of the phospholipids in the cell wall is relatively easy, occurring in the area between the double bonds (Figure 7.4).

Lysosomes membranes are also made up of phospholipid. When these are damaged the contents of the lysosomes are released into the cell at the wrong time.

Damage to Proteins

Generally, protein is less susceptible to free radical damage than lipids. The extent to which proteins are affected by free radicals very much depends on their amino acid make up. Sulphur-containing amino acids are the most susceptible to free radical damage (or certainly attack from an activated oxygen molecule). Proteins associated with metals, e.g. haem compounds found in enzymes, are also vulnerable to free radical damage (see Chapter 37 'Metabolic disorders', p. 296).

Two main reactions occur as a result of free radical damage to proteins:

- Cross-links are formed by sulphur-containing amino acids (see Figure 11.3, p. 83). This changes the protein structure, preventing it from acting as a receptor site.
- Amino acids are damaged, leading to a degradation of the protein that contains them.

• DNA and RNA

Free radicals:

- Interfere with the transfer from the template to the production of the protein (see Figure 11.6, p. 85).
- Cause deletions and mutations within DNA.
- Degrade the sugars and bases that form the backbone of DNA (see Figure 12.2, p. 90), breaking the DNA strands or forming unnecessary cross-links to proteins.

Body's Protection Against Free Radicals

Tissues are full of enzymes designed to protect against free radical damage.

Superoxide Dismutases (SOD)

Superoxide dismutases (SOD) can contain zinc and copper (Cu-Zn-SOD) and also manganese or iron. SOD converts superoxide to hydrogen peroxide and oxygen (Figure 7.5), and minimizes production of the hydroxyl radical that causes so much damage (it is the most potent of the oxygen free radicals). This system is nearly always the antioxidant defence in cells exposed to oxygen. It is extremely quick and can more than match the production of superoxide when working properly.

There are three forms of SOD in the human body:

- SOD1 in the cytoplasm: copper and zinc (Cu-Zn-SOD).
- SOD2 in the mitochondria: manganese is found in the liver but not in erythrocytes. Free radicals in the mitochondria are byproducts of oxidative phosphorylation, which produces energy.
- SOD3 extracellular: copper and zinc (Cu-Zn-SOD).

SOD is thought to protect from free radicals produced by the ageing process and ischaemic tissue damage. It also has an effect on inflammation.

Mutations in SOD1 have been linked to familial amyotrophic lateral sclerosis (ALS).

Catalases and Peroxidases

Catalases and peroxidases are enzymes that catalyse the decomposition of hydrogen peroxide to water and oxygen, preventing the formation of hydroxyl (•OH) radicals. Catalases react in the following way to rid the system of peroxide:

$$2H_2O_2 \rightarrow 2H_2O_2 + O_2$$

Peroxidases react differently, using a sulphur-containing compound called glutathione (see Figure 7.7):

$$SH_2 + H_2O_2 \rightarrow S + 2H_2O$$

Catalyse is present in all the major body organs. It is concentrated in the liver and erythrocytes but there is very little in the brain, heart and skeletal muscle.

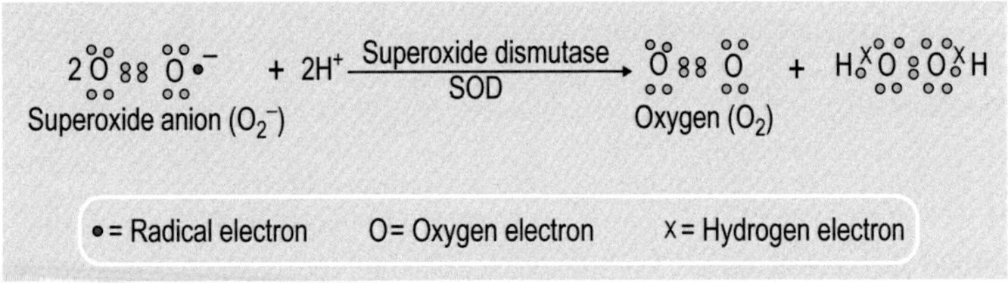

Figure 7.5 The action of superoxide dismutase (SOD).

Red blood cells can be very prone to damage if is there is a deficiency of glutathione as it is not possible to prevent the attack of peroxide on the plasma membrane, which results in red blood cell haemolysis.

Glutathione peroxidase is found largely in the liver and – to a much lesser extent – in the heart, lungs and brain, with very little activity in muscle. It contains selenium (see Chapter 13 'Vitamins and minerals', p. 100), a dietary source of which is required for its activity.

The reason that glutathione is so favoured by nutritionists is because it acts as a **cofactor** (a compound that works with an enzyme) for glutathione peroxidase.

Antioxidants

Antioxidants affect the oxidation of molecules. They oxidize but are able to remain stable. Antioxidants can therefore prevent free radicals from reacting with other compounds. They interact with the free radical mechanism at various points along the chain reaction. **If the number of free radicals is kept at a low enough level, oxidation will not occur.**

The type of molecule that can act as an **antioxidant can effectively juggle the configuration of electrons within its structure so that the overall effect is neutrality**. To be successful as an antioxidant, the molecule must:

- react with free radicals faster than they are capable of reacting
- form products, as a result of reacting with the free radical, that do not encourage oxidation
- be lipid soluble
- be capable of remaining stable after interacting with a free radical.

• Ascorbic acid

- Acts as a scavenger for oxygen. It is capable of taking an oxygen ion and converting it into harmless water. In other words, it gives two protons to the oxygen.
- Recycles alpha tocopherol after it has '**quenched**' (stopped) a free radical reaction. This is why nutritionists advise that vitamin C and E are taken together. The resulting ascorbate is then recycled by glutathione (see Figure 7.9).
- Is very soluble in water and is a very good reducing agent (it freely gives away electrons to other molecules of protons). Its small structure allows relatively good movement across a cell membrane.

• Flavonoids

- Are polyphenolic compounds (they all share a similar chemical structure containing two benzene rings on either side of a three-carbon ring; see Figure 21.14, p. 159).
- The capacity of flavonoids to act as antioxidants depends on their molecular structure (Figure 7.6).

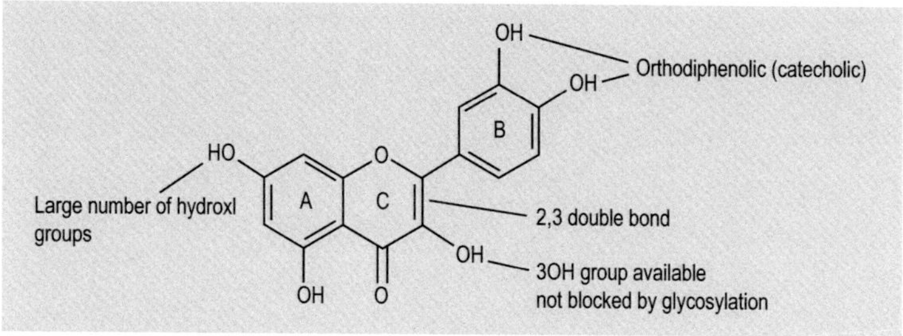

Figure 7.6 Anatomy of an ideal flavonoid antioxidant.

- The position of hydroxyl groups and other features in the chemical structure of flavonoids is important for their antioxidant and free-radical scavenging activities. Adjacent hydroxyl groups on the B ring increase their antioxidant activity (Wen Peng 2003). Quercetin, the most abundant dietary flavonol (see Chapter 21 'Phenols', p. 160), is a potent antioxidant because it has so many of the right structural features for free-radical scavenging activity.
- Flavonoids that lack the above key features do not possess antioxidant activity.
- They can prevent superoxide production.
- They can reduce free radicals.
- They are less bioavailable (the body is not as able to absorb and make them available for use) than ascorbic acid and tocopherol. The more hydroxyl groups they contain, the more hydrophilic they are and therefore the less lipid soluble.

Factors Increasing the Antioxidant Properties of a Flavonoid

- Large number of OH groups.
- Presence of a 2,3 double bond.
- Orthodiphenolic structure or catecholic (referring to the position of the hydroxyl groups on the B ring, which is the structure of a catechol; see Figure 5.3, p. 31).
- Reasonable fat solubility.

Factors Decreasing the Antioxidant Properties of a Flavonoid

- Glycosylation (sugar group) blocking the 3-OH group in the C ring.
- No hydroxyl group in the B ring.
- The presence of a methoxy group in the B ring (—OCH_3).

• Glutathione

- Is a **tripeptide** (three amino acids joined together) consisting of **glutamine, cysteine** and **glycine**. It can be made from these raw materials by the body.
- The —SH thiol (sulphydryl) group of the cysteine is the reactive part of glutathione. It reacts with another activated thiol (sulphydryl) group on another glutathione molecule and forms a disulphide bond (Figure 7.7)

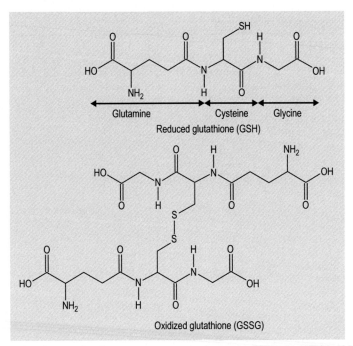

Figure 7.7 The structures of reduced glutathione and oxidized glutathione (GSSG).

- Is changed to oxidized glutathione (GSSG) as it becomes oxidized, thus removing hydrogen peroxide from the system. This bond formation keeps the glutathione stable.
- GSSG is then recycled by another enzyme.

$$H_2O_2 + 2\,glutathione \rightarrow GSSG$$

- Is found in most tissues, cells and subcellular compartments of higher plants. As a person gets older, glutathione levels decrease.
- Neutralizes singlet oxygen, superoxide and hydroxyl radicals (see Figures 7.1 and 7.2) and does not require an intermediary to act as a free radical scavenger.
- Is also responsible for regenerating ascorbate or reducing the disulphide bonds of proteins (see Figure 7.9).

Glutathione and Paracetamol (Acetaminophen) Poisoning

Paracetamol (acetaminophen) is toxic because its breakdown products form a compound that reacts with the glutathione. The breakdown product, N-acetyl-p-benzo-quinone imine; NAPQI) reacts with the sulphydryl groups of glutathione, which are used up by the excessive amount of breakdown product. When the glutathione is completely used up, the NAPQI begins to react with liver cell proteins, killing the cells. It causes necrosis in the liver cells and kidney tubules. This same principle occurs in mushroom or toadstool poisoning.

N-acetylcysteine, or methionine (both of which contain sulphur), can be used to reverse this situation as they are used by the cells to recycle GSSG back to useable glutathione.

Tocopherols

- The tocopherols (see Chapter 13 'Vitamins and minerals', p. 107) are a family of antioxidants.
- Alpha-tocopherol is considered to be the most active. It is a membrane stabilizer and antioxidant that scavenges oxygen free radicals, lipid peroxy radicals and singlet oxygen.
- Alpha-tocopherol has become almost synonymous with vitamin E, although technically the term 'vitamin E' refers to the other tocopherols as well.
- The tocopherols have an interesting structure in that part of it is lipid soluble whereas the other part works as antioxidant. It positions itself with the polar benzoquinone ring near the phosphate part of the membrane phospholipid with the rest of the molecule, which is **non-polar** and therefore **hydrophobic**, in the lipid layer (Figure 7.8).

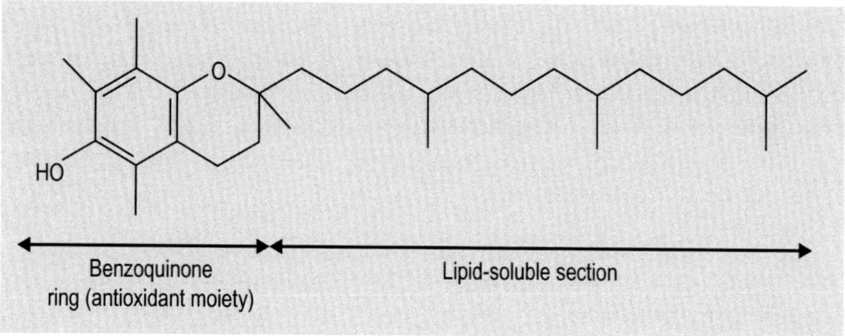

Figure 7.8 The structure of tocopherols.

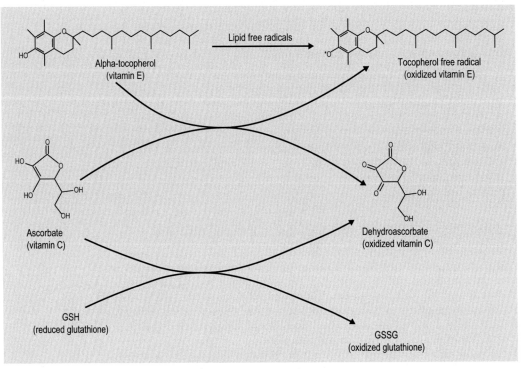

Figure 7.9 The interactions between vitamin E, vitamin C and glutathione.

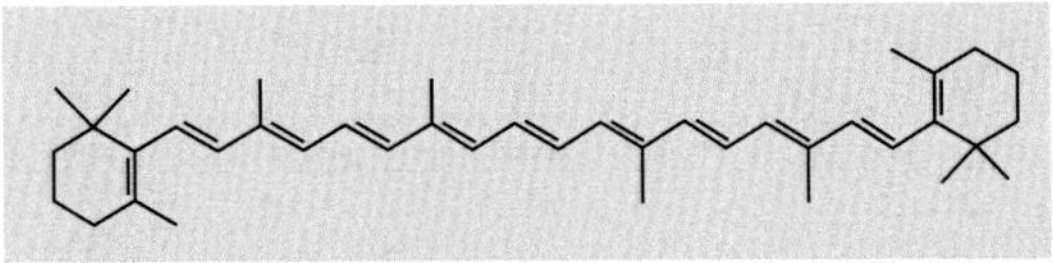

Figure 7.10 The structure of beta-carotene.

- The amount of alpha-tocopherol is particularly high in blood lipoproteins and the adrenal glands, which are particularly susceptible to oxidative damage.
- As the hydrophilic part of the tocopherol is near the edge of the membrane, **ascorbate** (vitamin C) has easy access to it and can easily regenerate it (Figure 7.9; and see Chapter 13 'Vitamins and minerals', p. 102).

● Carotenoids

- Carotenoids are tetraterpenes (see Figure 22.8, p. 174).
- There are two classes of carotenoids: carotenes and xanthophylls.
- The carotenoids are involved in photosynthesis (see Figure 9.1, p. 64).

Beta-carotene (Figure 7.10) is a more efficient scavenger of singlet oxygen than tocopherol. Not only does it have an aromatic part, it also possesses a polyunsaturated section (see Figure 10.1, p. 74). The mechanism of its antioxidant action is not properly understood. It has been demonstrated to quench singlet oxygen, scavenge peroxyl radicals and inhibit lipid peroxidation. There does not appear to be a mechanism to recycle beta-carotene.

Carotenes act by:

- reacting with lipid peroxidation products to terminate chain reactions
- scavenging singlet oxygen
- working synergistically with alpha-tocopherol to scavenge peroxy radicals.

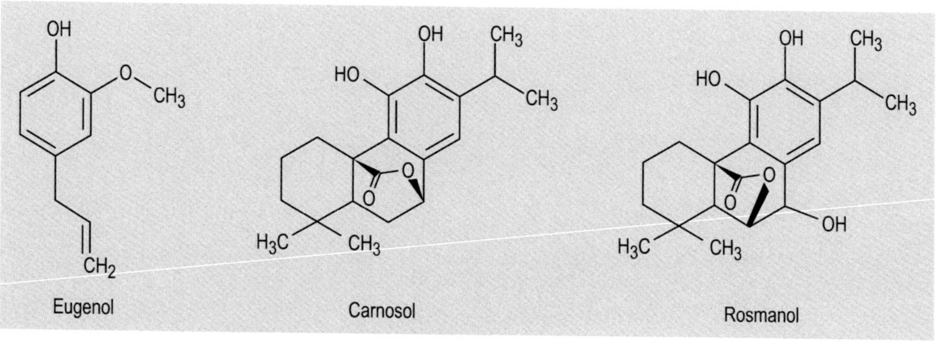

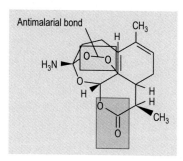

Figure 7.11 The phytochemicals that act as antioxidants.

Eugenol   Carnosol   Rosmanol

Antimalarial bond

Figure 7.12 The antimalarial bond in artemisinin is thought to create free radicals in the malarial parasite.

• Other Phytochemicals Acting as Antioxidants

Eugenol (found in cloves) and carnosol and rosmanol (Figure 7.11; these terpenes are found in rosemary leaves) inhibit oxidation.

Useful Free Radicals

Nitric Oxide

Nitric oxide (NO) is of great interest because it is a free radical that diffuses easily through the plasma membrane, thus affecting nearby cells. It is now thought to have substantial influence on the nervous system, and it might also be responsible for the damage incurred after a stroke. NO:

- relaxes blood vessels
- regulates the amount of neurotransmitter released by nerve endings
- plays a role in the cellular immune response.

Natural Antimalarials

Artemisinin in *Artemisia annua* (*Qing Hao*) (Figure 7.12) is a herbal example of a natural antimalarial (Klayman 1985, Olliaro et al 2001; see also Chapter 22 'Terpenes', p. 171).

Treatment of Herpes

In the treatment of herpes simplex, the lesions are painted with a dye that enters the infected cells, binds to the DNA or to the virus and is then illuminated. It destroys the DNA by free radical damage.

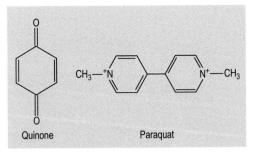

Figure 7.13 The structures of quinone and paraquat.

Diseases Associated with Free Radical Damage

Stroke

Free radical damage has been implicated in ischaemic brain disease (i.e. stroke). The brain and nervous system are particularly prone to oxidative injury because they are rich in lipids and the brain has only limited amounts of protective enzymes. Some areas of the brain are also rich in iron (e.g. the substantia nigra), which might enhance free radical action.

Porphyria

See Chapter 28 'Blood disorders' (p. 211).

Poisoning with Herbicides

A major class of herbicides works by interrupting photosynthetic electron flow in plants. They can do this because their structure (which is similar to that of the quinines) enables them to intercept electrons intended for flow down the electron chain (Figure 7.13; see Figure 21.7, p. 153). As human metabolism also uses quinines, it is possible that an accumulation of this type of pesticide will produce free radicals.

References

Klayman DL. Qinghaosu (artemisinin): an antimalarial drug from China. Science 1985;228:1049–1055.

Olliaro PL, Haynes RK, Meunier B et al. Possible modes of action of the artemisinin-type compounds. Trends in Parasitology 2001;17:122–126.

Wen Peng WI, Kuo S-M. Flavonoid structure affects the inhibition of lipid peroxidation in caco-2 intestinal cells at physiological concentrations. Journal of Nutrition 2003; 133:2184–2187.

Bibliography

Halliwell B, Gutteridge JM. Free radicals in biology and medicine. 2nd edn. Oxford. Clarendon Press; 1999.

Acids and bases

8

The concept of acids and bases is quite complex and there are several ways of approaching the subject in terms of pure chemistry. As this is a clinically oriented pharmacology book, the explanation will be limited to certain mechanisms, an understanding of which will help you appreciate the underlying principles and is necessary to underpin one of the most important principles of pharmacology. For this reason, all explanations of acids and bases will be given in terms of hydrogen ions or protons (the terms in this case are interchangeable) only.

The Involvement of Water in Acid–Base Reactions

As you have already seen, water is a very active molecule, forming and breaking hydrogen bonds between its molecules (see Figure 3.12, p. 19). This constant juggling of hydrogen bonds gives the water molecule the capability to break apart or disassociate.

Acid–base reactions occur in the presence of water as a result of this quality of disassociation of water into hydrogen ions (protons) and hydroxyl ions:

$$H_2O \leftrightarrow H^+ + HO^-$$

The environment of living tissues is largely water and when certain compounds enter this environment they can be encouraged to disassociate. The degree to which they dissociate depends on the number of hydrogen ions present. It is this balance of hydrogen ions that forms the basis for acid–base mechanisms.

$$R-ROOH \rightleftharpoons R-COO^- + H^+$$

Dissociation of an acid

$$R-NH_2 + H^+ \rightleftharpoons R-\overset{+}{N}H_3$$

Attachment of a hydrogen ion to a base

Figure 8.1 The action of acids and bases with regards to the hydrogen ion. Note that each reaction is reversible; this is a very important feature of these reactions in pharmacology.

Acids and Bases

Acids disassociate in water to form a hydrogen ion and the ion of the acid (Figure 8.1). In other words, in the right conditions, **acids tend to give away their hydrogen ions**, donating them to the aqueous solution.

The strength of an acid depends on the number of hydrogen ions in solution. The more hydrogen ions there are, the stronger the acid. Weaker acids such as ethanoic acid, otherwise known as vinegar or acetic acid, are weak acids because they are not very good at letting go of their hydrogens, compared to a strong acid like sulphuric acid, which is prepared to give away a very large amount. The difference in activity can be appreciated by the fact that putting sulphuric acid on your chips would result in them being disintegrated.

Bases accept hydrogen ions from aqueous solutions in the right conditions (Figure 8.1). A strong base is one that is very keen to grasp free hydrogen ions, whereas a weak base is not good at grasping free hydrogen ions. The result, regardless of strength, is a compound that has a positively charge ion.

Acids are thought of as proton donors (give away protons) whereas **bases are considered to be proton acceptors** (accept protons).

What is pH?

The pH range extends from 0 to 14. Although academics will argue that the situation is more complex than this, this range is more than adequate. The middle of this range – pH 7 – is considered neutral. Any number greater than 7 means it is a base and any number lower then 7 means it is an acid:

- pH 7–14 is a base: high pH
- pH 0–7 is an acid: low pH.

So, the higher the number, the stronger the base; the lower the number, the stronger the acid.

pH is a measure of the hydrogen ion concentration. It is usually calculated by measuring the concentration of hydrogen ions in a solution using something called logarithms. This is why it might seem a little strange that a solution with a low pH has a high concentration of hydrogen ions and one with a high pH has a low concentration of hydrogen ions. Discussion of how this logarithmic calculation is worked out is beyond the scope of the book, but the point is worth mentioning as this apparent contradiction can be confusing.

Why is the pH Important in Pharmacology?

Outside the cells, the pH regulates the rate of absorption of compounds. Inside cells, and in body fluids, pH or hydrogen ion concentration is very tightly controlled. This precision is necessary because almost all the enzymes in the body are influenced by the amount of hydrogen ions present in the solution around them.

What is pK?

The degree to which compounds are prepared to dissociate (break apart to form a hydrogen ion and a charged compound) can be measured and something called

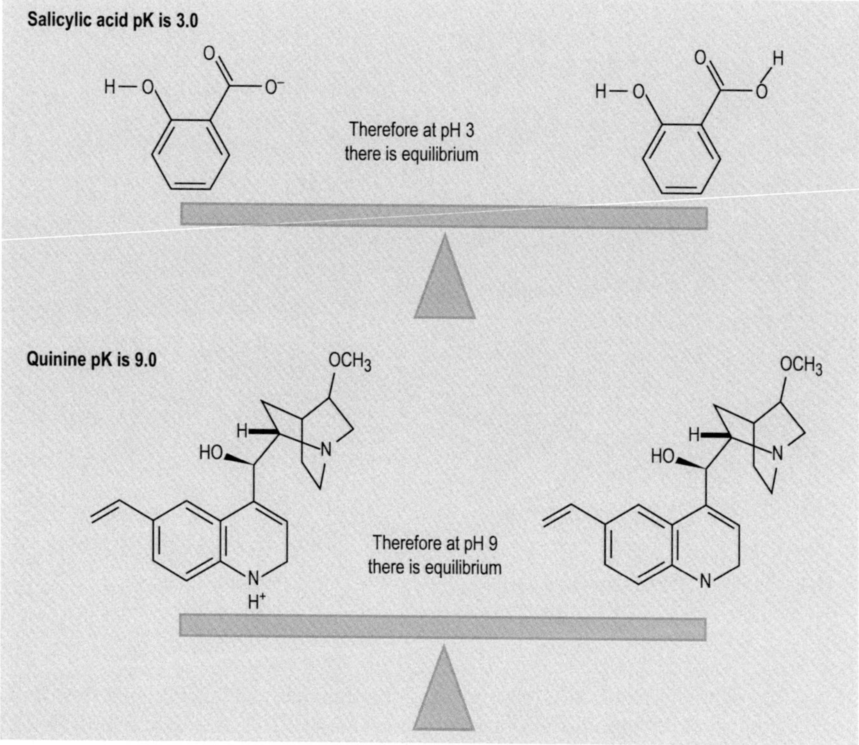

Salicylic acid pK is 3.0

Therefore at pH 3
there is equilibrium

Quinine pK is 9.0

Therefore at pH 9
there is equilibrium

Figure 8.2 The balance when the pH is the same as the pK value. There is an equilibrium between charged (polar) and uncharged (non-polar) compounds.

a **pK value** is used. This **dissociation constant** will tell you at exactly what pH a compound is half ionized and half not ionized. In other words, the pH at which the compound is in equilibrium.

How Are the pH and pK Values Relevant to Absorption?

The pK of salicylic acid is 3.0. At pH 3, 50% of the salicylic acid will be un-ionized and 50% will be in the form of salicylate ions (negatively charged), having lost its hydrogen (Figure 8.2).

As a further example, the pK of quinine is 9.0. At a pH of 9, 50% will be un-ionized quinine and 50% will be ionized (positively charged), having gained a hydrogen.

Putting the two compounds into a solution with a different pH (i.e. changing the concentration of hydrogen ions) will shift this equilibrium. Nowhere does the pH change more than in the progression through the gastrointestinal tract (GI tract), so this is used as an example below.

What Happens to Acids and Bases in a low pH?

The stomach has a pH of 1 (a low pH, a high concentration of hydrogen ions). With this many hydrogen ions, an acid with a pK value of 3 is not going to be able to give away its hydrogen ions (donate hydrogen ions) because there are too many in solution. Rather like a housing market flooded with properties makes it difficult for a vendor to sell their properties. However, a base with a pK of 9 will be only too happy to soak up the spare hydrogen ions. This is the same as a buyer having a great deal of choice when a house market is flooded with properties (a buyer's market).

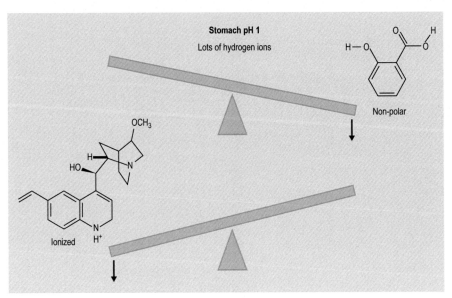

Figure 8.3 The balance of acids and bases at a low pH.

Therefore, in the acidic environment of the stomach, the salicylic acid stays in its configuration but quinine becomes positively charge due to the extra hydrogen ions (Figure 8.3). The **salicylic acid** is therefore **uncharged (un-ionized, non-polar)** and the **quinine** is **charged (ionized, polar).**

The **lining of the stomach consists of cell with a lipid membrane, which is non-polar.** Any **non-polar** compound, such as the salicylic acid in this case, is **easily absorbed across the membrane.** The **polar** quinine, however, is **not absorbed by the non-polar cell membranes.**

What Happens to Acids and Bases in a High pH?

There is a marked pH change further down the GI tract, with the pH becoming 7.8 in the small intestine. Now the previous situation becomes reversed, as a pH of 7.8 means that there is a much lower concentration of hydrogen ions in solution.

With so few hydrogen ions, an acid with a pK value of 3 will be able to give away (donate) almost as many hydrogen ions as it likes. A similar situation occurs in a housing market when there is a glut of people wanting to buy properties. It makes it so much easier for vendors to sell their property (vendor's market).

With a compound with a pK of 9 and a base, not many quinine molecules will be able to attach many hydrogen ions to it, because there are so few hydrogen ions. This is the same as having too many buyers for a very small number of properties.

By losing a hydrogen ion the **salicylic acid** therefore becomes **charged (ionized, polar**; Figure 8.4) and the **quinine**, by being unable to attach to a hydrogen ion is **uncharged (un-ionized, non-polar).**

Like the stomach, the lining of the small intestine is made up of cells with a lipid membrane, which is non-polar. Any **non-polar** compound, such as the **quinine** in this case is **easily absorbed across the membrane.** The **polar** salicylic acid, however, is **not absorbed by the non-polar cell membranes.**

How the Degree of Charge on a Compound will Affect its Absorption Rate into the Body

The environmental pH therefore has an effect on acids and bases, as different pHs can make them charged (ionized or polar) or uncharged (un-ionized or non-polar).

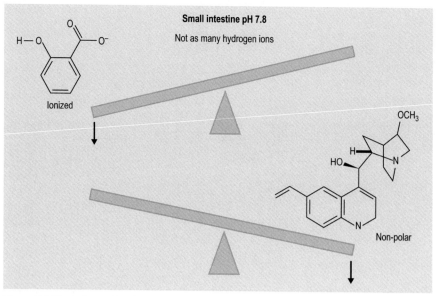

Figure 8.4 The balance of acids and bases at a high pH.

This in turn affects the absorption of an acidic or basic compound through a membrane that is largely non-polar due to its composition of non-polar lipids.

How the Degree of Charge on a Compound will Affect its Removal from the Body

The kidneys are a very active area when it comes to pH (see Figure 18.3, p. 135). The excretion of certain drugs can be altered depending on the pH of the urine.

The Importance of pH and pK

Under the right conditions, substances such as organic acids that have carboxyl groups (see Figure 5.1, p. 30) can ionize and form negatively charged COO^- ions and positively charged H^+ ions (or protons). This capacity of a molecule to lose or gain a proton is very important in maintaining stability of pH in the bloodstream and how easily a chemical is absorbed or removed from the body (see Chapter 18 'Drug excretion', p. 135). pH is kept very tightly controlled in the plasma.

Conjugate Acids and Bases

You might come across the terms 'conjugate acid' and 'conjugate base' in the literature. It is an interesting paradox that occurs in chemistry and one that you have already seen in action above. Figure 8.5 will enable you to follow the discussion more easily.

A **conjugate base** is formed when an **acid loses a hydrogen ion**. This situation effectively turns it into a base, as it now **lacks a hydrogen ion** and is **willing to accept hydrogen, just like a base**.

A **conjugate acid** is formed when a **base gains a hydrogen ion**. The compound is now an acid because it has **gained a hydrogen ion** and is **willing to donate it, just like an acid**.

Small intestine pH 7.8
Not as many hydrogen ions
Ionized
OCH₃
Non-polar

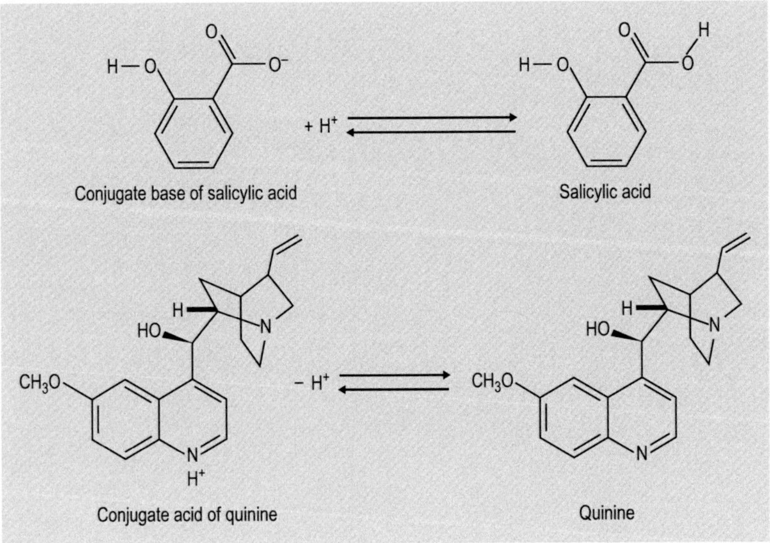

Figure 8.5 The principle of a conjugate base and a conjugate acid. Note that the reaction is reversible.

$\longleftarrow$ Excess H^+ ions

$$CO_2 + H_2O \rightleftharpoons H_2CO_3 \rightleftharpoons H^+ + HCO_3^-$$

Decrease H^+ ions $\longrightarrow$

Figure 8.6 The shift in equilibrium in the bicarbonate buffering system in the blood.

pKa and pKb

You might also see pKa and pKb in the literature. pKa is the dissociation constant for an acid and pKb is the dissociation constant for a base. Don't forget that although a base does not like to give away its protons, when it has acquired them it effectively becomes and acid and so will be prepared to disassociate.

How is pH – or Hydrogen Ion Concentration – Controlled in the Body?

- Acid–base buffer systems in the body fluids: hydrogen ions combine with an acid or base to prevent large changes in pH.
- The respiratory centre: regulates the removal of carbon dioxide from the blood.
- The kidneys (see Chapter 18 'Drug excretion', p. 134): capable of removing either acid or alkaline urine, which readjusts the pH in the body.

Bicarbonate Buffer System

When there are excess hydrogen ions (low pH; Figure 8.6, top arrow, right to left) the equilibrium is shifted to the left. To restore the correct hydrogen ion concentration (pH), the excess of hydrogen ions will react with the bicarbonate ions (HCO_3^-) eventually producing carbon dioxide and water.

When there is a decrease in hydrogen ions (high pH; Figure 8.6, bottom arrow, left to right), carbon dioxide will combine with water, eventually producing more hydrogen ions and bicarbonate ions. The respiratory centre will then increase respiration to remove excess carbon dioxide from the blood.

Control of pH by the Kidneys

There is a large flow of blood through the kidneys and – potentially – a large capability to remove fluids and solutes from the body (see Chapter 18 'Drug excretion', p. 135 and Chapter 26 'Cardiovascular disorders', p. 192). The kidneys are therefore a convenient way to control pH.

Large amounts of bicarbonate ions are continuously filtered into the kidney tubules. The amount of bicarbonate lost therefore acts to control the pH of the blood.

Section 2

Important primary metabolic components

Carbohydrates

9

Plant Metabolism

Two systems are at work in a plant:

1. **Primary metabolism**: products of photosynthesis, which provide the food necessary if the plant is to live, grow and reproduce.
2. **Secondary metabolism**: very diverse and thought to provide secondary functions for the plant, such as protection against animals that might eat it or preservation again microbial attack, thus preventing decomposition. In some cases, secondary metabolites interact with symbiotic organisms. For example, cyanogenic glycosides made by sugars linking to highly toxic cyanide are released when the plant is attacked by an insect or disease-causing organism.

Photosynthesis is the means by which plants use sunlight to produce sugar. Through various chemical reactions in the plant, this ultimately produces energy that the plant can use. Structures called **chloroplasts**, which are present in the leaves, enable plants to absorb light. The chloroplasts contain photosynthetic pigments called chlorophylls; **chlorophyll A** is the main photosynthetic pigment in all organisms except bacteria. Combinations of pigments in the plant increase the spectrum of light that plants can absorb for photosynthesis. **Carotenoids** (Figure 9.1; see Chapter 22 'Terpenes', p. 173) help to transfer this energy. Carbon dioxide and water combine to create chemical energy that can be stored.

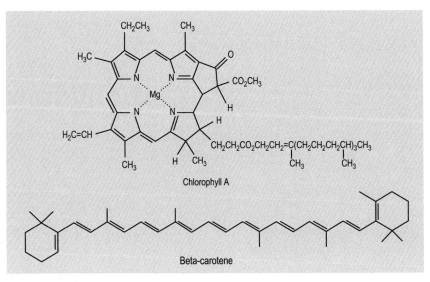

Figure 9.1 The structures of compounds (carotenoids) able to absorb light energy.

Formation of Carbohydrates

The energy that plants gain from the light is stored as carbohydrates. The classic equation for this is shown below:

$$6CO_2 + 12H_2O + light = C_6H_{12}O_6 + 6O_2 + 6H_2O$$

Function of Carbohydrates

- Energy storage (starch in plants and glycogen in animals): humans obtain some of their energy from carbohydrates that come from plants. Effectively, plants store carbohydrates as energy. When the carbohydrates are metabolized energy is released.
- Structural (cellulose cell walls or chitin exoskeletons; Figure 9.9, p. 70).
- Recognition (carbohydrates of glycoproteins and glycolipids; pp. 71–72).

Monosaccharides

Monosaccharides are the simplest form of sugar. They have more than one hydroxyl group and are based on a backbone of 3, 4, 5; or 6 carbons (triose, tetrose, pentose, or hexose, respectively). Figure 9.2 demonstrates the varieties of sugars of different numbers of carbons:

- Trioses: found in the initial stages after photosynthesis.
- Ribose, deoxyribose, fructose and glucose: can convert between a ring and straight structure.
- Glucose: usually referred to as blood sugar and used as a measure of how effectively the body deals with sugars.
- Fructose: very often used as a sweetener in drinks; in many cases it is derived from corn syrup.
- Ribose and deoxyribose: the sugar components of RNA and DNA.

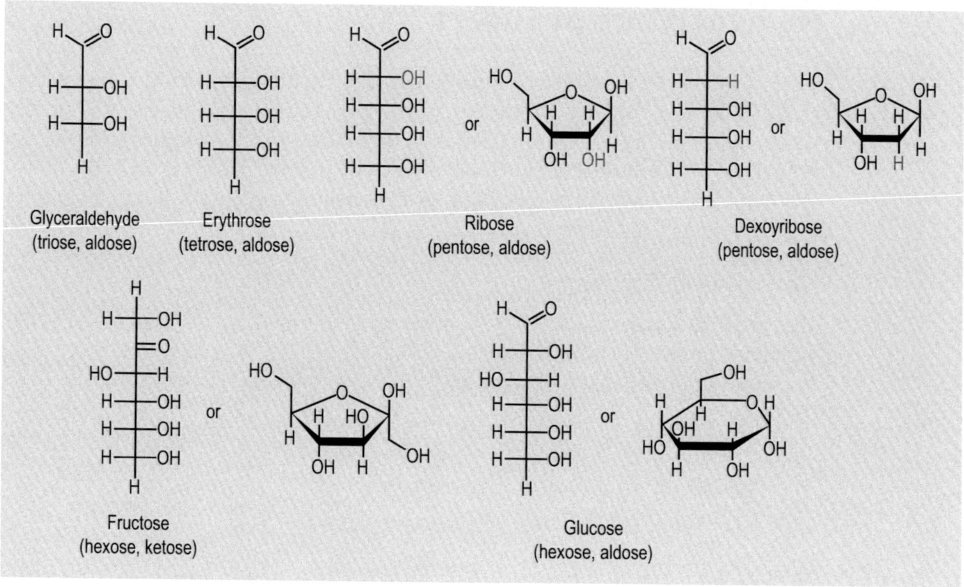

Figure 9.2 The variety of sugars.

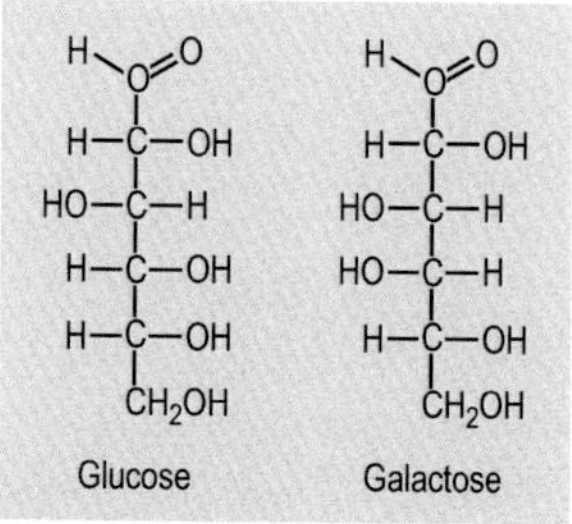

Figure 9.3 Comparison of glucose and galactose structures. These tend not to be in a position to rotate as mostly they are thought of a being in a ring structure.

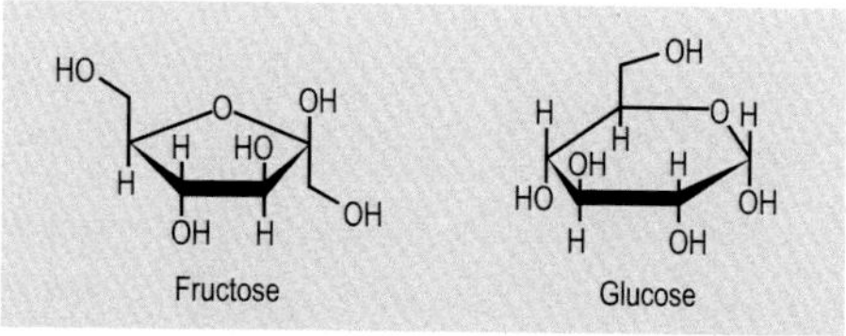

Figure 9.4 The differences between furanose (fructose) and pyranose (glucose) rings (note the thickened line indicating the ring coming out of the page towards you).

General Characteristics of Simple Sugars

- These simple sugars are polar (as a result of all the —OH groups) and therefore are readily water soluble. Because they are small, their passage through cell membranes is relatively easy and they are probably pulled through by simple osmosis (see Figure 16.1, p. 124) as the water is pulled though.
- Most (but not all) have a sweet taste; a sugar moiety is responsible for the sweet taste of a glycoside.
- Each carbon that supports a hydroxyl group, except for the first and last carbon (atoms) is a chiral centre (see Figures 6.3, 6.5, 6.6 and 6.7, pp. 36–39) and can therefore give rise to a number of isomers all with the same chemical formula (see Chapter 6 'Isomers', p. 35), for example, glucose and galactose have the same chemical formula but different chemical and physical properties (Figure 9.3).

Furanose and Pyranose

Sugars can form ring structures. There are two main types (Figure 9.4):

- Furanose: a five-membered-ring sugar molecule (fructose).
- Pyranose: a six-membered-ring sugar molecule (glucose).

Nomenclature of Sugars

When reading the literature on sugars, particularly those as part of the structure of glycosides (see Chapter 24 'Glycosides', p. 181) you might come across complex shorthand denoting the type of sugar or sugars to which the chemically active compound is attached. It is only really necessary to understand this if you want to pursue pharmacology to a very high level. Usually, it is enough to know you are looking at an active chemical attached to a glycoside.

Numbering Sugars

The carbon atoms in a sugar ring are numbered. This enables a chemist to see where functional groups are attached (Figure 9.5).

Abbreviations are used for some of the more common sugars, for example:

- Glc: glucose
- Man: mannose
- Gal: galactose
- Xyl: xylose.

Isomers

D and L (+) and (−) might be used to indicate which isomer the sugar is (see Chapter 6 'Isomers', p. 36).

Type of Ring Structure

p and f indicate pyranose and furanose rings.

• Alpha or Beta Sugars

Sugars in a ring are also known as either alpha or beta sugars:

- An —OH in the beta position is on the same side as the C6 carbon.
- An —OH in the alpha position is on the opposite side of the ring to the C6 carbon.

• 'Boats and Chairs'

Sugars that form a ring structure, such as glucose, have several options as far as shape is concerned. Figure 9.6 demonstrates these variations.

The chair structure is most commonly seen attached to various plant chemicals to form a glycoside. Its shape is more conducive to forming a compact shape than a boat structure, and it is considered the most stable form. The lower bold edge of the ring represents this part of the molecule projecting out of the page towards the reader.

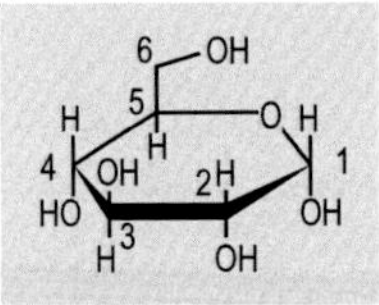

Figure 9.5 Numbering of a sugar molecule.

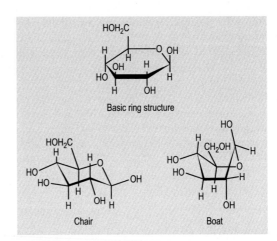

Figure 9.6 The different forms of cyclic sugar structures.

Disaccharides, e.g. Sucrose

- Composed of fructose and glucose (see Figure 4.7B, p. 26).
- This is the sugar that is used for human consumption and is found in cane and beet.
- Sucrose is a transportable form of energy and carbohydrate in the body.
- Disaccharides are sweet tasting.

Polysaccharides

- Consist of many monosaccharides and are known as polymers.
- Are sometimes referred to as glycans.
- Are created by a condensation reaction (see Figure 4.7B, p. 26).
- Are usually large, with a high molecular weight. They can be very branched, which, if the bonds between the individual sugars are orientated in a certain way, makes them difficult for the body to absorb and utilize.
- Tend to be insoluble in water and, unlike the mono- and disaccharides, do not taste sweet.
- Can be made up of the same or different types of sugar.
- Can either be used for storage (e.g. starch and glycogen; Figure 9.7) or for structure such as cellulose (which supports unlignified plants) or chitin (found in insect exoskeletons) (Figure 9.9).
- Very often, the active components of fungi (such as antibiotics) are complex polysaccharides (Figure 9.10).

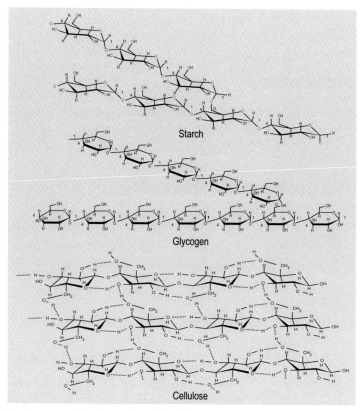

Starch

Glycogen

Cellulose

Figure 9.7 Structures of the polymeric sugars starch, glycogen and cellulose.

The Formation of Carbohydrate Polymers

Monosaccharides can join together by **condensation** (see Figure 4.7B, p. 26). When sugars are linked together the links can be one of two sorts: either at the fourth carbon (1–4 bond) or the sixth carbon (1–6 bond).

The bonds created between individual sugars can vary between the 1, 4 or 6 carbon atoms on each monosaccharide. This will lead to combinations that result in different chemical and physical properties (as shown in Figure 9.7).

Simple and Complex Carbohydrates

- Simple carbohydrates: one to three units of sugar linked together.
- Oligosaccharides: carbohydrates made up of two to ten monosaccharides.
- Complex carbohydrates: many sugar units linked together.

Why is Cellulose Difficult to Break Down?

When beta-glucose (the —OH is on the same side as the C6 carbon) forms the polymer cellulose, the linkage occurs through beta 1–4 glycosidic bonds. This arrangement allows the hydroxyl groups sticking off the sugar backbone to form hydrogen bonds (see Figure 3.13, p. 19, Figure 4.7B, p. 26 and Figure 9.7) with other strings of cellulose. This effectively 'glues' the strings together, so that as a whole the structure has a high tensile strength. This is important in plant cells walls because it makes them rigid. It also explains why cellulose provides fibre in the diet; cellulose is difficult to break down.

Carbohydrates such as starch or glycogen contain alpha 1–4 glycosidic bonds (the —OH is on the opposite side to the C6 glycosidic bond). This type of bonding creates coiling, which is not conducive to forming chains linked by hydrogen bonds.

Fat-free Foods

Foods that are called 'fat free' are not really fat free. Somewhere, the label will list some type of sugar in the ingredients. Sugar is transformed to fat in the body and stored if the sugar is not used up.

Polysaccharides with Special Uses

Pectins

Pectins are a complex group of polysaccharides that are commonly found in plants.

They are required in jam-making as they are what solidifies jam (Figure 9.8).

Mucilages

- These are highly branched structures composed of different sugars and acids.
- They are hydrophilic and their structure is therefore rather complex, enabling them to trap water inside their framework. This makes them swell, to form a gel, which is why mucilage swells when mixed with water. Try chewing linseed seeds; you will actually be able to feel the swelling taking place. Although animals find mucilage hard to break down, it is possible if the flora of the gut is normal. **This is one reason why it is important to have a healthy gut with the right bacteria.**

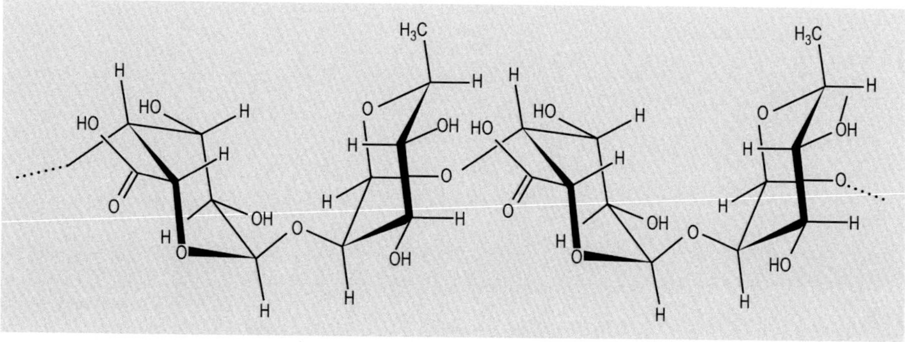

Figure 9.8 The structure of pectin.

- Mucilage is used by herbalist to soothe the gut wall. Its action is largely due to the mucilage acting as a barrier in the gut, allowing the gut wall to rest from the constant exposure to chemicals present that might irritate it. The mucilage might also hold other plant chemicals in place over the gut wall.

Plantago species (plantain, *Che Qian Zi*) contain **plantago-mucilage**, which works as outlined above. The seeds themselves, if smashed up and then eaten, have the dual effect of the mucilage protecting the gut wall and the husk acting as a bulking agent to help the movement of the gut wall.

Interestingly, Western medicine uses hydrocolloid dressings, which become gel-like on contact with water. This feature allows the dressing to sop up a moderate amount of exudate from the wound, while simultaneously sealing the wound from the outside world. Hydrocolloid dressings are often used when maggots are in place eating away necrotic tissue. They absorb the liquid produced and prevent the maggots from escaping.

Chitin

This is very similar to cellulose. It is the main component of fungal cell walls and arthropod exoskeletons (Figure 9.9).

Alginates

- Agar consists of agarose and agaropectin.
- Agarose can form a double helix, the central cavity of which can accommodate water molecules.

Gums

- Many of the gums used by the food industry are carbohydrate derivatives.
- These gums are formed by cutting into woody plant – effectively wounding them; the gums are thought to be the plant's way of sealing these injuries.

Antibiotics

Many important antibiotics are oligosaccharides or contain oligosaccharide groups (Figure 9.10).

Glycosaminoglycans

Glycosaminoglycans (GAGs) are:

- A family of sulphated, unbranched polysaccharides (repeating disaccharide units, with sulphur molecules).

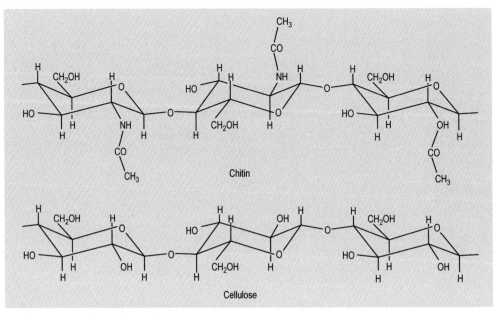

Figure 9.9 The structures of chitin and cellulose.

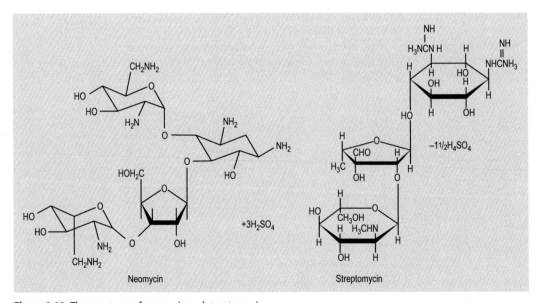

Figure 9.10 The structures of neomycin and streptomycin.

- The difference in the way they are arranged in space (stereochemistry; see Chapter 6 'Isomers', p. 35), length (number of sugars) and the position of the sulphurs creates a wide variety of molecules.
- GAGs are mainly found on the surface of cells or in the extracellular matrix.
- GAGs are very viscous and difficult to compress. They are ideally suited for their use of joint lubrication and are found as part of synovial fluid.
- Their rigidity gives structural integrity to cells; this is particularly noticeable in the cell walls of bacteria.

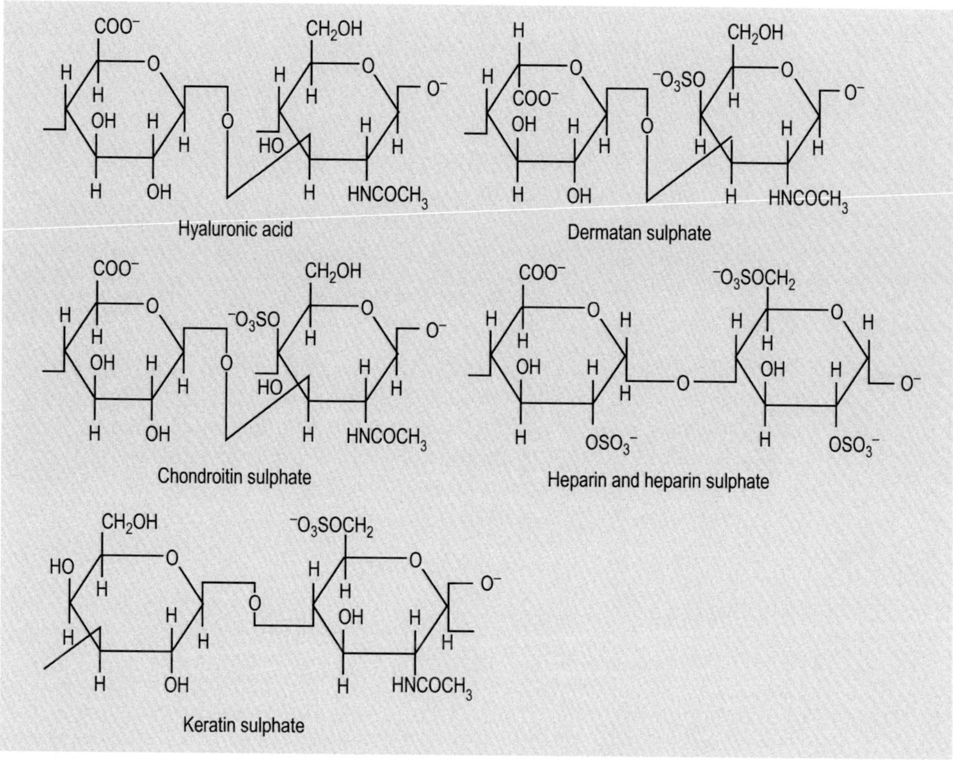

Figure 9.11 The various structures of glycosaminoglycans (GAGs). Notice the different position of bonds joining the sugars together.

Examples of GAGs (Figure 9.11):

- Hyaluronic acid (no sulphur): found in skin, cartilage and synovial fluid of articular joints for lubrication and the vitreous humor (fluid) of the eye.
- Chondroitin sulphate: found in cartilage, bone and heart valves.
- Dermatan sulphate: found in skin, blood vessels and heart valves.
- Heparin: used for its anticoagulant properties (see Chapter 28 'Blood disorders', p. 214).
- Keratin sulphate: along with chondroitin sulphate, this is part of the cartilage ground substance. It is also found in cornea and bone.

Glycoproteins

- Proteins attached to a carbohydrate core with saccharides.
- Found in all connective tissues.
- Found on the surfaces of many cells. The antigens that determine blood types belong to glycoproteins.
- Immunoglobulins (see Figure 30.3, p. 227) are glycoproteins, and therefore important for immune cell recognition.
- Their structures are extremely diverse, as GAGs vary greatly.

Proteoglycans

- A type of glycoprotein with one or more GAG chains attached to a protein core (originally, they were considered to be a separate group).

- Largely found in connective tissue.
- Major component of the filler substance between cells (extracellular matrix).

Glycolipids

- Lipids attached to carbohydrate core.
- Provide energy. Triglycerides (p. 203).
- Serve as markers for cellular recognition. The antigens that determine blood types belong to glycolipids.

Lectins

- Glycoproteins.
- Selectively bind carbohydrates.
- Can be toxic, e.g. castor bean lectins are very toxic in very small amounts. Kidney bean lectins are thought to cause food-poisoning-like symptoms.
- Currently being studied for role in treating cancer.

Lipids 10

These are generally water-insoluble organic substances found in cells. Lipids form the basis of a diverse range of compounds. Some examples are:

- fatty acids
- carotenoids
- terpenes
- steroids
- bile salts.

} These are ultimately derived from fatty acids.

Lipids have several functions. They are:

- structural components of membranes
- intracellular storage for metabolic fuel
- a transport mechanism for metabolic fuel
- precursors of many metabolic processes and hormones.

Characteristics of Fatty Acids

- All posses a long hydrocarbon chain (a compound consisting entirely of carbons and hydrogens) and a terminal carboxyl group.
- The chain can be saturated (without double bonds) or unsaturated (contains one or more double bonds) (Figure 10.1).
- They differ in chain length and in the position and number of their bonds.
- Nearly all of them have an even number of carbon atoms; those with 16 to 18 carbons are the most common.
- Unsaturated fatty acids have lower melting points than the saturated fatty acids (this becomes significant when considering whether they are solid or fluid at room temperature).

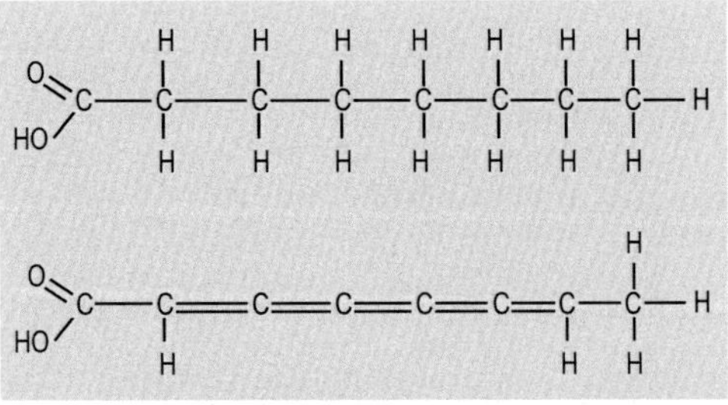

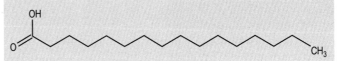

Figure 10.1 A saturated compound (top; containing only single bonds) and an unsaturated compound (below; containing some double bonds).

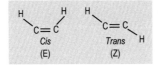

Cis
(E)

Trans
(Z)

Figure 10.2 Demonstrating the difference between *cis* (E) and *trans* (Z) fatty acids.

Figure 10.3 A fatty acid with the notation 16:0.

- The double bonds of nearly all the naturally occurring unsaturated fatty acids are in the *cis* formation (Figure 10.2).
- The most abundant unsaturated fatty acids in higher organisms are oleic, linoleic, linolenic, and arachidonic acids (see Figure 10.6).

Saturated Fatty Acids

Because they contain only single bonds, saturated fatty acids possess an enormous amount of flexibility, which allows them to bend into all kinds of shapes.

• Nomenclature of Saturated Fatty Acids

You might see a notation such as 16:0 (Figure 10.3).

- The methyl group at the end of the fatty acid is known as omega (ω).
- The number of carbon atoms is noted from the carboxyl end.
- The double bonds in fatty acids are numbered from the methyl or omega (ω) end.
- The first number indicates that the fatty acid has 16 carbon atoms.
- The second number indicates that there are no double bonds.

Unsaturated Fatty Acids

The *cis* conformations (see Figure 10.2) of the double bonds of unsaturated fatty acids have a bend in their structure of about 30 degrees. This creates significant structural features, particularly for membranes, and as components of membranes the fatty acids tend to have phosphate groups added to them to make phospholipids.

Cis fatty acids can be turned into *trans* forms by an industrial process. This creates fats with a much higher melting point, which are solid at room temperature and can be made into a spread (e.g. margarines). The natural formation of the bonds has been changed.

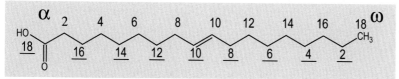

Figure 10.4 A fatty acid with the notation 18:1.

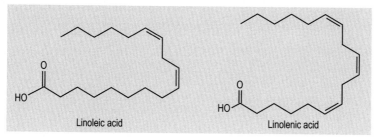

Figure 10.5 The configuration of linoleic and linolenic acids; both have *cis* configurations.

• Unsaturated Fatty Acids and the Relevance of its Nomenclature

Oleic acid is designated as 18:1 (Figure 10.4)

- The numbering runs from left to right, i.e. from the carboxyl group to the methyl group.
- The 1 indicates one double bond.
- The more precise designation is 18:1(n-9), which means that the last double bond is 9 carbon atoms from the terminal methyl group (numbers in bold and underlined).

This short-hand provides quite a bit of information at a glance to a pharmacist.

Linoleic Acid

- Linoleic or all-*cis*-9, *cis*-12-octadecadienoic acid – 18:2(n-6) – (see Figure 10.5).
- Has two *cis* double bonds: one 9 carbon atoms from the terminal methyl group (9 carbon atoms from the terminal carboxyl group), the other 6 carbon atoms from the terminal methyl group (12 carbon atoms from the terminal carboxyl group).
- Omega 6 fatty acid: this is where the term 'omega 6 fatty acids' comes from. The first double bond is at the sixth carbon from the methyl terminal group.

Linolenic Fatty Acids

There are two types (see Figure 10.6):

- alpha linolenic
- gamma linolenic.

Alpha linolenic acid or all-*cis*-9,12,15-octadecatrienoic acid:

- 18:3 (n-3)18 carbons.
- Three double bonds.
- First double bond 3 carbons from the methyl terminal group (15 carbon atoms from the carboxyl terminal end).
- Omega 3 fatty acid.

Gamma linolenic acid or all-*cis*-6,9,12-octadecatrienoic acid:

- 18:3(n-6)18 carbons.
- Three double bonds.
- First double bond 6 carbons from the methyl terminal group (12 carbon atoms from the carboxyl terminal end).
- Omega 6 fatty acid.

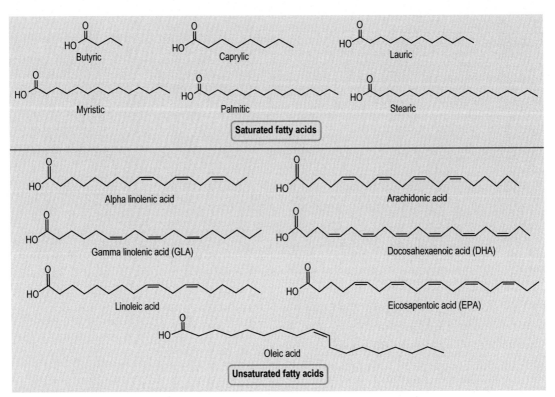

Figure 10.6 Various structures of fatty acids.

Structural Significance of *cis* Double Bonds

In natural unsaturated fatty acids, the *cis* bonds cause kinks and make them bend instead of sitting in a straight line (Figure 10.5). The kinking creates a more fluid membrane because the molecules cannot be packed close together, unlike the saturated fatty acids, which can lie in a line. The kinking also ensures that *cis* unsaturated fatty acids are fluid at room temperature (which is better for areas such as artery walls). *Trans* fatty acids are problematic because the lipids can lie flat, like a saturated fatty acid, and so cause solid areas of rigid plaque in places like the arteries.

General Information on Fatty Acids

Saturated Fatty Acids (Figure 10.6)

- **Butyric Acid**
  - Four carbons, no double bonds.
  - Found in rancid butter.
  - Formed by anaerobic bacteria.

- **Caprylic Acid**
  - Eight carbons, no double bonds.
  - Found in coconut milk and breast milk.

- **Lauric Acid**
  - 12 carbons, no double bonds.
  - Found in coconut milk and palm kernel oil.
  - Possesses antimicrobial properties.

- Myristic
  - 14 carbons, no double bonds.
  - Found in dairy products.

- Palmitic
  - 16 carbons, no double bonds.
  - Found in milk, cheese, butter, meat, palm oil and palm kernel oil.

- Stearic
  - 18 carbons, no double bonds.
  - Found in animal fats and vegetable oils.
  - Solid at room temperature.
  - Used to make soap, candles, plastics and cosmetics. Stearic acid is used to harden soaps.

Unsaturated Fatty Acids

- Arachidonic Acid (AA)
  - 20 carbons, four double bonds.
  - Found in phospholipids of cell membranes.
  - Precursor of eicosanoids, the prostaglandins (e.g. PGE2), leukotrienes and thromboxanes (see Figure 30.5, p. 229).
  - Essential fatty acid.
  - Very little or no arachidonic acid is found in plants.

- Eicosapentoic Acid (EPA) (Eicosapentaenoic)
  - 20 carbons, five double bonds.
  - Precursor for prostaglandin PGE3 (see chapter 30 'Inflammation and the immune system, p. 229).
  - Inhibits platelet aggregation and is therefore good for the cardiovascular system. However, supplements containing EPA should not be taken by anyone with a blood disorder).
  - Found in fish oils (cod, salmon, herring, sardine and mackerel) and human breast milk.
  - Omega 3 essential fatty acid.
  - Thought to act as an natural anti-inflammatory.

- Docosahexaenoic Acid (DHA)
  - 22 carbons, one double bond.
  - Omega 3 essential fatty acid.
  - Largely synthesized from alpha linolenic acid.

- Oleic Acid
  - 18-carbons, two double bonds.
  - Saturated form is stearic acid.
  - Found in animal fats and vegetable oils.
  - Found in olive oil and grape seed oil.

- Linoleic Acid
  - 18 carbons, two double bonds.
  - Essential fatty acid as an essential dietary requirement.

- Fatty acids derived from linoleic acid, particularly arachidonic acid, can adversely affect the body's anti-inflammatory processes.
- Found in pumpkin seeds, wheat germ, evening primrose oil and hemp seed oil.

Alpha Linolenic Acid

- 18 carbons, three double bonds.
- Omega 3 fatty acid.
- Essential fatty acid as an essential dietary requirement.
- Found in fish oil, flax seed oil, hemp seed oil.
- Linolenic acid in the form of precursors eicosapentoic acid [EPA; 20:5(n-3)] and docosahexaenoic acid [DHA; 22:6(n-3)] are found in fish oils.

Gamma Linolenic Acid (GLA)

- 18 carbons, three double bonds.
- Omega 6 fatty acid.
- Essential fatty acid.
- Precursor to prostaglandins (see Chapter 30 'Inflammation and the immune system', p. 229).
- Found in evening primrose oil, hemp seed oil, borage oil, blackcurrant seed oil.

Essential Fatty Acids

- Essential fatty acids are unsaturated fatty acids that are required in the human diet. They cannot be synthesized from other fatty acids and must be consumed to replenish stores in the body.
- They are essential for maintaining health.

Important Derivatives of Unsaturated Fatty Acids

Prostanoids

Prostanoids are biologically active lipids, which are synthesized from 20-carbon essential fatty acids or eicosanoids (see eicosapentoic acid, Figure 10.6). There are four main types of eicosanoid:

- prostaglandins
- prostacyclins
- thromboxanes
- leukotrienes.

Their function is discussed in more detail in Chapter 30 ('Inflammation and the immune system', p. 228).

Significance of Phospholipids

Membranes tend to be composed of phospholipids, which are lipids attached to a phosphate molecule:

- The phosphate part of the molecule is charged (polar and hydrophilic).
- The lipid part of the molecule is uncharged (non-polar and hydrophobic; see Chapter 4 'Bonds continued', p. 24).

A membrane forms because the polar, phosphate part collects near water and the lipid, non-polar part arranges itself in proximity to the other lipids in the molecule.

A cell membrane is a bilayer of phospholipids. In other words, two rows of phospholipids are arranged to accommodate the needs of the lipid and phosphate parts of the molecule (Figure 10.7).

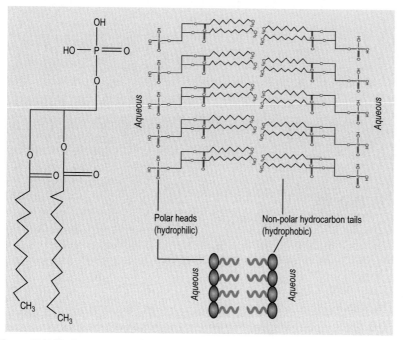

Figure 10.7 The incorporation of phospholipids into a cell membrane.

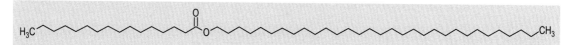

Figure 10.8 The configuration of a component of beeswax.

Utilizing the Characteristics of Phospholipids

Because membranes consist largely of lipids, only lipid-soluble substances, which are hydrophobic, can pass through them. This feature is utilized by pharmaceutical companies if they want a drug to be absorbed rapidly into the bloodstream.

There are ways of getting **polar substances** through a membrane but these usually involve a mechanism that requires energy; it is not a passive process, and will be covered in more detail later (see Chapter 16 'How do drugs get into cells?', p. 123 and Figure 31.1, p. 236).

A great deal of research is going into delivering drugs in liposomes – spherical aggregations of phospholipid bilayers. The drug is encased in the liposome, which has specially engineered qualities to make it favour attachment to a specified tissue or 'target organ'. In this way, it is hoped that highly toxic drugs, such as those used in chemotherapy, can be delivered more specifically and safely than the more inefficient 'shotgun' approach of general medication.

Waxes

Waxes (Figure 10.8) are classed as a type of lipid. They are:

- solid at room temperature, although usually malleable
- insoluble in water,

Waxes are very non-polar substances, and are therefore water resistant.

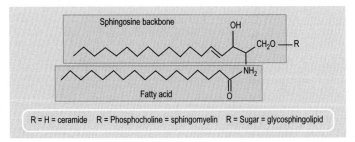

Figure 10.9 The basic structure of a sphingolipid (where the R group varies).

Glycolipids

See Chapter 9 ('Carbohydrates', p. 72) and Chapter 27 ('Problems with lipid metabolism', p. 203). Chylomicrons are large lipoprotein complexes and are synthesized in the cells of the small intestine. They are responsible for transporting lipid from the lumen to other tissues.

Sphingolipids

- Thought to provide a stable outer protective layer for a cell membrane.
- Found in neural tissue.
- Play an important role in signal transmission and cell recognition.
- The sphingosine backbone is attached to an R group, which varies, but provides a charge to that end of the molecule and a fatty acid.
- The three main types of sphingolipid are: ceramides, glycosphingolipids and sphingomyelins (Figure 10.9).
- These lipids are immensely complex.

Amino acids and proteins

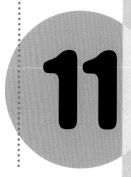

11

Amino Acids

- Amino acids are the 'building blocks' of living organisms.
- Two or more amino acids can be linked by **peptide bonds** (see Chapter 4 'Bonds continued', p. 26) to form compounds called peptides.
- **Peptides** can exist in the form of two or more linked amino acids; when many amino acids are linked, they form a **polypeptide** (see Chapter 4 'Bonds continued', p. 26).
- More than one polypeptide creates a **protein**.

Essential and Non-Essential Amino Acids

As with essential fatty acids (see Chapter 10 'Lipids', p. 78) not all amino acids can be synthesized by the body; some have to be taken in with food. They are generally considered essential in children as their metabolism is not mature enough to synthesize them.

Of the 20 standard amino acids that are encoded by DNA (there are considerably more amino acids than this but they are outside the scope of this book), 10 cannot be manufactured by the human body (**essential amino acids**); the remaining 10 can be synthesized and are therefore known as the **non-essential amino acids**. Plants contain all 20 amino acids. Their general structure is seen in Figure 11.2.

The essential amino acids (Figure 11.1) are:

- arginine
- histidine
- isoleucine
- leucine
- lycine
- methionine
- phenylalanine

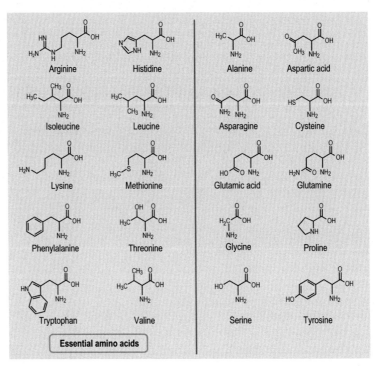

Figure 11.1 The 20 common amino acids.

- threonine
- tryptophan
- valine.

The non-essential amino acids are:

- alanine
- asparagine
- aspartic acid
- cysteine
- glutamic acid
- glutamine
- glycine
- proline
- serine
- tyrosine.

Proteins

Proteins serve several functions:

- Metabolic: enzymes.
- Structural: in tendons and muscles.
- Immune system: immunoglobulins.
- Receptors for hormones and neurological signalling.

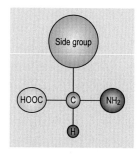

Figure 11.2 The general primary structure of amino acids.

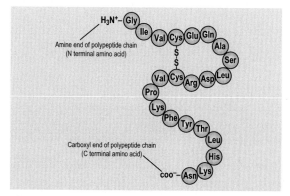

Figure 11.3 The primary structure of shown proteins as a peptide chain with a disulphide cross-link.

The Importance of Proteins

- Proteins are involved in just about every process in a living organism.
- They build cells and repair tissues.
- They provide structural support.

Protein Structure

• Primary (1°) Protein Structure (Figure 11.3)

Polypeptide Cross-Linking

The amino acid cysteine (cys) contains a sulphur group, which can form a cross-link with another sulphur, forming a **disulphide bond**. This cross-link strengthens the integrity of the polypeptide bond and lends itself to forming a more complex structure (Figure 11.3).

This type of bond has already been explored using the example of immunoglobulin (see Chapter 3 'Bonds found in biological chemistry', p. 15).

• Secondary (2°) Protein Structure

Alpha Helix

- The strands of protein can coil around themselves. This is the secondary structure.
- The secondary structure consists of an alpha helix where the side group orientates itself to the outside of the helix.
- The helix always twists in a clockwise direction; in other words, it is right handed.
- Hydrogen bonds (see Chapter 3 'Bonds found in biological chemistry', p. 19) are formed between the helices (Figure 11.4).

Beta Conformation or Beta Pleated Sheets

These consist of pairs of polypeptide chains lying side by side, stabilized by hydrogen bonds (Figure 11.4).

• Tertiary (3°) Protein Structure

To add even more complexity, the coils and sheets of polypeptides can fold in on themselves to create a tertiary structure (Figure 11.5); enzymes are an example.

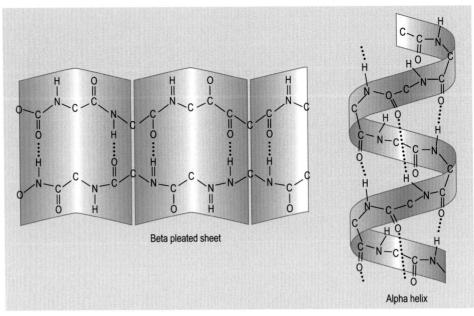

Beta pleated sheet

Alpha helix

Figure 11.4 The structure of a beta pleated sheet and an alpha helix.

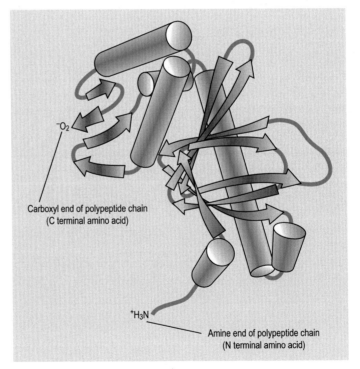

$^-O_2$

Carboxyl end of polypeptide chain
(C terminal amino acid)

^+H_3N

Amine end of polypeptide chain
(N terminal amino acid)

Figure 11.5 Protein tertiary structure (ribbons = beta pleated sheets; cylinders = alpha helices).

• Quaternary Structure

This is when tertiary structures that exist as whole units join together to form an even more complex protein unit. Examples are ion channels and haemoglobin.

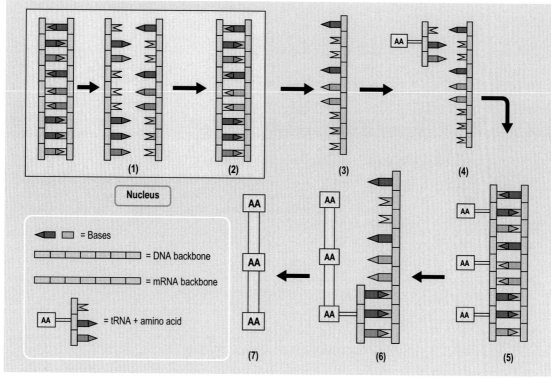

Figure 11.6 Protein synthesis. See the text for an explanation of the numbers.

The Significance of Protein Structure

Their tertiary structure gives proteins a very specific shape and is an important feature in the 'lock and key' function of enzymes, or receptor sites on cell membranes. Specificity can vary, in some cases sites can allow some variation in structure in other cases not.

This feature of 'correct fit' is utilized by pharmaceutical companies when creating new drugs, which are designed to have a close-enough structure to a receptor site to be able to fit into it, to either block or stimulate a reaction (see Chapter 19 'Pharmacodynamics: how drugs elicit a physiological effect', p. 137).

Factored into the combination of amino acids is the fact that they have chirality (see Chapter 6 'Isomers', p. 36), which also affects the shape of a receptor site and the shape into which the protein can fold. Natural amino acids are always L isomers.

Protein Synthesis

The numbers below refer to Figure 11.6.

1. DNA in the nucleus unzips. Unzipped DNA acts as a template for the synthesis of messenger RNA (mRNA).
2. The mRNA detaches from the template and the two DNA strands rejoin and 'zip up'. The base subunit of thymine in DNA is replaced with uracil in the mRNA (see Chapter 12 'Purines and pyrimidines', p. 90).
3. The newly formed mRNA migrates out of the nucleus and into the cytoplasm, where it latches onto a structure called a ribosome. Every three bases in the mRNA is the sequence for a particular amino acid.
4/5. Transfer RNA (tRNA) contains three bases, which line up to the complementary bases on the mRNA. Each tRNA with a particular sequence picks up a particular amino acid.

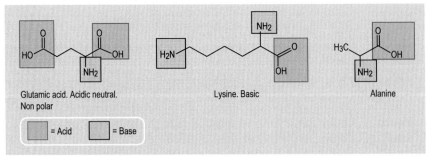

Figure 11.7 The characteristics of different amino acids.

6. As the tRNA attaches to the mRNA the amino acids link to each other with a peptide bond (see Chapter 4 'Bonds continued' p. 26). As the amino acids link, the tRNA detaches.

7. The polypeptide finally detaches from the mRNA.

This process explains why intact and correctly sequenced DNA is so important; a fault in it will result in defects in metabolism or the inability to produce polypeptides.

Viruses inject their own genetic material into a cell, changing the cell metabolism – by producing new enzymes – and gearing the cell to produce more viruses instead of its normal metabolism.

Some chemotherapy hopes to intervene to prevent cancer cells from multiplying by interfering with the above process in affected cells.

The Chemical Characteristics of Amino Acids and their Relevance to Pharmacology

Although they are called 'acids', amino acids can in fact have acidic, neutral or basic characteristics (Figure 11.7).

Amino acids possess a —COOH and an —NH$_2$ element. They are able to lose a hydrogen from the —COOH part and grasp a hydrogen on the —NH$_2$ part (see Chapter 8 'Acids and bases', p. 54). Potentially, this leaves the amino acid negatively charged at the carboxyl end (—COO$^-$) or positively charged at the amine end (—NH$_3^+$) or both.

From Figure 11.7 it is possible to see that some amino acids are more predominantly acidic or basic than others (lysine, with two amine groups, is predominantly basic and glutamic acid, with two carboxyl groups, is predominantly acidic), whereas other amino acids such as alanine are effectively neutral.

This ability to juggle (**buffer**) with the hydrogen ions in a solution is a very important aspect of amino-acid chemistry as it enables them to act as buffers, preventing the body from becoming too acidic or too basic. But this is not the only important function of amino acids. Enzymes are proteins and proteins are made up of a very large number of amino acids.

Figure 11.5 demonstrates how a protein folds in on itself. The amino acids that are part of this protein will have COO$^-$ and NH$_3^+$ groups sticking out in various positions. The substances temporarily bonding with the enzyme will have a need for hydrogen ions or will want to give them up (see Chapter 8 'Acids and bases', p. 54). The right substrate for the enzyme will fit exactly to the right bonds in the correct orientation.

With some amino acids, such as alanine (see Figure 11.7), changing the environment can change its character as it has both an acid and base element in equal quantities. This is significant, as various enzymes will be activated only at a specific pH.

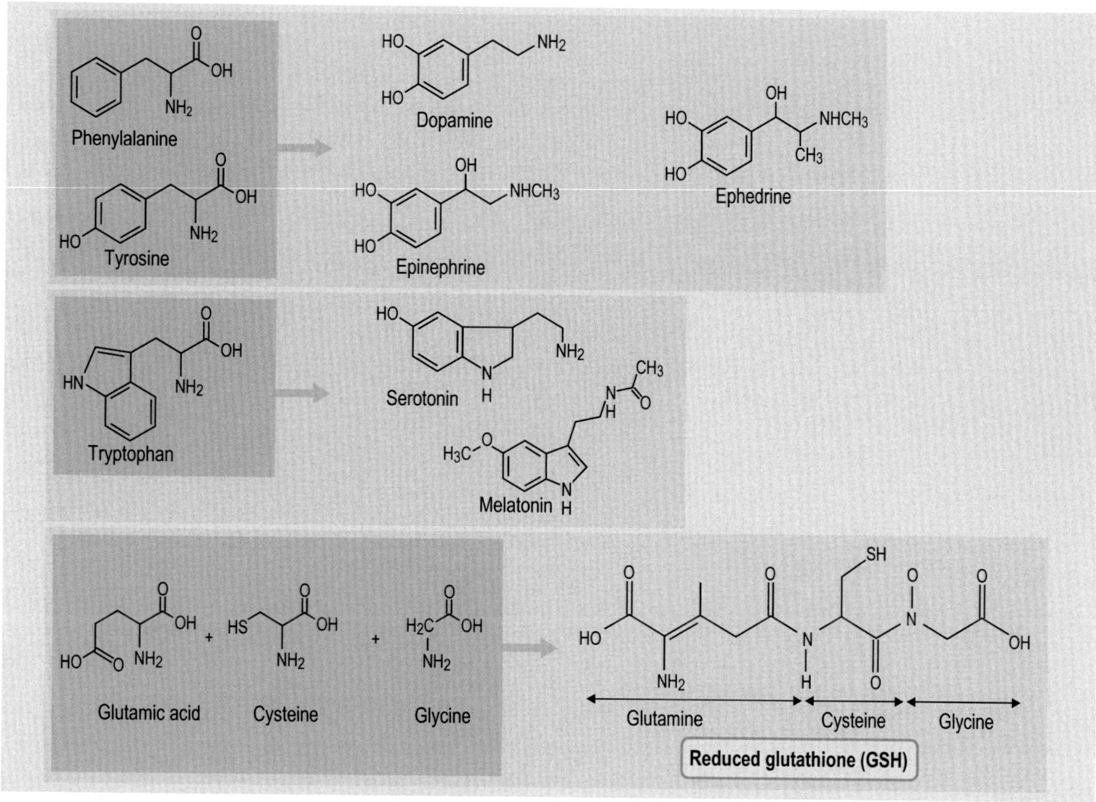

Figure 11.8 Some natural derivatives of amino acids.

This is how the **lock and key** system of receptors and enzymes works, and this characteristic is used by pharmaceutical companies when developing drugs that mimic these substances; the combinations are seemingly limitless. It is also how hormones or neurotransmitters work and explains why proteins are so important in living organisms.

Derivatives of Amino Acids

Amino acids are found in many different natural substances. Some examples are shown in Figure 11.8.

Purines and pyrimidines

Purines and pyrimidines are known as **nitrogenous bases**. The two groups have different features (Figure 12.1):

- Purines: a six-membered and a five-membered nitrogen-containing ring fused together.
- Pyrimidines: a six-membered nitrogen-containing ring.

These nitrogenous bases are crucial not only to the storage and transmission of genetic information, but also as a means of storing mobile energy. They can be synthesized in the body from basic components. The degraded bases can be salvaged and reused (see Chapter 37 'Metabolic disorders', p. 295).

Nucleosides and Nucleotides

When a sugar is added to a nitrogenous base, a **nucleoside** is formed (Figure 12.2).
When phosphate groups attach to the nucleoside, a **nucleotide** is formed (Figure 12.2) with one phosphate (**monophosphate**), two phosphate (**diphosphate**) or three phosphate (**triphosphate**) groups attached.

Nucleotides

Nucleotides are very important chemicals. They:

- Store genetic information in the nucleus in the form of DNA.
- Transmit genetic information in the form of messenger RNA.
- Are responsible for the storage of energy in chemicals adenosine triphosphate (ATP) and guanosine triphosphate (GTP).
- Are involved in signal transduction, which is the movement of signals from outside the cell to its inside (see Figure 19.5, p. 141).
- Act as secondary messengers in cellular communication in the form of cyclic adenosine monophosphate (cAMP).
- Are required for coenzyme function (coenzymes enable enzymes to work properly), e.g. nicotinamide adenine dinucleotide phosphate ($NADP^+$).

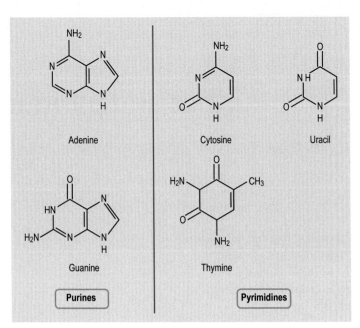

Figure 12.1 The structure of purines and pyrimidines.

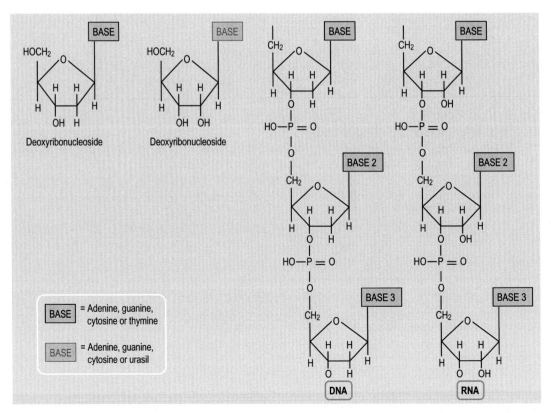

Figure 12.2 The basic structure of nucleosides and their inclusion in the nucleotide structures of RNA and DNA.

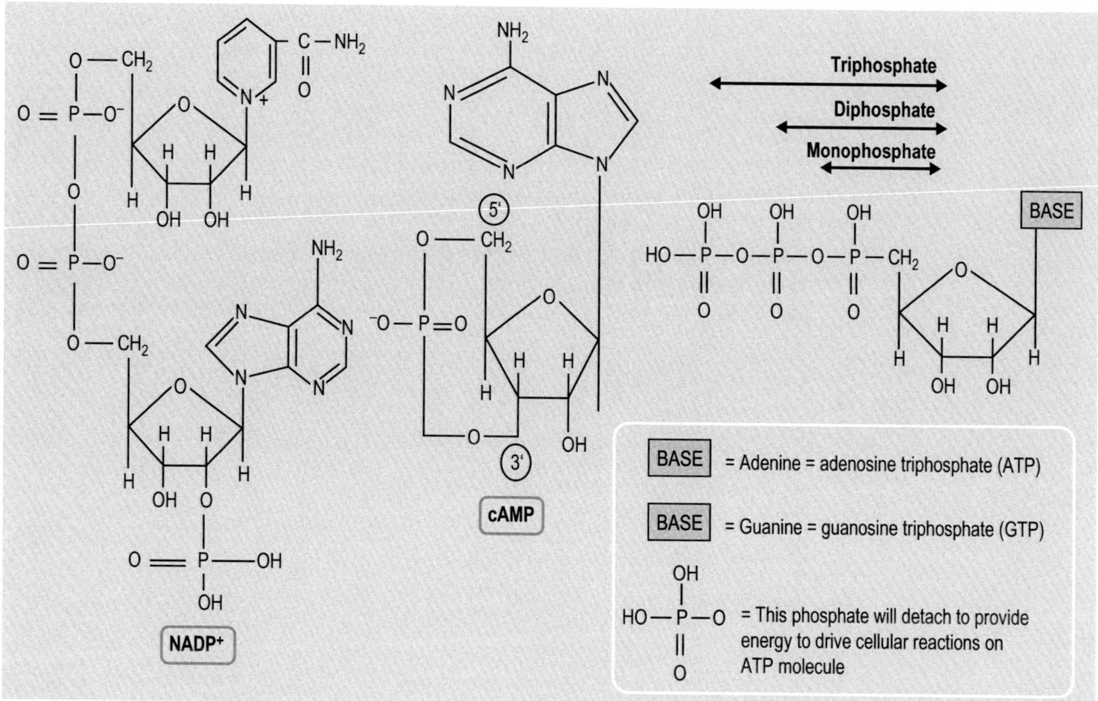

Figure 12.3 The structure of the coenzyme nicotinamide adenine dinucleotide phosphate (NADP⁺), the secondary messenger cyclic adenosine monophosphate (cAMP) and the energy carrier adenosine triphosphate (ATP), all of which are derived from purines and pyrimidines.

Adenine and thymine base pair

Guanine and cytosine base pair

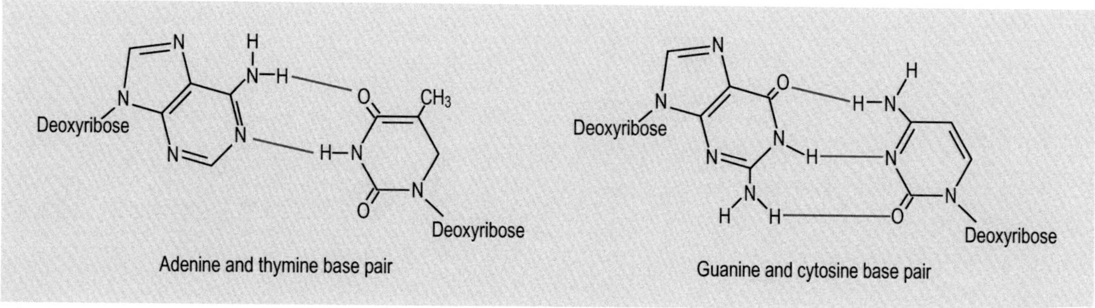

Figure 12.4 Hydrogen bonding between the nitrogenous bases in DNA. This is where alkylating agents used for chemotherapy work.

The Importance of Hydrogen Bonds in DNA (Figure 12.4)

The two strands of the DNA structure are held together by hydrogen bonds between the nitrogenous bases (see Chapter 3 'Bonds found in biological chemistry', p. 18) (Figure 12.4). This allows the structure to be pulled apart and put back together in protein synthesis (see Figure 11.6, p. 85).

Metabolism of Purines and Pyrimidines

Every body organ has a different capacity to synthesize purines and pyrimidines. The liver is responsible for synthesizing the majority of purines from their basic components (***de novo* synthesis**).

Those purines and pyrimidines that are not resynthesized are removed from the body and their breakdown results in the production of uric acid, primarily by the liver, which is excreted by the kidneys. A defect in this process will result in a clinical condition, as in the case of gout (see Chapter 37 'Metabolic disorders', p. 295).

DNA and RNA

It is important to note that although there is a turnover of RNA within a cell, this does not occur with DNA. Instead, enzymes excise the damaged parts during a process of repair. If this process goes wrong then cell metabolism malfunctions. This is considered when treating viral infections and using chemotherapy to damage the viral or aberrant cell DNA (see Chapter 39 'Chemotherapy', p. 309).

Vitamins and minerals

13

This chapter provides an overview of the vitamins and minerals encountered in pharmacology, and their relevance to practice.

Reference Values

- **Recommended daily allowance (RDA):** the average daily intake that is recommended as being sufficient to meet the nutrient requirements of 97% of healthy people; it differs for children, adults, and different sexes.
- **Estimated average requirement (EAR):** the average daily dietary intake estimated to meet the requirements of 50% of healthy individuals; it differs for children, adults and different sexes.
- **Adequate intakes (AI):** the recommended average daily intake when there is insufficient scientific data available to determine an RDA. AIs meet or exceed the amount needed to maintain an adequate nutritional state in nearly all members of a specific age and sex.
- **Tolerable upper intake levels (UL):** the maximum daily intake likely to result in no adverse health effects. If intake above this level is reached the potential risk of adverse effects might increase.

There is now a move to change all these, amalgamating them into the **dietary reference intake (DRI),** which takes into account the above values.

People at Risk from Deficiencies

Any condition of the gastrointestinal tract that reduces absorption can put the individual at risk of a vitamin deficiency (see Chapter 15 'Methods of administration', p. 119). Other causes include:

- The very young, who have an underdeveloped metabolism.
- The very old, who have reduced hydrochloric acid production in the stomach and a generally less efficient metabolism. Elderly individuals might also not eat properly, either as a result of problems with food preparation or because of their inability to take in food.
- Patients with gastrointestinal conditions that reduce absorption, e.g. Crohn's disease.
- Patients with chronic liver conditions that will affect the bile, e.g. cirrhosis.
- Alcoholics.
- Patients on chemotherapy, which damages the lining of the gastrointestinal tract.
- Individuals who follow special diets, e.g. vegetarians, vegans.
- Fad diets for weight loss.

Metals

- Usually occur in the form of trace elements, which occur in the body in very small or 'trace' amounts. They generally constitute less than 0.001% of the body mass and are incorporated into structures such as haemoglobin.
- They are also used in enzyme reactions.

Essential Trace Element Minerals

- Iron.
- Copper.
- Zinc.
- Chromium.
- Manganese.
- Selenium.
- Molybenum.
- Iodine.
- Fluorine.

Other Trace Minerals not Considered Essential

- Silicon.
- Nickel.
- Boron.
- Vanadium.
- Arsenic.
- Cobalt.

A trace element is needed by an organism in very small quantities to maintain correct physiological function.

Two Important Elements

Magnesium

- Found in plants in chlorophyll (see Chapter 9 'Carbohydrates', p. 64).
- Structural role: found in bone and in cell membranes. Magnesium is usually combined with calcium in supplements to improve absorption.
- Involved in almost all metabolic process in the body (e.g. carbohydrate and lipid metabolism and detoxification) as a cofactor (a helper molecule required by an enzyme; see Chapter 19 'Pharmacodynamics: how drugs elicit a physiological effect', p. 139).
- Necessary for muscular contraction of skeletal, smooth and heart muscle.
- Protein synthesis: is required for a number of steps in the synthesis of DNA and RNA.

Thus adequate levels of magnesium in the body are important.

• Facts about Magnesium

- Stress makes magnesium move from the cells to the bloodstream and promotes accelerated magnesium secretion.
- Magnesium deficiency will result in increased secretion of adrenal hormones (adrenaline/epinephrine and noradrenaline/norepinephrine).

• Dietary Sources of Magnesium

- Buckwheat.
- Blackstrap molasses.
- Pulses and soy beans (including tofu).
- Broccoli and green leafy vegetables.
- Oats, whole barley, and millet.
- Fruit.
- Nuts and seeds.
- Seafood and fish.

• Magnesium as an Adjunct to Orthodox Medication

- Magnesium has been shown to play an important part of acute asthma management.
- Intravenous magnesium sulphate is used for patients with pre-eclampsia.
- Magnesium is important in the prevention of osteoporosis.

• Signs and Symptoms of Magnesium Deficiency

- Nausea.
- Irritability, confusion, tremors and nervousness.
- Muscle weakness: magnesium deficiency can result in problems with muscular tetany or heart arrhythmia.

Calcium

- Structural: the most common mineral in the body.
- 99% of calcium in the body is found in the bones and teeth; the rest is in blood and soft tissue.
- Necessary for muscle contraction (see Chapter 31 'The nervous system', p. 237). Low levels of calcium can lead to tetany.
- Effective in reducing blood pressure in some types of hypertension, e.g. high blood pressure during pregnancy.
- Is a cofactor.

- ● Calcium Metabolism

See Figure 37.1 (p. 290).

- ● Dietary Sources

- Dairy products.
- Nuts.
- Dark green leafy vegetables (high in calcium, but it is not easily absorbed).
- Blackstrap molasses.
- Seafood and fish.

- ● Interaction of Food Substances with Calcium

Calcium is absorbed along the entire length of the gastrointestinal tract. Absorption can be affected by:

- Phytates: found in whole grains; can combine with calcium (see Chapter 15 'Methods of administration', p. 120).
- Oxalates: interfere with the uptake of calcium in the same food source. Spinach contains calcium but this is chemically bound to the oxalates that are also present in the spinach and is therefore not available for absorption. Similar foods are rhubarb and sweet potatoes.
- Phosphorus: ingested largely in soft drinks. Phosphorus-rich foods tend to increase the calcium content of digestive secretions. This results in a higher than usual calcium loss through removal by the faeces. Although the effect of drinking fizzy drinks is still unclear, the large quantities consumed by some children are currently causing concern.
- Caffeine: the extent to which caffeine affects the loss of calcium through the urine is contested, as there are so many factors affecting bone metabolism. A genetic factor might be important in determining the amount of loss (Rapuri et al 2001).
- Fibre: dietary fibre binds with calcium to form an insoluble complex.
- Sodium: increased sodium intake results in an increased loss of calcium in the urine. This is possibly due to competition between sodium and calcium by active transport mechanisms in the kidney or the effect of sodium on the parathyroid hormone (PTH) secretion (see Chapter 37 'Metabolic disorders', p. 289). Dietary sodium is thought to have considerable potential for influencing bone loss.
- High protein intake: increases the absorption of calcium from the gastrointestinal tract, which then increases the amount of calcium present in the urine.
- High intake of calcium: can reduce iron absorption from both haem (meat) and non-haem (green leafy vegetables, legumes, whole grains, dried beans and nuts) sources.

- ● Kidney Stones and Calcium

See Chapter 36 ('Urinary tract infection', p. 283).

Trace Elements

Iron

Iron is essential to plants and animals and is usually found incorporated in a protein complex called a haem, where it forms the nucleus of the haem complex. This complex is an essential component of:

- Haemoglobin: two-thirds of the iron in the body is in the form of haemoglobin.
- Myoglobin (the primary oxygen-carrying pigment of muscle): responsible for carrying oxygen in the muscle.
- Cytochromes: which form part of the electron transfer mechanism in oxidative phosphorylation (see Figure 2.5, p. 10).

- Cofactors: required by enzymes (e.g. cytochrome p450, which is used in detoxification in the liver and has a central haem core) (see Chapter 17 'Metabolism', p. 129 and Chapter 19 'Pharmacodynamics: how drugs elicit a physiological effect', p. 139).

Iron is also required to deal with bacterial infection; in this situation the body stores as much iron as possible in the storage molecule ferritin inside the cells, so as to deprive the bacteria of it.

• When can Iron Deficiency Occur?

- Patients with low dietary intake of iron, particularly haem iron: vegetarians and vegans.
- Pregnancy.
- Women and teenagers with heavy menstrual loss (postmenopausal women do not lose much iron and therefore have a low risk of iron deficiency).
- Patients with kidney failure, especially those on dialysis. Due to kidneys not being able to create enough erythropoietin (see Chapter 28 'Blood disorders', p. 209).
- Conditions that lead to chronic malabsorption: Crohn's disease; chronic inflammation of the small intestine will affect absorption of not only iron but also other nutrients.
- Deficiency of vitamin A: vitamin A helps mobilize iron from its storage site; a deficiency of vitamin A will therefore reduce the body's ability to use stored iron. This leads to a strange situation in which haemoglobin levels are low, giving the impression of iron deficiency anaemia, even though there is an adequate store of iron.
- Preterm and low birthweight infants.

For symptoms of iron deficiency anaemia, see Chapter 28 'Blood disorders' (p. 209).

• Sources of Iron

Iron comes from two sources:

- **Haem**: meat, fish and poultry.
- **Non-haem**: fruit, vegetables, beans, nuts, soy beans and whole grains.

Haem iron is absorbed much more easily than non-haem iron. Only 1–7% of non-haem iron is absorbed when eaten on its own. Non-haem iron absorption can also be decreased by the following:

- Excessive consumption of high-fibre foods that contain phytates (see Chapter 15 'Methods of Administration', p. 120): phytates can inhibit absorption.
- Large amounts of tea or coffee, ingested at the same time as a meal: polyphenols bind the iron.
- Large of amounts of highly processed foods with simple carbohydrates (see Chapter 9 'Carbohydrates', p. 64) (Kant 2003).
- High-dosage calcium supplementation.

There are, however, ways of increasing non-haem absorption:

- By eating foods that contain vitamin C in the form of ascorbic acid, e.g. oranges, grapefruits, tomatoes, broccoli.
- By eating non-haem food with haem food.
- Alcohol (in moderation) can help the absorption of iron, which is why there are tonics, both in Western society and in Chinese medicine, that are administered in alcohol.
- By cooking a non-haem food in an iron cooking vessel.
- Supplementation by an iron–amino acid chelate (the iron is attached to the amino acid to increase absorption).

Copper

Copper is a cofactor in various metabolic processes:

- Energy production: oxidative phosphorylation (see Figure 2.5, p. 10).
- Scavenging free radicals: copper is a cofactor of superoxide dismutase (SOD; see Chapter 7 'Free radicals', p. 46 and Chapter 19 Pharmacodynamics: how drugs elicit a physiological effect', p. 139).

Copper is also involved in:

- The production of collagen and elastin: the connective tissues of the body.
- The formation of bone (see Chapter 37 'Metabolic disorders', p. 290).
- Neurotransmitter synthesis: conversion of **dopamine** to **norepinephrine (noradrenaline)** (see Figure 31.6, p. 242).
- Neurotransmitter degradation: degradation of the monoamine neurotransmitters (see Chapter 31 'The nervous system', p. 242).
- Pigment formation.
- Gene regulation.

● Interaction with Food Substances

- Zinc: high intakes of zinc increase the synthesis of a cell protein that binds to metals like copper and has a greater affinity for copper than zinc, making it unavailable for use.

● Copper Deficiency

Blood disorders (see Chapter 28 'Blood disorders', p. 209 and Chapter 41 'Scientific tests', p. 331):

- Macrocytic anaemia: the average size of the erythrocytes is larger than normal.
- Neutropenia: abnormal decrease in the number of the white blood cells.
- Decrease in mean platelet volume: decrease in platelet size.
- Osteoporosis.

Less common:

- Loss of pigmentation.
- Neurological symptoms.
- Impaired growth.

● Dietary Considerations

- Cow's milk is low in copper: cow's milk infant formulae are supplemented with copper.
- Premature infants, particularly those with a low birth weight, might have difficulties absorbing nutrients.
- Malabsorption syndromes such as coeliac disease, short bowel syndrome, cancer of the small intestine (see Chapter 15 'Methods of administration', p. 119).

● Sources of Copper

- Nuts.
- Grains.
- Blackstrap molasses.
- Seafood and fish.

Zinc

- Enzyme activator, therefore important for general metabolic processes.
- Scavenging free radicals: zinc is a cofactor of superoxide dismutase (SOD; see Chapter 7 'Free radicals', p. 46 and Chapter 19 'Pharmacodynamics: how drugs elicit a physiological effect', p. 139).

- **Dietary Sources of Zinc**
  - Meat.
  - Pulses.
  - Nuts.
  - Whole grains.
  - Pumpkin and sunflower seeds.

- **Deficiency**
  - Hair loss.
  - Skin lesions.
  - Wasting.
  - Associated with benign prostatic hyperplasia.

Note that phytates can interfere with the absorption of zinc (see Chapter 15 'Methods of administration', p. 120).

Chromium

- The naturally active form of chromium is trivalent Cr^{3+} (i.e. will accept three electrons).
- Encourages insulin in its activity of stimulating glucose uptake by cells. The whole involvement of chromium, however, is not fully understood. As type 2 diabetes (non-insulin dependent diabetes; NIDDM) might be due to a decreased insulin sensitivity of cells, chromium is thought to assist this condition, but the assumption is still controversial.

- **Dietary Sources**
  - Meats.
  - Whole grains.
  - Broccoli, green beans, spices (e.g. cinnamon).
  - Foods with a high concentration of sucrose and fructose (simple sugars) are low in chromium and have been found to promote chromium loss.

Manganese

- Carbohydrates, amino acid synthesis: cofactor.
- Formation of cartilage and bone: cofactor for synthesis of proteoglycans (see Chapter 9 'Carbohydrates', p. 71) and needed for the formation of cartilage and bone.
- Suppression of free radicals: cofactor of superoxide dismutase (SOD; see Chapter 7 'Free radicals', p. 46 and Chapter 19 'Pharmacodynamics: how drugs elicit a physiological effect', p. 139).
- Healing of wounds: cofactor in enzymes required for tissue repair.

- **Nutrient Interactions**
  - Magnesium: can interfere with manganese absorption.
  - Iron: manganese may share common absorption and transport pathways.
  - Calcium: milk does not appear to affect manganese absorption. There are mixed ideas as to how much calcium supplementation affects the absorption of manganese.
  - Tannins: may reduce the absorption of manganese.

- **Dietary Sources**
  - Green leafy vegetables.
  - Nuts.

- Whole grains.
- Seaweed.

• Foods that can Inhibit Manganese Absorption

- Oxalates (see above).
- Phytates (see Chapter 15 'Methods of administration', p. 120).

• Toxicity

Usually through inhalation:

- Inorganic: combustion products from cars or trucks, dusts present in steel or battery factories.
- Organic: petrol additives, some pesticides, some tests for cancer contain a manganese compound.
- Neurological symptoms and Parkinson-like symptoms
- Occupation can be an important factor in the case history.

Toxicity due to ingestion:

- Due to over supplementation, but is extremely rare.

• Patients with a Predisposition to Manganese Toxicity

Manganese is eliminated from the body in bile. Chronic liver disease will, therefore, affect the production of bile and decrease excretion of bile.

Selenium

Suppression of free radicals: selenium is a cofactor for glutathione peroxidase (see Chapter 7 'Free radicals', p. 47 and Chapter 19 'Pharmacodynamics: how drugs elicit a physiological effect', p. 139).

• Dietary Sources

- Meat: particularly liver and kidneys.
- Seafood.
- Grains.
- Nuts.

Molybdenum

A cofactor in various metabolic processors (see Chapter 19 'Pharmacodynamics: how drugs elicit a physiological effect', p. 139):

- Breakdown of nucleotides (precursors to DNA and RNA).
- Metabolism of sulphur-containing amino acids.
- Metabolism of drugs.

• Food Sources

- Green leafy vegetables.
- Pulses.
- Grains.
- Lentils.
- Meat.
- Milk.

• Deficiency

Lin Xian in Northern China has unusually low concentrations of molybdenum in the soil and has one of the highest incidences of oesophageal cancer in the world (Yang 2000).

Iodine

Vital for the normal function of the thyroid gland (see Chapter 37 'Metabolic disorders', p. 288).

• Dietary Sources

- Seafood and fish.
- Seaweed.
- Iodized salt.

• Deficiency

- **Goitre**: Iodine is generally widely available and found in drinking water and food but in certain areas of the world (e.g. Central Asia) there is iodine deficiency and supplementation in salt or bread is necessary.

Fluoride

- 95% of the total fluoride found in the body is in the bones and teeth.
- Helps to form rigid lattice in bone.

• Dietary Sources

- Tea.
- Fish that can be eaten with their bones intact.

• Deficiency

- Dental caries.

Boron

Appears to be involved in calcium and magnesium metabolism, therefore deficiency might be a factor in osteoporosis.

Cobalt

See vitamin B_{12} (p. 105).

Silicon, Nickel, Arsenic and Vanadium

Deficiencies induced under laboratory conditions indicate depression in growth and impaired reproduction. As they are all readily available in the general diet, these nutritional requirements are normally easily met.

Phosphorus

- Needed for bone and teeth formation.
- Present in membranes as part of phospholipids.
- Necessary for energy production and cell signalling. Found in compounds such as ATP and GTP.
- Easily absorbed in gut.

• Dietary Sources

- Dairy products.
- Fish.
- Nuts.
- Whole grains.

Water-Soluble Vitamins

Vitamin C and the B-Complex Vitamins

- Water-soluble vitamins: are easily excreted in the urine in small amounts, therefore the potential for toxicity is normally very low.
- No stable storage form: have to be provided continuously in diet (except for vitamin B_{12}, which can be stored in human liver for several years).
- Vitamin C and all the B-complex vitamins except cobalamin (vitamin B_{12}) can be synthesized by plants.
- All water-soluble vitamins except vitamin C serve as coenzymes or cofactors in enzymatic reactions.

Vitamin C (Ascorbic Acid)

- Active form ascorbate or ascorbic acid.
- Antioxidant.

• Absorption of Ascorbic Acid

The absorption of ascorbic acid occurs actively as well as passively (see Chapter 16 'How do drugs get into cells?' p. 123). When the concentrations of ascorbic acid are low, active transport predominates, whereas at high concentration the active transport system becomes saturated leaving only passive diffusion. Therefore, slowing down the rate of stomach emptying (see Chapter 15 'Methods of administration', p. 117) or providing a slow-release form of ascorbic acid should increase its absorption.

• Dietary Sources

- Fruits: particularly citrus fruits and juices.
- Vegetables: potatoes are a common source.
- Green and red peppers.

• Deficiency

Scurvy: a group of symptoms including tiredness, muscle weakness, joint and muscle aches, bleeding gums and skin rash.

• High Doses

- High doses of vitamin C will cause diarrhoea due to the increased concentration of vitamin C in the gut pulling water into the gut by osmosis.
- Very high doses of vitamin C can precipitate an acute sickle-cell crisis in patients with sickle-cell disease.
- If a patient has iron-overload (as is the case with porphyria; see Chapter 28 'Blood disorders', p. 211) vitamin C should be avoided. This might be due to the ability of the ascorbate to stimulate iron-dependent peroxidation of membrane lipids under certain conditions (see Figure 7.4, p. 45).

B-Complex Vitamins

These are divided into those associated with:

- Energy production: thiamin (vitamin B_1), riboflavin (vitamin B_2), pantothenic acid (vitamin B_5), niacin (nicotinic acid), pyridoxine (vitamin B_6) and biotin.
- Haematopoietic (blood cell formation) vitamins: cobalamin (vitamin B_{12}) and folic acid.

• B Vitamins Involved with Energy Production

B$_1$ (Thiamin)

- Coenzyme in carbohydrate metabolism and some amino acids (see Chapter 19 'Pharmacodynamics: how drugs elicit a physiological effect', p. 139).
- Need to increase in pregnancy.
- Prevents inflammation of nerves (beri beri).

Dietary Sources

- Unrefined cereal grains.
- Organ meats – heart, kidney, liver.
- Brewer's yeast.
- Nuts and seeds.

Signs and Symptoms of Deficiency

- Neuropathy.
- Muscle wasting.
- Confusion.
- Anorexia.
- Enlarged heart.

Deficiency likely to occur when patient is consuming:

- Highly processed white flour.
- White rice.
- Sugar.

Vitamin B$_2$ (Riboflavin)

- Necessary for healthy eyes, skin, lips and tongue.

Dietary Sources

- Dairy products.
- Meats.
- Fish.
- Green leafy vegetables.

Signs and Symptoms of Deficiency

Oral (buccal) cavity lesions, e.g. angular stomatitis (inflammation at the corners of the mouth).

Vitamin B$_3$ (Niacin or Nicotinic Acid)

Forms part of the nicotinamide adenine dinucleotide (NAD) structure (see Figure 12.3, p. 91 and Chapter 19 'Pharmacodynamics: how drugs elicit a physiological effect', p. 139).

Dietary Sources

- Meat.
- Eggs.
- Liver.
- Fish.
- Wheat germ.
- Yeast.

Note: Although vitamin B3 is found in maize, it is largely in a bound form and therefore not available as a nutrient. This is worth bearing in mind in patients consuming large quantities of maize in the diet and very little meat.

Signs and Symptoms of Deficiency

- Pellagra: leads to a triad of dermatitis, diarrhoea and dementia.
- Oral lesions and a red tongue: might be the only noticeable symptoms.

Large doses of nicotinic acid have been found to lower both cholesterol and triglyceride levels in the bloodstream, as it is responsible for inhibiting their synthesis.

Note: nicotinamide is usually preferred to nicotinic acid as a supplement because there is less chance of gastric irritation.

Vitamin B$_5$ (Pantothenic Acid)

Involved in synthesis and oxidation of fatty acids and other important energy-producing reactions (see Chapter 19 'Pharmacodynamics: how drugs elicit a physiological effect', p. 139).

Dietary Sources

- Meat.
- Eggs.
- Whole grains.
- Legumes.
- Royal jelly.

Signs and Symptoms of Deficiency

Very rare because it is so easily obtained from food.

Vitamin B$_6$ (Pyridoxine, Pyridoxal and Pyridoxamine)

- Necessary for normal cell membrane function and stability: assists in the balancing of sodium and potassium, hence neurological problems with a deficiency (see Figure 31.1, p. 236).
- Promotes red blood cell production.
- Prevents the formation of homocysteine (see Chapter 36 'Metabolic disorders', p. 296).

Dietary Sources

This vitamin is easily destroyed by food processing:

- Meats are the best source.
- Fruits.
- Vegetables.
- Whole grains.

Signs and Symptoms of Deficiency

- Tissue changes: including glossitis (inflammation of the tongue), stomatitis.
- Neurological: depression, headaches, nausea, weakness, tingling and pain in the extremities.
- Microcytic hypochromic anaemia: see Chapter 28 'Blood disorders', p. 209).
- Elevated homocysteine levels: see Chapter 37 'Metabolic disorders', p. 296).

Vitamin H (Biotin)

- Involved in fatty acid and amino acid metabolism.
- Contains sulphur.
- Synthesized in the lower gastrointestinal tract by **commensals**.

Dietary Sources

- Liver.
- Egg yolk: egg white contains a biotin-binding glycoprotein (see Chapter 9 'Carbohydrates', p. 71), so excessive consumption can potentially create a biotin deficiency.
- Grains.
- Soy.
- Yeast.

Signs and Symptoms of Deficiency

- Rare.

● Haemopoietic B Vitamins

Vitamin B_{12}

Vitamin B_{12} is bound to a protein that is removed in the stomach. Intrinsic factor, a protein produced by the parietal cells in the stomach wall, then combines with the vitamin B_{12} complex. This protects the complex against bacteria and degradation by digestive enzymes, and improves its absorption through the small intestine wall. Vitamin B_{12} can be absorbed without intrinsic factor but not as easily. Once absorbed, the intrinsic factor is cleaved off.

Its structure is similar to that of chlorophyll (see Figure 9.1, p. 64) and the haem structure found in red blood cells, but with cobalt instead of magnesium or iron.

Dietary Sources

- Meats.
- Seafood and fish.
- Dairy products (but not to such a great extent as the above).

Given the right environment, the bacteria of the colon can synthesize vitamin B_{12}.

Deficiency

- Pernicious anaemia: vitamin B_{12} deficiency leads to large red blood cells (**macrocytic, megaloblastic anaemia**; see Chapter 28 'Blood disorders', p. 210). Although apparently having a normal structure, they are far more fragile than normal blood cells and therefore easily prone to rapidly breaking down.
- Overt vitamin B_{12} deficiency can take quite a few years to become evident.
- Neurological: paraesthesia, peripheral neuropathy.

Reasons for Vitamin B_{12} Deficiency

Autoimmune inflammation of the stomach creates a progressive destruction of the cells in the stomach wall, which leads to decreased secretion of the enzymes and acid required to release the vitamin B_{12} complex from its dietary protein. Antibodies bind to intrinsic factor, inhibiting its attachment to vitamin B_{12} and therefore its absorption. There is also a neurological element involved.

As vitamin B_{12} is found only in animal food sources, it might be necessary for vegans to use vitamin B_{12} supplementation.

Drug Interactions Specific to Vitamin B_{12}

- Proton pump inhibitors (e.g. omeprazole; see Figure 35.3, p. 277): decrease the stomach acid secretions necessary for the efficient absorption of vitamin B_{12}. This does not appear to affect supplements. The H2-receptor antagonists (Tagamet, Zantac, etc.) have also been found to reduce vitamin B_{12} absorption, but the inhibition of secretions is not as prolonged as with the proton pump inhibitors. For this reason, H_2 receptor antagonists (see Figure 35.2, p. 276) are less of a problem as regards to vitamin B_{12} deficiency.
- Neomycin (antibiotic).
- Colchicine (antigout).
- Metformin (type 2 diabetes).

Supplementation of vitamin B_{12} is possible because the vitamin B_{12} is not bound to protein and enters the body through an alternative pathway to that required for vitamin B_{12} ingested in the normal diet.

Vitamin B_9 (Folic Acid, Folate)

- Folic acid is the active form of folate; vitamin C is involved in the conversion.
- Helps to prevent spina bifida.
- Involved in homocysteine metabolism (see Chapter 37 'Metabolic disorders', p. 296).

Dietary Sources

- Liver.
- Seafood and fish.
- Fresh, raw, dark green leafy vegetables: folate can be lost in cooking.
- Legumes.
- Whole grains.

Importance of Vitamin B_{12} and Folic Acid

- Vitamin B_{12} and folic acid are required for the synthesis of DNA: the erythroblasts, the precursor to the red blood cells, are unable to form normal red blood cells if these vitamins are deficient.
- Vitamin B_{12} is responsible for activating folic acid to its active form.

Fat-Soluble Vitamins

- Vitamins A, D, E and K.
- Are absorbed from the gut along with dietary fats, so in any condition in which the fat is substantially reduced in the diet (e.g. a low-fat diet) or in cases where the patient is consuming very little fat absorption, this can be impaired.
- Can be stored in the fat and therefore **possibly reach a level of toxicity if they are not utilized.**
- Require at least 10 g per day of fat in the diet to be absorbed efficiently.

Vitamin A

Required for:

- Bone growth.
- Immune system.
- Good vision.
- Fertility.

• Dietary Sources

Can be obtained in two forms:

1. Carotene (see Figure 22.8, p. 174):

    *   A precursor found in dark green leafy vegetables (spinach), orange non-citrus fruit (mangoes, papayas, apricots) and orange vegetables (carrots, pumpkins).
    *   Converted to vitamin A in liver.
    *   Low toxicity.
2. Retinol:

    *   Is preformed vitamin A found in liver, butter and egg yolks.
    *   Has a tendency to become toxic if allowed to build up.

• Deficiency

*   Increase in infection.
*   Night blindness.

Vitamin D

Two types:

* D_2 (cholecalciferol): of plant origin.
* D_3 (ergocalciferol): manufactured in the skin. Sunlight starts the conversion of a cholesterol-related vitamin D precursor in the skin to an active form.

Needed for:

*   Bone formation: in calcium metabolism, works in conjunction with parathyroid hormone (see Figure 37.1, p. 290).
*   Regulating blood pressure.
*   Tumour suppressant.

• Dietary Sources

*   Eggs.
*   Butter.
*   Fortified food products such as milk or margarine.

Phytates can interfere with vitamin D absorption (see Chapter 15 'Methods of administration', p. 120). Storage, cooking and processing do not appear to degrade vitamin D.

• Deficiency

*   Rickets.

Deficiency is usually not a problem except in societies where it is customary to completely cover the body and to consume foods that are high in phytates, e.g. products made from flour.

Vitamin E (Alpha Tocopherol)

Two groups of compounds have vitamin E activity (Figure 13.1):

*   Tocopherols: there are four types – alpha, beta, gamma and delta (according to number and position of methyl groups on the aromatic ring). Unsaturated side chain (see Figure 10.1, p. 74). The alpha type has highest activity; the synthetic isomer considerably less (see Figure 6.7, p. 39).
*   Tocotrienols: saturated side chain (see Figure 10.1, p. 74).

• The Role of Vitamin E

- Essential for reproduction: probably due to its antioxidant effect.
- Antioxidant effect: protects polyunsaturated fatty acids, other cell-membrane components and low-density lipoprotein from oxidation by free radicals (see Figure 7.4, p. 45 and Figure 7.9, p. 50).

• Interactions with Anticoagulant Medication

- Large doses of vitamin E inhibit the clotting action of vitamin K (see Chapter 28 'Blood disorders', p. 215).

• Dietary Sources of Vitamin E

- Green leafy vegetables.
- Whole grains: milling of whole grains removes the outer husk and the germ. Bleaching of flour destroys most the vitamin E content.
- Various oils.

Vitamin E is heat stable but can be destroyed by high temperatures, such as those used in frying food.

• Deficiency

Deficiency is rare.

- Neurological problems: there might be muscle weakness, problems with balance, loss of vibratory perception and problems with reflexes.
- Retinal defects.
- Possible infertility.

Vitamin K

- Antihaemorrhagic factor: essential for the formation of prothrombin (see Figure 28.1, p. 212). Therefore a patient with deficiency has increased clotting times.
- Involved in bone formation.

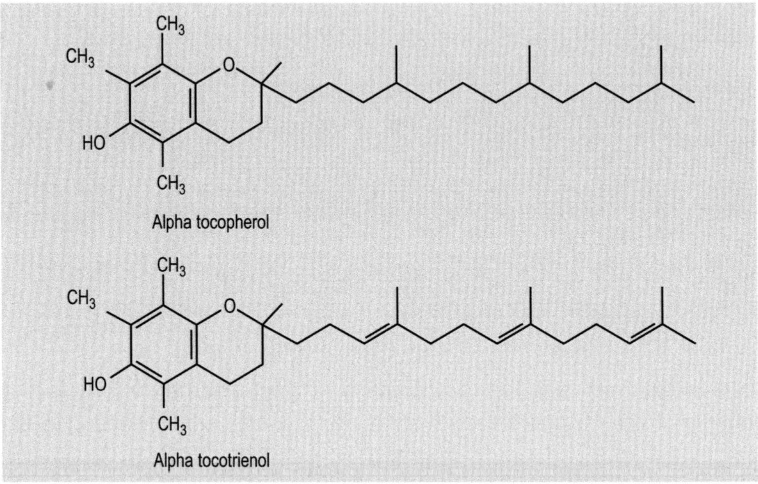

Figure 13.1 Demonstrating structures of alpha tocopherol and tocotrienol.

- **Dietary Sources**
  - Green leafy vegetables.
  - Vegetable oils (olive, soybean).

Deficiency occurs due to:

- Bile unable to enter gut: e.g. obstructive jaundice.
- Some malabsorption syndromes: e.g. coeliac disease or after small intestine resection.
- Reduced commensal flora: vitamin K is synthesized by bacteria in the jejunum and ileum. This is worth noting in any situation where the bacteria may be compromised, e.g. long-term antibiotic treatment, chronic alcoholism.

Choline

- By strict definition, choline is not a vitamin.
- Involved in lipid metabolism.
- Involved in the synthesis of structural components of cell membranes (see Figure 10.7, p. 79).
- Involved in nerve function see Figure 10.9, p. 80).
- Used to form betaine, which is used to render homocysteine harmless (see Chapter 37 'Metabolic disorders', p. 296).

- **Dietary Sources**

Choline is a component of phosphatidylcholine (lecithin), which is found in eggs, liver and soybeans.

- **Signs and Symptoms of Deficiency**

Very difficult to become deficient due to amount consumed under normal circumstances.

References

Kant AK. Reported consumption of low-nutrient-density foods by American children and adolescents: nutritional and health correlates, NHANES III, 1988 to 1994. Archives of Pediatrics and Adolescent Medicine 2003;157(8):789–796.

Rapuri PB, Gallagher JC, Kinyamu HK, Ryschon KL. Caffeine intake increases the rate of bone loss in elderly women and interacts with vitamin D receptor genotypes. American Journal of Clinical Nutrition 2001;74(5):694–700.

Yang CS. Vitamin nutrition and gastroesophageal cancer. Journal of Nutrition 2000; 130(2S suppl):338S–339S.

Bibliography

Bendich A, Deckelbaum RJ. Preventative nutrition. The comprehensive guide for health professionals. 3rd edn. Totowa, New Jersey: Humana Press; 2005.

Peckenpaugh NJ. Nutrition essentials and diet therapy. 9th edn. Philadelphia: Saunders: 2003.

Sanders T, Emery P. Molecular basis of human nutrition. New York: Taylor and Francis; 2003.

United States Department of Agriculture. National Agricultural Library. DRIs for vitamins, electrolytes and water, elements and macronutrients. Online. Available: http://desearch.nal.usda.gov/cgi-bin/dexpldcgi? gry1383539189; 1 [accessed 2 March 2008].

World Health Organization (WHO). Vitamin and mineral requirements in human nutrition. 2nd edn. Geneva: WHO; 2004.

Section 3

Pharmacokinetics and pharmacodynamics

Pharmacokinetics and pharmacodynamics: introduction

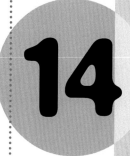

A good grasp of the principles of pharmacokinetics and pharmacodynamics are vital for understanding the actions of orthodox drugs, herbs and supplements. Without such an understanding, you will at best give ineffectual remedies, at worst be responsible for a foreseeable adverse reaction.

Certainly, as orthodox medication becomes more diverse and complex in its actions, it is necessary to keep up to date with possible interactions. Studying the interactions of the chemical constituents of drugs, herbs and supplements with the body and each other should also include a good basic understanding of the physiology of the system involved. So no aspect of pharmacology should ever be studied in isolation.

The terms 'pharmacodynamics' and 'pharmacokinetics' are often used interchangeably. This is usually due to a lack of understanding of the definitions:

- **Pharmacokinetics**: studies what a body does to chemicals (in drugs, herbs, supplements).
- **Pharmacodynamics**: studies the effects of chemicals (drugs, herb or supplements) on the body.

Four basic processes are involved in pharmacokinetics:

1. **Absorption**: how and where the substance enters the body.
2. **Distribution**: where the substance goes when it is absorbed.
3. **Metabolism**: breakdown or detoxification of a drug.
4. **Excretion**: removal of the substance or its breakdown products from the body.

The chemical make-up of the drug or herbal remedy influences:

- Where and how they are absorbed.
- Where they are distributed to.
- Where and how they are metabolized.
- How quickly they are removed from the body.

For ease of reading and comprehension, pharmacokinetics has been divided into:

- Routes of administration: how you get drugs into the body.
- Distribution: how drugs get into cells.
- Metabolism: how the body deals with drugs.
- Excretion: how the body gets rid of drugs.

Pharmacodynamics is covered in Chapter 19. Usually, this section of pharmacology involves calculations. These have been omitted as they are not necessary for the scope of this book.

For the sake of simplicity the term 'drug' will also mean remedy or supplement unless another term is more appropriate.

Bibliography

Neal MJ. Medical pharmacology at a glance. 5th edn. Oxford: Blackwell Science; 2005.

Rang HP, Dale MM, Ritter JM. Pharmacology. 6th edn. Edinburgh: Churchill Livingstone; 2007.

Waller DG, Renwick AG, Hillier K. Medical pharmacology and therapeutics. 2nd rev. edn. Edinburgh: Elsevier-Saunders; 2005.

Methods of administration

15

A drug can be administered in different ways. Supplements and herbs are generally administered **orally**, although other forms of delivery are possible:

- **Enteral**: administered through the gastrointestinal tract, including the mucosa of the mouth, stomach, small intestine, colon and rectum.
- **Parenteral**: not administered via the gastrointestinal tract but one of the following:
  - respiratory tract: including nasal cavity and lungs
  - vagina
  - topically/transdermally: absorption through skin
  - subcutaneous injection
  - intravenous injection
  - intramuscular injection
  - spinal injection.

Enteral Administration

Oral administration is the most common way to get drugs or remedies into the body. The gastrointestinal tract is essentially a long tube with a varied and complex ecosystem.

Advantages

- Ease of administration: patients are used to ingesting food, so this form of administration is generally acceptable.
- Ease of absorption: in many places, the lining of the digestive tract is only one cell thick and moist, which is ideal for absorption.
- Large surface area for absorption: the gastrointestinal tract is very long, which allows substances to be absorbed over a long period of time.

115

- Each area of the digestive tract has different qualities: this allows a wide range of remedies to be absorbed.

- **Disadvantages**
  - Some patients find administration difficult due to taste, texture, etc.
  - The variety of environments encountered by the substance in the passage down the gut can prevent proper delivery, for example, insulin cannot be ingested as its structural integrity is destroyed in the stomach.

Sublingual Administration

- **Advantages**
  - Rapid access to the bloodstream.
  - Easy to use.
  - Initially bypasses liver: nitroglycerine (for angina) has a very short half-life and is rapidly metabolized by the liver. For this reason, it is given under the tongue to get to the heart quickly and at a high enough dosage.

- **Disadvantages**
  - Short action: the drug might be almost entirely removed in the liver.

Administration via the Stomach

- **Advantages**
  - Large surface area for absorption.

- **Disadvantages**
  - Thick mucous layer slows absorption time.
  - Drug only in place for a short period of time.

Administration via the Small Intestine

- **Advantages**
  - Large surface area for absorption.

- **Disadvantages**
  - Blood from small intestine passes directly to the liver.
  - Intestinal microflora might inactivate drug.

Administration via the Colon

- **Advantages**
  - Direct access to the treatment site.
  - Less hostile environment with less diversity and intensity of activity than the stomach and small intestine

- **Disadvantages**
  - Requires complex delivery system to enable the drug to be released at this stage in the gut.

Administration via the Rectum

This is a possible method of delivering herbal remedies.

- **Advantages**
  - Bypasses liver.
  - Common way to getting anti-inflammatories into the body as it bypasses the gut and therefore any irritation of the gut lining. It can also be used for drugs that can produce nausea if taken orally.
  - Also used in treatment of haemorrhoids.

- **Disadvantages**
  - Possible adverse reaction as dosage not tempered by liver metabolism.
  - There might be problems with patient compliance.

Factors Affecting Absorption Through the Gastrointestinal Tract

- **Surface Area**

Absorption of a drug or remedy is greatest in the small intestine due to the large surface area created by the villi.

- **Gut Motility**

The more active the stomach movement, the shorter the transit time. This decreases the amount of drug or remedy that can be absorbed in the stomach.

- **Gastric Emptying**

The faster this occurs, the faster the drug or remedy can reach the small intestine and start to be absorbed.

Factors Increasing Gastric Emptying

- Fasting.
- Anxiety.
- Antacids.
- Hyperthyroidisms increase gastric emptying.
- Fluids: giving herbs with plenty of fluid will speed up the time it takes to reach the main area of absorption, the small intestine.

Factors Decreasing Gastric Emptying

- Fatty foods.
- Large, bulky foods: get in the way of the drugs and the gut wall.
- Hyperacidity.
- Peptic ulcers.
- Hypothyroidism.
- Clinical depression.

Different Types of Oral Delivery System

- Tablet.
- Capsules.
- Powders.

- Decoction.
- Tincture.
- Syrup.

Tablet

- **Advantages**
  - Convenience and palatability.
  - Patient compliance.

Placing a coating on the tablet:

- Prevents the tablet cracking or breaking while being transported.
- Allows controlled release of an active ingredient.
- Masks the taste.
- Prevents tablet breaking up in the gastrointestinal tract before it reaches the appropriate area.
- Makes tablet easier to swallow.

- **Disadvantages**
  - Can be difficult to swallow.
  - Might not easily be broken down.
  - Other substances will be present, such as flowing agents or fillers; some patients might have sensitivity to these.

Capsules

- **Advantages**
  - Convenience and palatability.
  - Compliance.
  - Granulated preparation quickly provides a large surface area for absorption.

- **Disadvantages**
  - Can be difficult to swallow.
  - Contents might be released too rapidly; patient might experience discomfort in the stomach.
  - Other substances present as bulking agents, e.g. potato starch or cornflower starch, to which some patients may be sensitive.

Powder

- **Advantages**
  - Large surface area for easy absorption.
  - Easy to prepare.

- **Disadvantages**
  - Bulking agents: as above.
  - Taste: with some powders there might be a gritty texture because the powder does not dissolve completely.

Decoction

- **Advantages**
  - Relatively pure liquid.
  - Easy to swallow.

- Well-used, proven traditional extraction; less traditional methods of extraction, e.g. in alcohol, might affect the nature of active pharmacological ingredients or not extract them at all.

- **Disadvantages**

  - Poor patient compliance because of preparation time and taste.

Tincture
- **Advantages**
  - Easy to swallow.

- **Disadvantages**
  - Poor patient compliance due to taste.
  - Alcohol: will exclude patients with alcohol addiction.

Syrup
Advantages
  - Easy to swallow.
  - Large surface area for easy absorption.

- **Disadvantages**
  - Stability of the preparation might be an issue.
  - Possible problems with patient compliance because of taste; either the syrup is too sweet or the taste of the preparation comes through.
  - Dental caries.
  - Other substances might be present.

General Gastrointestinal Tract Health

A healthy gastrointestinal tract is essential to maintain the right pH. Different pHs activate different enzymes. Certain enzymes will only work in a limited pH range. The pH of the gut changes along its length.

The pH can affect the degree of disassociation of a substance, resulting in increased absorption if the substance remains fully associated and non-polar (see Figures 8.2, 8.3 and 8.4, pp. 55–57). Drugs are designed for certain pHs, if these are not correct (due to poor gut health) then the drugs will not be as effective.

A healthy gastrointestinal tract ensures the correct content of commensals, as these are an important part of the gut chemistry, particularly the enterohepatic cycle (see Chapter 17 'Metabolism', p. 131). If there is an imbalance then drugs might not be utilized properly or might remain in the body for an extended period of time, resulting in toxicity.

Factors Affecting Absorption
- Disease affecting the lining of the gastrointestinal tract: e.g. Crohn's disease, in which flattening of the villi leads to a decrease of the surface area available for absorption.
- Short bowel syndrome: surgical removal of the small intestine due to diseases such as advanced Crohn's disease and carcinoma of the small intestine.

- Alcohol abuse: damages not only the liver but also the lining of the gut. Vitamin B_{12} deficiency is a common side effect of this problem (see Chapter 13 'Vitamins and minerals', p. 105).
- Parasitic infections: parasites can absorb nutrients (this is particularly relevant in vitamin and mineral supplementation).
- Disease affecting the gall bladder: substantially affects fat absorption. The bile salts are responsible for creating **micelles** – small globules – that make it much easier for the gut wall to absorb the fats and provide a larger surface area for enzymes to work on (see Figure 4.5, p. 25).
- Chronic liver disease e.g. cirrhosis: affects the function of the gall bladder.
- Other diseases such as myasthenia gravis, anorexia, chronic gastritis and pancreatitis also affect absorption.
- Poor blood flow: the small intestine has a very good blood supply. Combined with the increased surface area formed by the villi, this explains why the most absorption occurs here.
- Presence of food: certain foods increase or decrease the absorption of drugs in the gastrointestinal tract.
- Certain chemicals found in foods can interfere with absorption by creating an insoluble complex. **Phytates** found in cereals are an example of this as they can bind minerals such as zinc, iron and calcium (see Chapter 13 'Vitamins and minerals', pp. 95, 96, 98) and interfere with remedy absorption.
- Milk and other dairy products reduce the effectiveness of tetracyclines.
- Fat will reduce the motility and emptying time of the stomach.

Parenteral Administration

Nose

- **Advantages**
  - Rapid absorption due to the use of fine sprays.
  - Rapid access to cerebral tissues.
  - Rapid local action.

- **Disadvantages**
  - Difficult to remove if there is a reaction.

Mucous Membranes

- The mouth, rectum, vagina and nose all contain mucous membranes. As these are thin and moist and absorption is usually fairly efficient.
- Drugs given orally and absorbed from the gastrointestinal tract are carried via the hepatic portal vein to the liver, where they are at least partly, if not completely, metabolized. In some cases, the drug is removed from the system before it has time to work. This factor is appreciated by pharmaceutical chemists, and is the reason that glyceryl trinitrate, given for angina, is taken sublingually.
- Aromatherapy can quickly affect the mental state of a patient, as volatile oils breathed in through the nose are rapidly absorbed into the mucous membranes and from there have rapid access to the brain.

Lungs

This is a possible method of delivering herbal remedy, e.g. steam bath for respiratory conditions.

- **Advantages**
  - Large surface area.
  - The nature of mucous membranes encourages absorption.
  - High perfusion rate (good blood supply).
  - Prompt response because drugs absorbed quickly.

- **Disadvantages**
  - Particles of medication can cause lung damage.

Vagina

Possible method of delivering herbal remedy for the local treatment of conditions such as thrush.

- **Advantages**
  - Quick local action.

- **Disadvantages**
  - Difficult to remove if there is a reaction.

Topical/Transdermal

Qualities required for absorption by this method:

- Must be lipid soluble.
- A thin layer must be applied over the affected area, e.g. over joints and face.
- Areas that facilitate absorption contain plenty of hair follicles and sweat glands (neck, shoulders, extremities and back of hands).
- If substance is to be carried further than the local area, the rate of blood supply to the area of application needs to be reasonable.
- Carriers are usually used to get a remedy through the skin. **Glycerol** is easily absorbed but is hydroscopic (attracts water from the environment) and therefore has a drying effect. **Lanolin** mixes the best of both worlds; while being easily absorbed by the lipid layer of the skin it is able to take on board a large amount of water, by forming an **emulsion**. This is because part of it is **ionic** and therefore **hydrophilic** and part is **non-polar** and **hydrophobic** and therefore **fat soluble** (see Chapter 4 'Bonds continued', p. 24).

- **Advantages**
  - Large surface area.
  - Easy to use and works locally if dermatological condition, wound, etc.
  - Good patient compliance.

- **Disadvantages**
  - Local reaction.
  - Remedies absorbed this way are not quickly metabolized by the liver.
  - Generally, the chemicals in remedies need to be fat soluble if they are going to be effective. The skin is generally water resistant but soaking the area for some time will improve absorption, which is why herbal baths are used to assist faster absorption. Occlusive dressings or ointments can do this on a small scale. This is important to note in terms of Chinese medicine; where a skin condition is deemed to be damp this type of dressing will exacerbate the condition.

Subcutaneous Injection

- Must be lipid soluble.
- Insulin injections delivered this way avoid enzyme destruction in gastrointestinal tract.
- Iscador (*Viscum album* preparation) delivered this way.

- **Advantages**
  - Quick to administer.

- **Disadvantages**
  - Not the most desirable way to administer a drug.
  - Fibrous tissue build-up if site is used repetitively.

Intramuscular Injection

Must be lipid soluble.

- **Advantages**
  - Extended release of drug.

- **Disadvantages**
  - Painful to administer.

Intravenous Injection

- **Advantages**
  - Instant access to blood stream. Drug thought to be 100% bioavailable because it goes directly into the circulation and all of it may have an effect.

- **Disadvantages**
  - Uneven delivery.
  - Easy to overdose.

Spinal Injection

- **Advantages**
  - Rapid insertion of drug into area.

- **Disadvantages**
  - Difficult to reverse process if there is a reaction to the drug.

How do drugs get into cells?

16

Absorption at the Cellular Level

- Cell membranes are effectively selective biological barriers that inhibit the passage of certain molecules.
- Cell membranes are largely made up of two layers of phospholipids.
- Globular proteins – of varying size and make-up – are embedded within the membrane. These tend to be for transport and regulatory functions.

Drugs or remedies cross cell membranes by the following methods:

- passive diffusion
- facilitated passive diffusion
- active transport
- pinocytosis.

Passive Diffusion (Absorption)

- Accounts for the greatest amount of chemical transport across the cell membrane.
- Uses no energy.
- Transfer occurs down a chemical gradient; in other words, chemicals move from an area of high concentration to an area of low concentration (**osmosis**) (Figure 16.1); This can be from the gastrointestinal tract to the bloodstream, where the concentration of the substance is lower.
- Chemicals absorbed this way tend to be fat soluble and non-polar, features that allow them to pass across the phospholipid membrane. Some polar molecules can pass through but they must be very small.
- Small molecules will penetrate the membrane more easily, and therefore more rapidly, than a large molecule.
- Because there is rapid removal of substrates due to the circulation flowing rapidly past the site, absorbed chemicals become distributed over a wide area of the body.

As the pH varies through the digestive tract, so do the characteristic of many compounds (see Chapter 8 'Acids and bases', p. 55). This leads to certain compounds

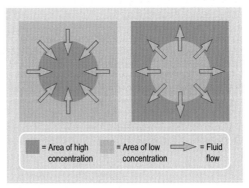

Figure 16.1 Passive diffusion into a cell.

being more non-polar than others. This then affects how easily they can pass through the membrane. The condition of the digestive tract is therefore an important factor in chemical absorption.

Facilitated Passive Diffusion

- Does not work against a concentration gradient but is a type of enhanced osmosis.
- There is possibly some type of carrier that combines reversibly with the molecules on one side of the membrane and transfers them over to the other side. Such carriers are specific for certain molecules.
- The whole process is limited by the number of carriers present, so it is possible for the system to reach saturation, at which point it will be unable to work any faster.
- The process seems to require no energy.

• Passive Diffusion Through Protein Channels and how these Channels are 'Gated'

Sodium, potassium and calcium salts, which are vital to the function of cells, need to be able to pass through cell membranes down a concentration gradient. Such a mechanism is provided by proteins, which can be seen by electron microscopy across the cell membranes. These channels can be placed in an open position or closed because they are '**gated**'. In other words, a barrier can go across the channel when required to prevent the flow of the ions.

Various medications can affect the patency (openness) of these sodium, potassium and calcium channels, e.g. calcium-channel blockers (which, as the name suggests block the calcium channels and prevent the flow of calcium) and potassium channel activators (which keep the potassium channels open to allow the flow of potassium out) in heart medication.

Control of the opening and closing can be done in one of two ways:

- voltage gating
- chemical gating or ligand gating.

Voltage Gating

Usually found in neurons, in which a rapid change in voltage is responsible for the generation of an action potential being passed along the axon. Muscle tissue is also sensitive to voltage change. In this respect, the protein gates act like an electromagnet, opening and closing depending on the charge that is present.

Whether these gates are open or closed will dictate the quantity of chemical allowed through the membrane. In this situation, a massive influx of sodium creates an action potential; the opening of the potassium gates, changing the charge back again, stops the action potential.

Voltage gating is covered in more detail in Chapter 31 (see Figure 31.2, p. 237).

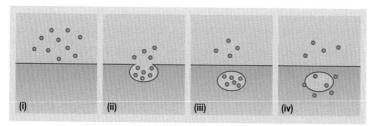

Figure 16.2 Pinocytosis by a cell membrane (see text for explanation).

Chemical Gating or Ligand Gating

Some protein channels are opened when a specific chemical substance (a ligand) binds to them. This causes a change in shape of the protein, thus opening and closing the channel, depending on what shape they are. The neurotransmitter acetylcholine works in this way. This method of gating allows a nerve impulse to be transmitted from one neuron to the next until it reaches its target organ.

Note: this is not the same as active transport (see Figure 31.1, p. 236) or facilitated diffusion (see p. 124), as the substances pass down a concentration gradient. It is basically controlled osmosis.

Active Transport

Active transport requires a carrier mechanism, that uses energy to move a drug or remedy up a concentration gradient. The rate of movement does not depend on concentration but on the capacity of the carrier mechanism. The sodium–potassium pump is a form of active transport (see Figure 31.1, p. 236).

Pinocytosis

The mechanism by which white cells engulf bacteria and amoebae engulf their prey is well known. The engulfing process is usually by cells that are part of a cell membrane. In this case, the substance is much smaller than that engulfed by the white cells or amoeba and is dissolved in water. The process is often referred to as 'cellular drinking', which suggests that the substances that are taken in by the cell are dissolved in liquid.

Pinocytosis probably plays a minor role in drug transport, except for protein drugs (Figure 16.2):

(i) Solute (substance dissolved in water) outside the cell, at the cell surface.
(ii) 'Pocket' forms round solute.
(iii) 'Pocket' closes, trapping solute inside cell.
(iv) Solute is dispersed in cell.

Distribution of the Drug

Three main factors that have to be considered in drug distribution:

- blood flow
- transport across the cell membrane
- extent of binding to plasma and tissue proteins.

The Importance of Blood Flow

The perfusion rate in different tissues varies as follows:

- High perfusion rates: hormone-producing glands and other tissues that secrete chemicals, the brain, lungs, heart, kidneys and liver, actively dividing cells.

- Moderate perfusion rates: skin, muscles and fatty tissues.
- Low perfusion rates, poorly supplied: teeth, bone, ligaments and tendons.

Other factors will also affect the drug or remedy distribution:

- Patient activity.
- The size of the organ (an enlarged organ will usually have a much higher blood flow).
- Actively dividing cells require a good blood supply (hence the order of perfusion rate listed above).
- Local tissue temperature.

Any tissue that is actively dividing or unusually enlarged will usually enjoy a higher rate of blood flow. This situation is taken advantage of in chemotherapy; actively dividing cells require a good blood supply, and following this logic will therefore receive more of the drug than elsewhere. Conversely, if the blood flow is disrupted in any way, the decreased perfusion rate will reduce the chances of the right amount of drug or remedy getting to the area where it is needed.

This principle is helpful when dispensing herbal remedies, where a herb is included to increase blood flow to an area requiring treatment.

Plasma Protein Binding

A drug or remedy can be bound to circulating plasma proteins (usually albumin) or it can move around freely in an unbound state. If the remedy is bound then it is not free to be used and is said to be inactive, therefore only the unbound remedy works. As these unbound molecules leave the circulation, molecules are released from the blood proteins because the concentration of free molecules is lower (see Figure 16.1, p. 124).

Note: plasma protein binding is extremely important for the effectiveness of a drug or remedy, and also for its potential toxicity.

The Practicalities of Blood–Protein Binding

Blood proteins are reasonably non-specific in their binding habits, which means they are not choosy as to what they bind to. Therefore, different drugs or remedies will compete for the same binding site. Displacement can be a problem if the protein prefers one molecule to another and throws off one chemical in favour of another. It is therefore a potential site for **drug–herb interaction**:

- Warfarin: is usually bound to plasma proteins and is very easily displaced, which is why patients on warfarin who receives other medication have to have their warfarin levels checked very carefully.
- Berberine (found in *Huang Lian*, *Huang Bai*): can increase bilirubin levels by displacement of bilirubin from albumin, by the berberine (Chan 1993).

Effect of Membrane Barriers on Absorption

Generally, small molecules up to a molecular weight of 500 kDa are absorbed through capillary walls even if they are ionized, because the cell junctions are not entirely sealed and are in fact a little 'leaky'. However, other barriers are not so easy to get through.

Blood–Brain Barrier

- A very well protected barrier: the glial cells are tightly packed, making a very effective barrier to prevent molecules seeping through (Figure 16.3).
- Lipid-soluble molecules can pass through the membrane relatively easily. Ionized (polar) molecules find this membrane difficult to pass through, because it is un-ionized (non-polar).

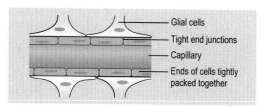

Figure 16.3 The blood–brain barrier.

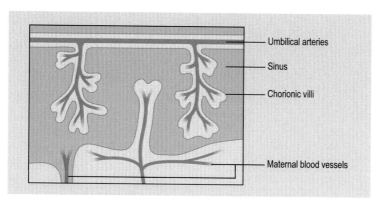

Figure 16.4 The blood–placenta barrier.

• Blood–Placenta Barrier

- A complex structure.
- The fetal capillaries are enclosed by the chorionic villi (the tiny finger-like projections extending from the chorion to the uterine lining). They are separated from the maternal blood vessels by a large cavernous sinus (Figure 16.4).
- Permeability of this barrier is of great interest to both pharmacists and herbalists.
- Generally, the placental membranes offer very little resistance to chemical molecules and only act as a barrier to ionized molecules with a molecular weight greater than 50.

Reference

Chan E. Displacement of bilirubin from albumin by berberine. Biology of the Neonate 1993; 63(4):201–208.

Metabolism

17

The Liver

- One of the most metabolically active areas in the body.
- The main site of detoxification in the body.
- The detoxification process has two phases: phase I (involves an enzyme complex called cytochrome P450) and phase II.
- This processing, which allows chemicals to be made water soluble and excreted from the body, can make it difficult to achieve a sufficient concentration of remedy in the body.
- Liver disease causes great problems because harmful substances are not prepared for removal from the body.

The First-Pass Mechanism

All orally administered remedies (apart from the very small amounts absorbed through the mucous membranes in the mouth) pass through the liver before they reach the tissues. Some drugs (such as nitroglycerin) are almost completely removed by the liver at the first pass (i.e. on the first go). Others take a little longer because they are not completely removed by this system (due to the enterohepatic cycle or they are just more difficult to remove). Other drugs rely on this system to activate their components, as the liver will change the chemistry of the drug.

The more resistant a drug is to the first-pass mechanism, the longer its **half-life** (i.e. the time it takes for a remedy to halve its dosage in the body). It is difficult to say how herbal remedies are affected by the first-pass mechanism because the constituents and their interactions are so complex. However, some elements of the first-pass mechanism will be involved in the metabolism of herbal remedies.

Liver Enzyme Induction and Inhibition

Enzymes can be encouraged to speed up or slow down. For example, cytochrome p450 (the enzyme involved in phase I in the liver), of which there are several variations, can be particularly affected.

• Enzyme Induction

Many substances already present in the body, or that can be introduced (e.g. nicotine, caffeine, alcohol, dioxin, oranges, tangerines and excess protein from high-protein diets) will speed up the metabolism. Chemicals such as hormones will also increase the activity of enzymes.

Hypericum (St John's wort) increases the rate of action of cytochrome P450.

• Enzyme Inhibition

Certain flavonoids and furanocoumarins (see Chapter 21 'Phenols', p. 156) inhibit cytochrome P450. Naringenin (found in grapefruits) is a well-known flavonoid that inhibits cytochrome P450; bergapten and quercitin also have this effect. Such inhibition can be a greater problem than enzyme induction, as an unusual rise of a drug or remedy in the system beyond its therapeutic limit can be harmful to the body.

Note: water-soluble chemicals tend to be less toxic than lipid-soluble chemicals because they can be so easily removed via the kidneys. Lipid-soluble compounds, if not dealt with by the detoxification pathways in the liver, tend to be stored in fatty tissues and released at a time when fat stores are utilized, for example if the patient fasts. This is why fasting can make patients ill.

The Gastrointestinal Tract

There are largely two factors at work here:

- digestive enzymes
- intestinal flora (commensals).

Digestive Enzymes

These are involved in the hydrolysis of conjugated chemical substances (*remember*: the conjugate group can be a sugar) so that the active ingredients are made available for entry into the bloodstream.

This process is **capacity limited**; in other words, there are only so many enzymes and when their sites are all taken up, and no longer available, the rest of the drug or remedy remains unconjugated, no matter how high the dose. The cells of the gastrointestinal tract lumen are not the only type of cells to have this function.

Intestinal Flora

Certain intestinal flora (commensals) can remove conjugate groups, returning the chemicals to their non-polar state and allowing them to be more easily absorbed by the cells of the gut wall. The composition of the microbes is important and can be adversely affected by:

- Diet: too much sugar can produce an overgrowth of the wrong type of microbe.
- Disease: can affect the lining of the gastrointestinal tract or the gastrointestinal environment.
- Drugs: antibiotics kill not only harmful bacteria but useful bacteria as well.

The correct balance of microbes in the gut is therefore the key factor in the **enterohepatic cycle** (see below). Healthy cells in the lumen are also important as there is some active transport of the unconjugated bile salts.

• Other Aspects of Intestinal Flora

The enzymes produced by intestinal bacteria synthesize vitamin K, biotin, folic acid, thiamine and vitamin B_{12}.

In individuals who are deficient in lactase (the enzyme responsible for breaking down the lactose in milk), the undigested lactose is fermented by bacteria residing in the colon. Fermentation can be vigorous fermentation, resulting in flatus and possibly diarrhoea.

Enterohepatic Cycle or Circulation

Some chemicals metabolized in the liver are excreted in the bile, which passes into the intestinal lumen, to be once again reabsorbed by the intestinal cells and returned to the liver (Figure 17.1). This enterohepatic circulation prolongs the time the drug can spend in the body, because it is recycled.

Conjugated compounds are polar and therefore require active uptake by the cells in the lumen of the gastrointestinal tract; unconjugated compounds are non-polar and are more easily absorbed by the non-polar bilipid cell membrane (see Chapter 3 'Bonds found in biological chemistry', p. 24). When conjugated compounds are returned to the gastrointestinal tract, the conjugate group can be cleaved from the drug, allowing the non-polar drug to be reabsorbed. In the enterohepatic cycle, these conjugates are cleaved from the drug by the commensals (the microbes present in the small intestine).

Bile salts and cholesterol tend to be recirculated between the gut and the liver in this way, as do a variety of chemicals and drugs, for example:

* oestrogens
* many steroids
* metabolites of vitamin D
* digitalis
* morphine
* colchine
* choramphenicol.

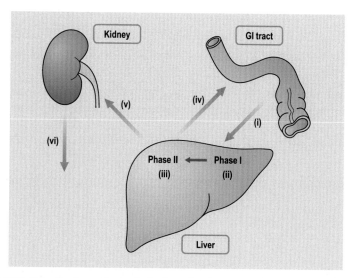

Figure 17.1 Detoxification pathways in the liver, showing removal and the enterohepatic cycle. (i) Drug is absorbed from the gastrointestinal tract, passing to the liver via the hepatic portal vein. (ii) Drug encounters phase I enzymes (variations of cytochrome P450), which prepare it for phase II. (iii) Phase II adds a compound to the drug (conjugation), making it more polar and therefore water soluble. (iv) Conjugated drug is recycled to the gastrointestinal tract, where bacteria cleave off conjugated compounds (the enterohepatic cycle). Some of the drug is removed from body via the faeces. (v) Conjugated, water-soluble drug passes to the kidney to be removed in urine (vi).

This phenomenon has been extensively studied with morphine, a lipid-soluble drug. Morphine becomes conjugated in the intestine but the intestinal flora is capable of removing the conjugate. This significantly prolongs the activity of morphine and, over a period time, increases the dosage in the body. Cardiac glycosides found in herbs such as *Convallaria majalis* and *Crataegus* species are involved in the same process.

It is very important to take the enterohepatic mechanism into consideration because it can maintain the concentration of a drug or remedy in the body, even increasing it with further ingestion. This results in the possibility of toxicity, although many drugs are designed to take advantage of this phenomenon.

Drug excretion

Drug excretion can occur by several means:

- via the kidneys
- in the bile
- through the lungs
- in saliva, tears, perspiration
- in breast milk.

Kidneys

- The greatest proportion of drug excretion occurs through the kidneys.
- The liver makes most drugs and remedies water soluble for removal via the kidneys (see Figure 17.1, p. 131).
- One-fifth of the plasma reaching the kidney glomerulus is filtered through the pores in the glomerular cell membrane. The rest passes through the blood vessels around the renal tubules (Figure 18.1).
- Substances with a low molecular weight and not bound to plasma proteins can easily pass through the cell membranes into the tubules.
- Active secretion against a concentration gradient also takes place in the tubules.

The factors affecting the rate at which the drug or remedy is excreted by the kidneys are:

- kidney disease
- pH of urine
- change in renal blood flow
- concentration of drug or remedy in plasma
- its molecular weight.

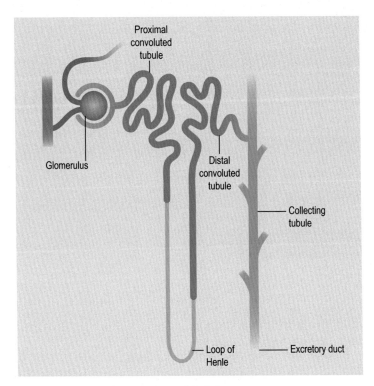

Figure 18.1 A nephron: the functional unit of the kidney.

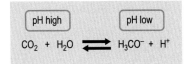

Figure 18.2 The buffering equation.

Kidney Disease

Useful complexes such as plasma proteins (see Chapter 16 'How do drugs get into cells?', p. 126) can be lost, increasing the amount of unbound remedy in the body, with resulting toxicity. Other compounds may be lost in the urine as the reuptake is reduced.

pH of Urine

The pHs of the urine and blood are interrelated. **Tubular secretion**, which takes place in the kidneys, is an active process whereby certain molecules and ions are removed from the blood and actively secreted into the tubules. From the buffering equation (Figure 18.2), it is possible to see that:

- When the pH of the blood decreases, more hydrogen ions need to be secreted (thus removing them) to maintain the balance.
- If the pH increases, fewer hydrogen ions need to be secreted (they need to be retained).

The kidneys are capable of absorbing fluctuations in pH and will adjust the removal or retention of hydrogen ions as necessary. **This is why the pH of the urine can vary so widely but the blood pH is maintained within very narrow limits**.

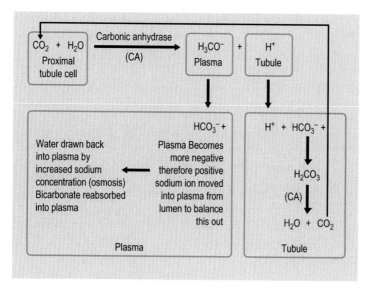

Figure 18.3 Reactions in the kidney involving the enzyme carbonic anhydrase (CA).

Any reduction in tubular secretion due to disease may result in serious ion imbalances in the body. Blood is buffered through a balance between carbon dioxide (CO_2) and bicarbonate concentrations (HCO_3^-).

The kidneys act when the blood becomes too acidic (right-hand side of the equation) or too basic (left-hand side of the equation) by altering the amount of water lost through urination. The buffering mechanism is associated with sodium balance, which is also controlled by the kidneys (Figure 18.3) and involves an enzyme called carbonic anhydrase (CA; see Chapter 26 'Cardiovascular disorders', p. 198).

The erythrocytes also contain carbonic anhydrase, which acts as described above to enable them to carry carbon dioxide in the form of the bicarbonate ion (see Chapter 28 'Blood disorders', p. 209).

There are also other buffers in the blood, such as the plasma proteins, but the kidneys have the most dramatic effect as regards pH balance in the blood.

• How Does pH Affect Drug Excretion?

The filtrate passing into the first part of the renal tubule has the same pH as plasma, roughly neutral. As the pH of urine can be anything from 4.5 to 8.0, this will affect the rate of drug excretion (see Chapter 8 'Acids and bases', p. 55).

Take, for example, a drug that is weakly acidic: the lower the pH (e.g. 4.5), the more free hydrogen ions will be available and the weakly acidic drug molecules will be unlikely to give up their hydrogen molecules. They will therefore remain non-polar (uncharged) and be reabsorbed, through the non-polar cell membranes.

In very alkaline urine (e.g. 8.0), the acidic drug molecules will tend to be removed as they will have more readily given up their hydrogen molecule and become polar (charged), making their reabsorption through the non-polar (uncharged) cell membranes more difficult. They are also more easily removed by the ionic active process.

For a more alkaline drug the converse will occur.

Meat eaters tend to have slightly acidic urine (due to the type and amount of protein in their diet) and vegetarians have slightly alkaline urine. A patient's diet might therefore be a consideration in the treatment plan.

Change in Renal Blood Flow

Perfusion rates are as important for removal as the distribution of a drug or remedy (see Chapter 16 'How do drugs get into cells?', p. 125). Any change in renal blood flow due to kidney (or another) disease will increase the time it takes for a substance to leave the body.

Concentration of Drug or Remedy in Plasma

Normally, a high concentration of unbound substance will ensure its removal if it is small and water soluble. Many drugs are bound to plasma proteins (see Chapter 16 'How do drugs get into cells?', p. 126). How tightly they are bound then affects how easily they can be removed when they reach the kidneys. This can be controlled by pH or the amount of free substance in the plasma.

Kidney disease affects the degree to which a substance is removed from the body. Changes in pH affect polarity and the abnormal exit of plasma proteins from the kidneys to which these substances might be attached.

Molecular Weight

The larger the chemical, the more difficulty it has passing through a cell membrane even if it is lipid soluble.

Bile

Drugs can be actively removed into the bile for removal from the body. Because this is done against a concentration gradient, and requires an active process, there might be competition for receptors. The drugs in question will be conjugated to achieve their removal, but might then take part in the enterohepatic cycle (see Chapter 17 'Metabolism', p. 131). However, this process is not 100% effective and some substance is removed from the body in the faeces.

Lungs

These account for very little excretion, although small amounts of alcohol will undergo pulmonary excretion.

Saliva, Tears and Perspiration

All will excrete some chemicals, particularly if the drugs are lipid soluble.

Breast Milk

Some chemicals are excreted through breast milk, particularly volatile oils. Although the amounts are likely to be small this process is worth noting because the baby's digestive system might be affected.

Pharmacodynamics: how drugs elicit a physiological effect

19

Proteins play an integral role in controlling body functions through their roles as:

- enzymes
- receptors
- carrier molecules.

The chemical composition of protein molecules allows for great variation in three-dimensional structure, creating sites which, generally speaking, will interact only with specific molecules that are able to fit into the particular site (see Figure 11.5, p. 84). Most drugs act by interfering with this process at the molecular level, fitting into sites intended for the original protein molecule.

The 'Lock and Key' Hypothesis

The simplest way to consider the action of a chemical on an enzyme or receptor is the concept of the 'lock and key.' A bond is made with the enzyme or receptor (Figure 19.1). If the protein is an enzyme, a chemical reaction will take place; if it is a receptor, it might trigger a chemical reaction or start a chain of events leading to a physiological response.

This is a very simplistic explanation and there might be a certain moulding of the site to the substrate or ligand, as the protein structure is not completely immobile, but generally speaking the 'lock and key' mechanism is a reasonable concept.

Enzymes

- **Enzymes are proteins that catalyse chemical reactions**: in other words, enzymes affect the rate of a reaction but they themselves remain unchanged at the end of the reaction.
- Molecules (**substrates**) attach to the enzyme that converts them to something else.

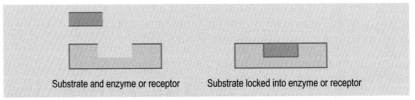

Substrate and enzyme or receptor   Substrate locked into enzyme or receptor

Figure 19.1 The 'lock and key' mechanism.

- **Most reactions in cells require enzymes to take place at a reasonable speed**: left to their own devices, without the assistance of enzymes, reactions would take place far too slowly.
- **The enzyme reaction site is fairly specific** (see Figure 11.5, p. 84), which is why metabolic pathways are associated with specific enzymes.
- The efficiency with which enzymes catalyse a reaction depends on how many of them are available, as a reaction will be limited by the number of sites provided by the enzymes (capacity limited). **When no more binding sites are left, the reaction has reached its optimum level.**
- Enzyme activity can be affected by molecules other than substrates, which can slow down or stop a reaction. These molecules are called **inhibitors**. Poisons and drugs are often enzyme inhibitors.

Enzyme Inhibition

Most enzyme receptor sites are not completely specific (there is some structural leeway given the number of combinations possible and the mobility of the protein) and a relatively similarly shaped molecule might be able to achieve a 'close fit'. This creates competition for molecules of a similar shape and the original molecule might find itself unable to find a binding site because it is already occupied. Many drugs are designed to take advantage of this phenomenon.

The various ways in which enzyme function can be affected are not dissimilar to the ways receptor function can be affected. These principles are worth bearing in mind when looking at chemicals that act directly on receptor sites.

● Competitive Inhibition

- Competitive inhibition [Figure 19.2(i)] is reversible: another molecule competes with the normal substrate and takes its place in the site.
- However, when the normal substrate concentration exceeds that of the competing molecule, the situation is more favourable and the normal substrate replaces the competing molecule.
- While the competing molecule is in place it blocks the normal action of the enzyme.
- Competitive inhibition can be reversed by increasing the substrate concentration.

● Non-Competitive Inhibition

- Non-competitive inhibition [Figure 19.2(ii)] is reversible.
- The inhibitor, which is not a substrate, attaches itself to another part of the enzyme, thereby changing the overall shape of the site for the normal substrate so that it does not fit as well as before, which slows or prevents the reaction taking place.
- This type of inhibition decreases the turnover rate of an enzyme rather than interfering with the amount of substrate binding to the enzyme. The reaction is slowed rather than stopped. Non-competitive inhibition, therefore, cannot be increased by increasing the substrate.

● Irreversible Inhibition

- The inhibitor becomes covalently linked or bound to the enzyme so tightly that is very difficult to detach it from the enzyme [Figure 19.2(iii); see Chapter 3 'Bonds found in biological chemistry', p. 13].
- The situation cannot be reversed.

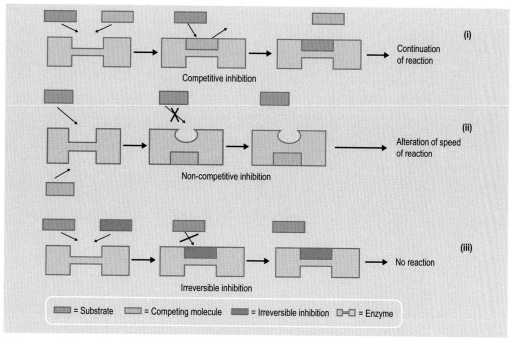

Figure 19.2 Competitive (i), non-competitive (ii) and irreversible (iii) inhibition.

Cofactors

- Some enzymes require a non-protein moiety to be active.
- Inorganic cofactors are metals such as zinc.
- If the cofactor is organic it is called a coenzyme, e.g. $NADP^+$ (see Figure 12.3, p. 91). Coenzymes also transport chemicals from one group to another.
- Many coenzymes are derived from vitamins, e.g. niacin $NADP^+$, pantothenic acid (coenzyme CoA) (see Chapter 13 'Vitamins and minerals', pp. 103, 104).
- Cofactors are a very small part of the overall part of the enzyme.

139

• Apoenzymes

When an enzyme requires a cofactor but this is not attached, the cofactor is called an **apoenzyme**.

The Logic Behind Drug Design

- Drugs can act as inhibitors of enzymes [Figure 19.3(i)].
- The drug molecule can undergo a chemical change to form an abnormal product, which alters the normal chemical pathway [Figure 19.3(ii)].
- Some drugs require enzymes to convert them from the inactive form that has been ingested to an active metabolic form [Figure 19.3(iii)].

Receptors

Receptors are specialized areas in cell walls that interact with molecules (**ligands**). Ligands can be hormones, neurotransmitters or drugs or chemicals from remedies and are found in:

- postsynaptic membranes, e.g. neurotransmitters
- cell membranes, e.g. hormones.

Receptors work in a similar way to enzymes with regard to the attachment of chemicals to the receptor sites. In many cases, the receptors are linked up to intermediary systems such as G proteins (Figure 19.5, p. 141).

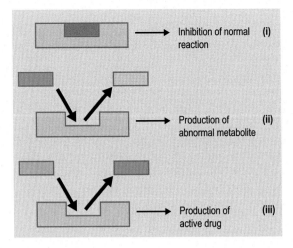

Figure 19.3 Ways in which medication is designed to interact with enzymes.

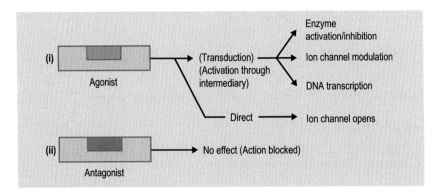

Figure 19.4 Action of receptors.

This time, however, the attachment of a molecule will activate the site, producing a physiological effect through a series of chemical reactions (**agonist**) [Figure 19.4(i)] or block the site and therefore the active response of the cell to the chemical (**antagonist**) [Figure 19.4(ii)].

Some drugs can have a dual action, simultaneously behaving as an agonist for one receptor and an antagonist to another, e.g. buprenorphine (see Chapter 32 'Analgesia and relief of pain', p. 252).

Receptors are effectively sensors for the chemical communicating system in the body, which coordinates the function of all the different cells in the body.

Agonists

These molecules can activate a site by binding to it. Many hormones and neurotransmitters work in this way. They will either work directly as in the case of ion channels (see Figure 19.6) or through an intermediary (**transduction**), for example a G protein (Figure 19.5). The response from the stimulated cell can lead to:

- enzyme activation or inhibition
- ion channel modulation
- DNA transcription.

Antagonists

When they bind to a site, antagonists do not stimulate a physiological response, e.g. antihistamines bind to the histamine receptors thus reducing the histamine response. Antagonists can either be competitive or non-competitive. Many drugs act either as **agonists** or **antagonists**.

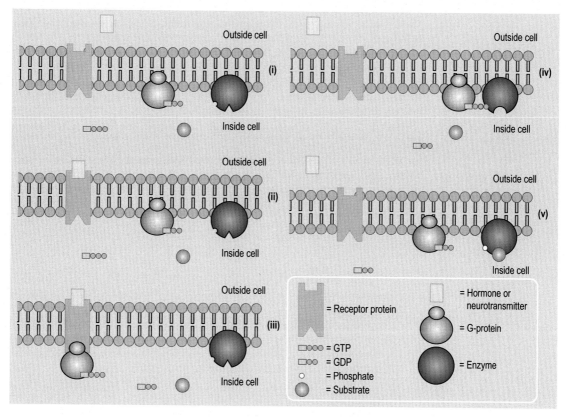

Figure 19.5 The action of G protein. (i) A hormone or neurotransmitter attaches itself to a cell membrane or synaptic receptor. The receptor is composed of a protein embedded in the phospholipid membrane that straddles the membrane. (ii) This changes the shape of receptor site of the receptor protein inside the cell. (iii) The G protein moves laterally along the membrane and binds to the now activated receptor site. (iv) This triggers an exchange of guanosine diphosphate (GDP) for guanosine triphosphate (GTP). (v) The G protein moves laterally to the inactive enzyme, releasing a phosphate into a receptor site, activating the receptor site of the enzyme ready for the substrate. (vi) The substrate attaches. Once the reaction has taken place the enzyme loses the phosphate molecule.

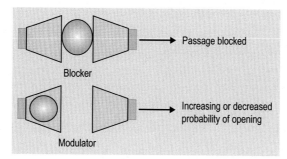

Figure 19.6 An ion channel.

G Proteins

G proteins act as an intermediary to a stimulation of a receptor. These transmembrane proteins convert the action of ligand binding into an intracellular signal.

G protein receptors are very diverse in their use, capable of being stimulated by photons from light in some cases, or chemicals such as histamines in others. They are therefore used by the visual and olfactory mechanisms, the autonomic system, in the regulation of the immune system and in adjusting behaviour and mood.

The extent to which they are involved in the human body has resulted in a large proportion of orthodox medication being designed with them in mind.

How the signalling though the membrane works in not clearly understood, but the inactive G protein, bound to the receptor when inactive, detaches itself when the receptor alters shape as a result of stimulation, and then acts as an intermediary by switching on an enzyme in the cell. When this is done, the receptor either activates another G protein or returns to an inactive state.

Ion Channels

Ion channels are composed of protein and control the flow of ions in and out of cells (Figure 19.6; see Chapter 16 'How do drugs get into cells?', p. 124 and Figure 31.2, p. 237). They differ according to:

- the type of ion they allow through (e.g. Na^+, K^+, Cl^-)
- the way they are regulated
- their structure.

There are several kinds:

- Non-gated (resting channels): continuously open, allowing a leakage of ions.
- Chemically gated:
  - Direct: the drug directly binds to parts of the channel protein. This might amount to a simple physical blocking of the channel by the drug molecule. Local anaesthetics can work in this way, blocking the sodium–potassium gate.
  - Indirect: activated by a G protein and other intermediaries.
- Ligand gated: linked directly to a receptor and opened only when the receptor is occupied by an agonist.
- Voltage gated: see Figure 31.2 (p. 237). The gate is controlled by a voltage sensor, which opens or closes the gate according to the level of the membrane potential.

Carrier Molecules

Ions and small molecules need to be transported across the lipid membranes of cell walls (Figure 19.7(i)). The carrier is a protein, which has a recognition site that makes specific for particular substrates. These can be blocked [Figure 19.7 (ii)] or made to take a false substrate, which then accumulates in the cell [Figure 19.7 (iii)] and affects the cell metabolism in some way.

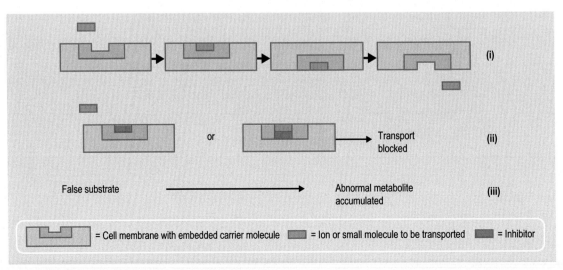

Figure 19.7 Carrier systems and how they can be affected by drugs.

Feedback Loops

The physiological processes of the body are controlled by feedback loops. The presence or absence of a substance in the body is fed back into the system that produces it, turning production on or off to maintain the correct level of that substance in the body.

The endocrine system is an example of a feedback loop system. It comprises a group of glands situated at various locations around the body, that secrete chemical messengers (hormones), which circulate in the bloodstream to affect distant organs or other glands. A classic feedback loop occurs within the female reproductive system to produce the menstrual cycle and the induction and shutdown of labour (see Figure 38.1, p. 300).

Factors Affecting a Patient's Response to a Drug

Age

Drug metabolism is poor in the elderly, babies and small children. In older people this is because metabolic processes are becoming less efficient; in babies and young children, some enzymatic pathways are not fully formed.

Body Weight

The larger the person, the more drug or remedy that person can process.

Nutritional Status

Patients with metabolic diseases, gut disease or who are malnourished for any reason will have altered drug or remedy distribution and utilization.

When plasma protein levels become reduced, a larger amount of free, unbound drug is available for activity (see Chapter 16 'How do drugs get into cells', p. 126).

Loss of body fat will also release stored chemicals into the bloodstream. Many drugs are lipid soluble and a depletion of body fat will mean a reduced capacity to take chemicals out of circulation, as there is less storage available.

Food–Drug Interactions

As already discussed, certain foods can affect absorption (see Chapter 15 'Methods of administration', p. 120).

Disease Process

- **Liver diseases**: such as hepatitis, cirrhosis and liver failure reduce the metabolism of drugs or remedies and can result in a toxic overload due to the build-up of chemicals in the system.
- **Circulatory diseases**: such as heart failure and peripheral vascular disease reduce distribution and transport of drugs. Associated with the circulatory system the renin–angiotensin system (see Figure 26.6, p. 197) of the kidneys will affect the blood pressure, so kidney disease becomes more of an issue than simple excretion.
- **Gastrointestinal tract**: any disease of the gastrointestinal tract will lead to poor absorption of remedies and an alteration in the enterohepatic cycle due to the amount of normal commensals being affected.
- **Kidney disease:** affects the pH balance. Destruction of the glomerular membrane will result in loss of plasma proteins, which will increase the level of unbound chemicals (see Chapter 16 'How do drugs get into cells?', p. 126).

Adverse Reactions

See Chapter 40 'Toxicology' p. 317.

Section 4

Plant pharmacology

Introduction to plant pharmacology: secondary metabolites

20

Two systems are at work in plants:

- **Primary metabolism**: principally, products of photosynthesis, which provide the food that enables the plant to live, grow and reproduce. Primary metabolites are thus necessary to keep the plant healthy and alive. They comprise the sugars, lipids, amino acids and nucleotides that are used to produce the polymers essential for the plant's structure and metabolism and that are part of our normal diet.

- **Secondary metabolism**: very diverse, and thought to provide a secondary function for the plant such as protection against animals that might eat it or against bacteria, viruses, fungi or parasites. For example, some plants produce cyanogenic glycosides (see Chapter 24 'Glycosides', p. 181), which are made when sugars link to highly toxic cyanide. These are released when the plant is attacked by an insect or disease-causing organism. Whatever the reason for secondary metabolites, they are extremely useful as medicines, food, flavourings, colourings, perfumes, aromatherapy oils and dyes.

Approximately a quarter of prescription drugs contain at least one chemical that was originally isolated and extracted from a plant.

The diversity of secondary metabolites is astounding, and very often families of plants produce similar secondary metabolites, with similar chemical characteristics. So, whenever possible, these plant families, with examples, are listed in the various chemical groups. For example, terpenes can act as antibacterials and hormonal-like substances, depending on the type of terpene.

Based on the principle 'structure dictates function', being able to recognize structure goes a long way to being able to make an educated guess as to what function the compound performs. Many secondary metabolites originate from a similar compound, which is transformed at the last minute by an alternative pathway, for example, shikimic acid is the starting point for phenol-based compounds (see Figures 21.1 and 21.2, pp. 149 and 150).

Bibliography

Bruneton J. Pharmacognosy, phytochemisty, medicinal plants. Andover: Intercept; 1999.

Dewick PM. Medicinal natural products. A biosynthetic approach. 2nd edn. Chichester: John Wiley; 2004.

Lewis WH, Elvin-Lewis MPF. Medical botany. Plants affecting human health. 2nd edn. Edinburgh: John Wiley; 2003.

Mills S, Bone K. The principles and practice of phytotherapy. Modern herbal medicine. Edinburgh: Churchill Livingstone; 2000.

Pengelly A. The constituents of medicinal plants. Wallingford, UK: Cabi Publishing; 2004.

Phenols

21

Phenols constitute probably the largest group of plant secondary metabolites, varying in size from a simple structure with an aromatic ring to complex ones such as lignins. Although many of the essential oils are terpenes, some are phenolic compounds, for example thymol from *Thymus* spp. (thyme) (Figure 21.1). Many simple phenols are responsible for taste, for example eugenol in cloves. They are called the **phenylpropanoids** because they originate from phenylalanine (see Figure 11.1, p. 82) and they have a six-carbon (C6) and three-carbon (C3) structure (Figure 21.2). They comprise several groups:

- simple phenols
- quinones
- naphthoquinones

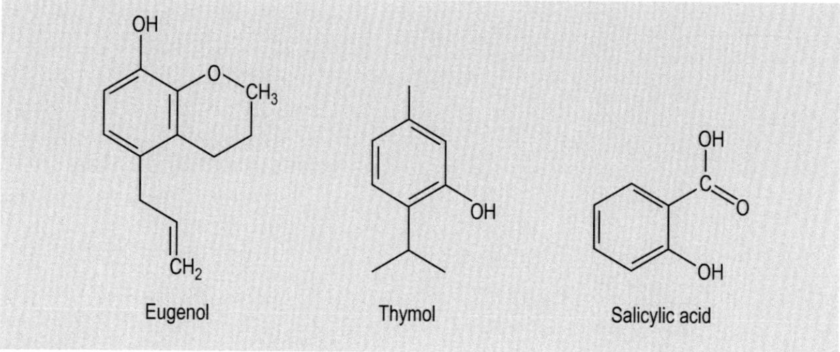

Eugenol   Thymol   Salicylic acid

Figure 21.1 The structure of simple phenols.

- anthraquinones
- xanthones
- coumarins, including furanocoumarins and chromones
- flavonoids
- tannins
- lignin and lignans.

Many of these are attached to sugars that have to be cut or cleaved before activity (see Chapter 24 'Glycosides', p. 181).

Shikimic Acid

The starting point for the production of phenylpropanoids is shikimic acid (Figure 21.2). Shikimic acid (or shikimate) is the precursor for:

- Amino acids: e.g. phenylalanine, tryptophan and tyrosine (see Figure 11.1, p. 82).
- Aromatic aldehydes: e.g. vanillin.
- Simple aromatic acids: e.g. gallic acid.

The shikimic acid pathway is absent in mammals.

Abridged Phenylpropanoids

These possess no side chain or a side chain with one carbon atom (Figure 21.3).

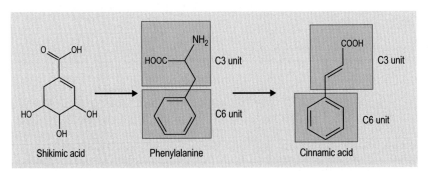

Shikimic acid   Phenylalanine   Cinnamic acid

Figure 21.2 Showing the development of simple phenylpropenes from shikimic acid and demonstrating the C3 and C6 units.

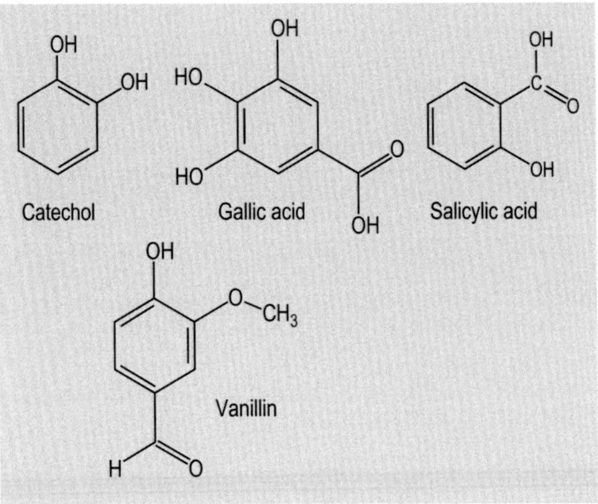

Catechol   Gallic acid   Salicylic acid

Vanillin

Figure 21.3 Abridged phenylpropanoids.

Simple Phenols

These are based around:

- Benzoic acid derivatives: e.g. salicylic acid, hydroquinone, catechol, vanillin.
- Cinnamic acid derivatives: e.g. rosmarinic acid found in *Rosmarinus* spp. (rosemary) and *Melissa officinalis* (lemon balm).
- Benzoic, cinnamic, salicylic and rosmarinic acids (Figure 21.4) are carboxylic acid derivatives (see Figure 5.1, p. 30).

Phenols are are found in:

- Ericaceae: *Arctostaphylos uva-ursi* (bearberry, uva-ursi).
- Rosaceae: *Filipendula ulmaria* (meadowsweet, Queen of the meadow), *Agrimonia* spp. (agrimony, *Xian He Cao*), *Crataegus* spp. (hawthorn, *Shan Zha*).
- Vitaceae: *Vitis* spp. (grape).
- Asteraceae: *Cichorium intybus* (chicory).
- Labiatae (Laminaceae): *Mentha* spp. (mint, *Bo He*).
- Boraginaceae: *Pulmonaria officinalis* (lungwort), *Lithospermum erythrorhizon* (*Zi Cao*).

Action of Phenols

- Antiseptic.
- Bactericidal.
- Fungicidal.
- Antihelminitic.
- Mild anaesthetic.
- Calmative.

Phenols have a benzene ring with at least one hydroxyl group attached to it. Other compounds attached to the benzene ring change its function.

Hydroxycinnamates

- Derivatives of cinnamic acid (Figure 21.5).
- Have become of great interest due to their antioxidant properties.

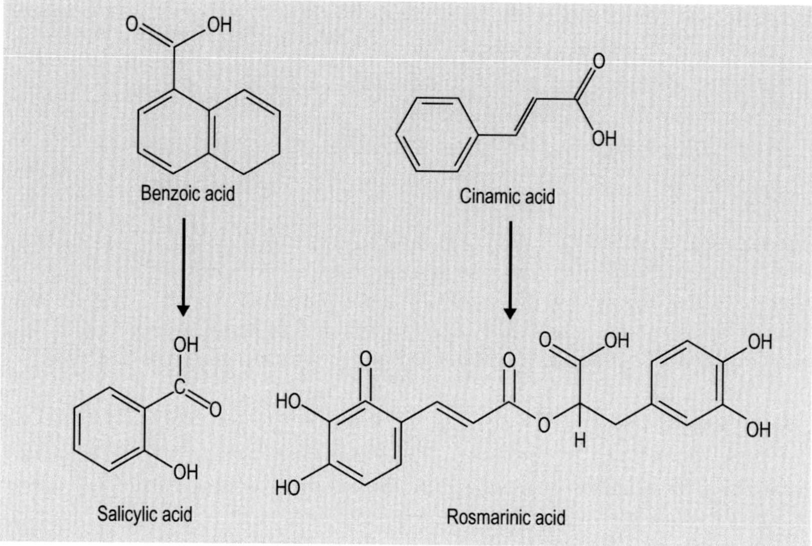

Figure 21.4 Demonstrating derivations of phenolic acids from benzoic and cinnamic acid.

Pharmacology A handbook for complementary healthcare professionals

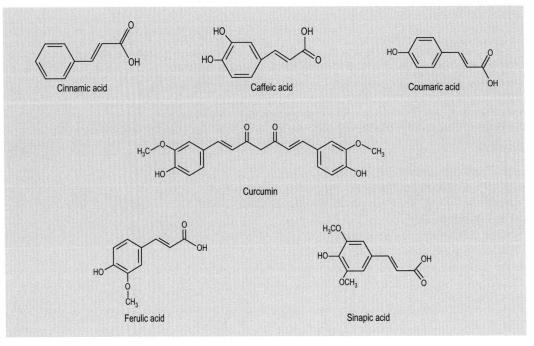

Figure 21.5 Chemical structures of cinnamic acid and the hydroxyl derivatives.

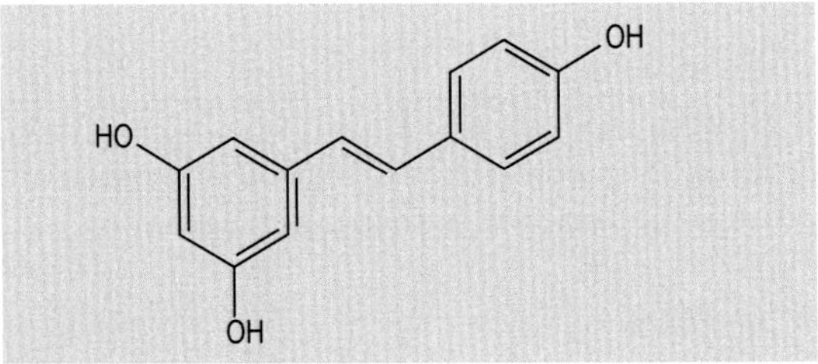

Figure 21.6 Chemical structure of resveratrol.

Examples are:

- Caffeic acid: coffee, apples, blueberries.
- Coumaric acid: spinach, cereals.
- Curcumin: *Curcuma* spp. (turmeric, *Jiang Huang, E Zhu*).
- Ferulic acid: coffee, cereals, citrus juices.
- Sinapic acid: broccoli and other brassicas, citrus juices.

Stilbenes

These are found in the heartwood of plants. They are thought to be responsible for 'French paradox' whereby deaths from heart disease in France are lower than in other countries. Resveratrol (Figure 21.6), a component of red wine, acts not only as an antioxidant and an anti-inflammatory but also as an antitumour agent. It is found in blueberries, bilberries, cranberries, and in the skins and seeds of grapes.

Quinones

Derived from the oxidation of phenols, quinones are closely involved in photosynthesis because they have the ability to gain and lose electrons, which enables the conversion of light energy in a form of energy a plant can use (see Chapter 2 'Atoms', p. 10). They are able to carry electrons between the components that are involved in light reactions (Figure 21.7). Quinones are very lipid soluble.

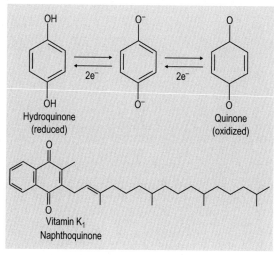

Figure 21.7 Comparison of quinones and naphthoquinones.

Naphthoquinones

- Naphthoquinones are effectively quinones with another aromatic ring fused onto them. They usually occur as glycosides.
- Vitamin K is an example of a naphthoquinone.
- They have antibacterial and antitumour effects.

Naphthoquinones are not widespread but are found in:

- Bignoniaceae: *Kigelia pinnata, Tabebuia* spp. (*Pau d'arco*).
- Ebenaceae: *Diospyros* spp. (persimmon, *Shi Di*).
- Droseraceae: *Drosera* spp. (sundew).
- Juglandaceae: *Juglans* spp. (walnut, *Hu Tao Ren*).
- Plumbaginaceae: *Plumbago* spp. (leadwort, *Bai Hua Dan*).
- Boraginaeceae: *Borago* spp. (borage).

Their appearance is sporadic throughout these groups.

Anthraquinones

- Yellow–brown or orangey red in colour.
- Can be found free and as glycosides (see Chapter 24 'Glycosides', p. 181). Most commonly occur as O- or C-glycosides.
- The basic aglycone (see Chapter 24 'Glycosides', p. 182) has a central quinone with a phenol group either side (Figure 21.8).
- There are variants of anthraquinones such as anthranols (alcohols) and anthrones (ketones).

• Action of Anthraquinones

- Laxative.
- Antibacterial.
- Antiviral.

They can be found in:

- Rhamaceae: *Picramnia* spp. (cascara), *Frangula alnus* Miller, *Rhamnus frangula* (alder buckthorn), *Ziziphus jujube* [*Dao Zao* (fruit), *Suan Zao Ren* (seed)].
- Leguminosae: *Cassia obtusifolia* (*Jue Ming Zi*).

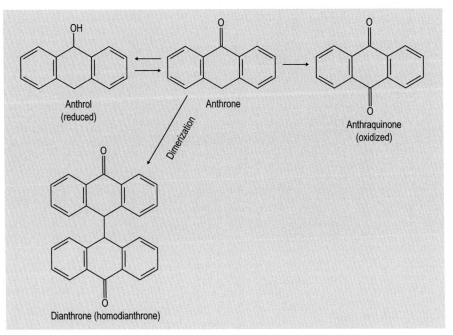

Figure 21.8 Diagram showing the relationship between anthraquinones, anthrones, dianthols and dianthrones.

- Liliaceae: aloe vera.
- Polygonaceae: *Rumex* spp. (docks and sorrels), *Rheum palmatum* (*Da Huang*).
- Fabaceae: *Senna alexandrina* (senna).
- Guttiferae (Hypericaceae): *Hypericum perforatum* (St John's wort).
- Rubiaceae: *Cephaelis* spp. (ipecacuanha).
- Polygonaceae: *Rheum palmatum* (*Da Huang*).
- Ericaceae: *Arctostaphylos uva-ursi* (bearberry, uva-ursi), *Vaccinium myrtillus* (bilberry).
- Euphorbiaceae: *Ricinus communis* (castor oil plant).

They also occur in a number of fungi and lichens.

Relationship Between Anthraquinone Derivatives

Anthrones tend to be unstable. The dianthols exist only as glycosides. Anthrones can exist as dianthrones, which creates a stable compound. This occurs when a herb containing an anthrone compound is dried. There are two types of dianthrone:

- **Homodiathrones** (Figures 21.8 and 21.9): the two dianthrones are the same.
- **Heterodianthrones** where the two dianthrones are different.

These compounds were originally thought to exert their laxative effect by irritating the gut wall. However, this is now thought to be incorrect and the effect is more likely to be due to stimulation of the peristaltic action and inhibition of water and electrolyte reabsorption by the gut.

Hypericin is two of the same anthrone joined together to form a homoanthrone.

Pharmacokinetics of Anthraquinone Action

The glycosides of anthraquinones and dianthrones are polar (see Chapter 3 'Bonds found in biological chemistry', p. 15) and therefore not easily absorbed across the phospholipid membranes of the cells of the gut wall. Once the bacteria have cleaved the sugar off, the compound becomes non-polar and is absorbed across the non-polar cell membrane of the gut wall cells.

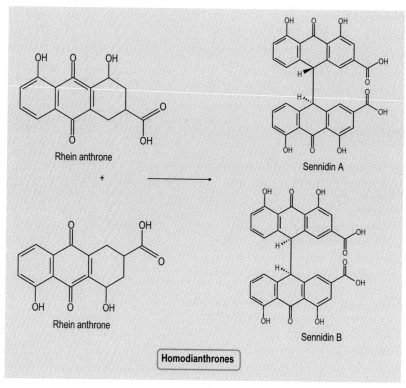

Figure 21.9 Two of the same anthrones forming a dianthrone (homoanthrones).

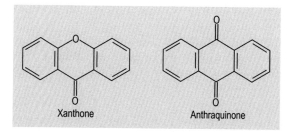

Figure 21.10 Comparison of the chemical structures of xanthone and anthraquinone.

155

Excessive consumption of anthraquinones can cause severe disruption of the colon with resultant pain and diarrhoea. The length of use of herbs containing anthraquinones should therefore be limited.

The action of an anthrone (Figures 21.8 and 21.9) is excessively vigorous, which is why certain herbs, such as *Frangula* (buckthorn bark), have to be stored before use. The storage time allows the anthrones to become oxidized so that they form the less reactive anthraquinone glycosides.

Xanthones

Contribute to the yellow colour of the gentian root. Xanthones (Figure 21.10) are mainly found in:

* Gentianaceae: *Gentiana* spp. (gentian, *Long Dan Cao*).
* Hypericaceae: *Hypericum* spp. (St John's wort).

Chemical Activities

- Antifungal.
- Antibacterial.
- Inhibition of platelet aggregation.
- Anti-inflammatory.

Coumarins

- Are lactones: compare with sesquiterpene lactones such as artemisinin (see Figure 22.5, p. 171).
- Coumarin variants (Figure 21.11) are common in plants both as aglycones and glycosides.
- 1000 natural coumarins have been isolated. Coumarin itself is found in about 150 species belonging to over 30 different families.
- The coumarin is probably present as a *trans*-O-glycoside (see Chapter 24 'Glycosides', p. 181).

Coumarins are commonly found in:

- Compositae (Asteraceae): *Artemisia* spp.
- Fabaceae: *Trifolium* spp.
- Rutaceae: *Ruta graveolens* (rue) as furanocoumarins.
- Umbelliferae (Apiaceae): *Apium graveolens* (celery), *Ledebouriella* spp. (*Fang Feng*) as pyranocoumarins.
- Leguminosae: sweet clover, melitot, woodruff.

Anticoagulant Actions

Coumarin itself is not an anticoagulant. However, it can be converted into the dicoumarol (usually when the plant is damaged), which is an anticoagulant (Figure 21.12). Dicoumarol interferes with the activation by vitamin K of clotting, as it is similar in structure to vitamin K, and competes with the enzyme involved in vitamin K

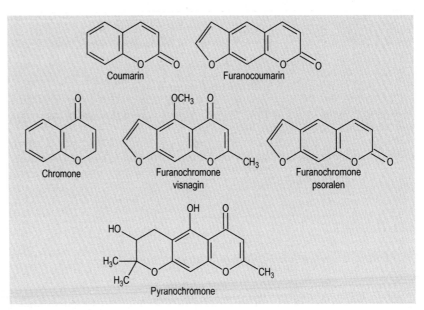

Figure 21.11 Structures of various coumarins.

production (see Figure 28.1, p. 212). Dicoumarol is similar in structure to vitamin K, so is able to inhibit vitamin K production.

Psoralens (Furanocoumarins)

Psoralens are coumarins that possess a furan ring (see Figure 21.11, and compare with the structure of furanose sugar in Figure 9.4, p. 65), which is why they are also called furanocoumarins. This extra ring on the coumarin structure means that they absorb light readily, so consideration of the exposure a patient who is given herbs containing furanocoumarins will be getting to sunlight is important.

Ingestion of *Psoralea corylifoliae* (*Bu Gu Zhi*) has been documented as having an association with skin reaction to sunlight because it contains the furanocoumarin psoralen. However, skin reactions are rare. This effect has been utilized in the treatment of psoriasis. Psoralens are ingested by the patient, who is then exposed to UVA in PUVA treatments.

Psoralens are commonly found in:

- Rutaceae: *Ruta graveolens* (rue).
- Umbelliferae: *Apium graveolens* (celery fruits contain rutaretin and apiumentin), *Angelica archangelic* (angelica), *Petroselenium crispum* (parsley).

Chromones

- Structural isomers coumarins. Compare their structures in Figure 21.11; the oxygen in the chromone is in a different position to that in the coumarin.
- Display antibacterial activity.

Flavonoids

- Polyphenols: slightly larger than the quinones and are found in all vascular plants. They can be found in foods such as fruits, vegetables, teas and wines.
- Phenylpropene (six- and three-carbon units; source shikimic acid) + six-carbon unit. Three molecules of malonyl-coA = triketide unit (see Figure 21.3). Their basic structure is based on a skeleton of 15 carbon atoms (C15).
- All flavonoids have the same biosynthetic origin.
- **Carotenoids are often confused with flavonoids** because they both end with –oid. Comparison of structures will clearly show the difference between the two (see Figure 9.1, p. 64 and Chapter 22 'Terpenes', p. 174).

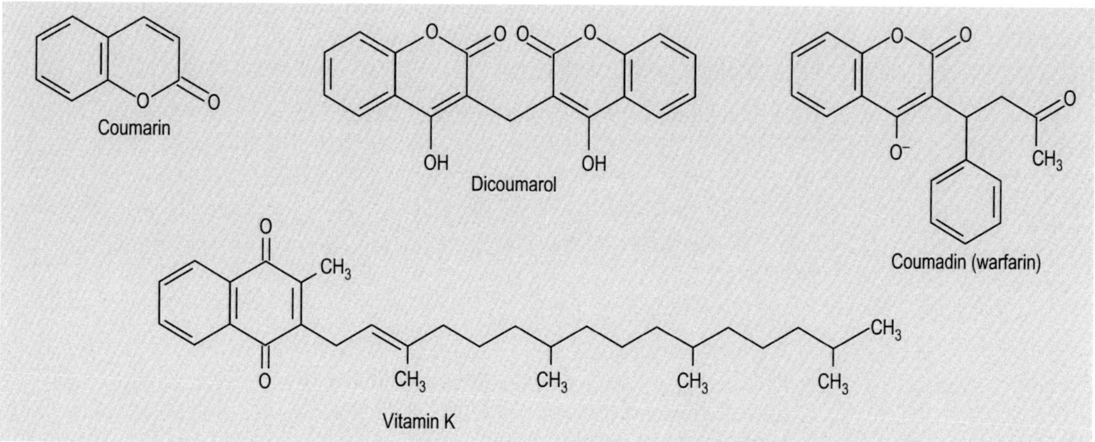

157

Figure 21.12 Comparison of chemical structures of coumarin, dicoumarol, coumadin (warfarin) and vitamin K.

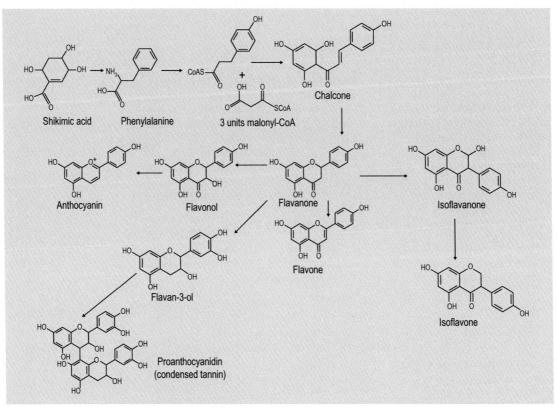

Figure 21.13 The synthesis of flavonoids from shikimic acid.

- Antioxidants: the ability of flavonoids to act as antioxidants depends on their molecular structure. The arrangement of the hydroxyl groups and other groups is important for the antioxidant activities. **Catechin-based quercitin is very good at free radical scavenging** for this reason (see Figure 7.6, p. 47).
- **Water soluble.**
- Are very often attached to sugars.
- **Are not present in algae.**
- Anti-inflammatories: flavonoids influence arachidonic acid metabolism and hence have an anti-inflammatory effect (see Figure 30.5, p. 229).
- Flavonoids are resistant to boiling and fermentation (Kim et al 1998).

Formation of Flavonoids

The formation of flavonoids is illustrated in Figure 21.13. The structures of different flavonoids are shown in Figure 21.14.

Colours Associated with Flavonoids

Colour is dependent on the placement of the hydroxyl groups around the basic skeleton:

- Chalcones: yellow or colourless.
- Flavanones: colourless.
- Flavones: pure flavones are colourless but the more hydroxyl groups that are present, the more intense the yellow colour. Flavones are co-pigments that protect anthrocyanins.
- Flavonols: colourless co-pigments that protect anthrocyanins.

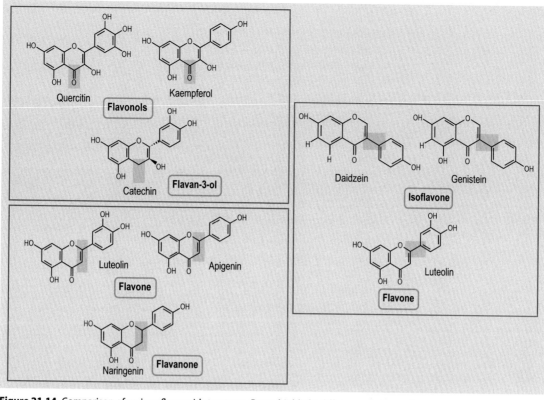

Figure 21.14 Comparison of various flavonoid structures. Boxes highlight differences between the groups.

- Anthocyanidins: red, blue, purple, violet.
- Isoflavones: colourless.
- Catechins: colourless.

• Chalcones

Found in:

- Cannabinaceae: *Humulus lupulus* (hops).
- Compositae: *Cartharmi tinctoria* (*Hong Hua*).
- Leguminosae: *Glycyrrhiza* spp. (*Gan Cao*).
- Piperaceae: *Piper methysticum* (*Kava kava*).
- Intermediate compounds in the biosynthesis of flavonoids.
- The numbering system is slightly different to the flavonoids in that rings A and B (see Figure 5.5, p. 31) are reversed.

Properties

- Antioxidant.
- Antifungal.
- Antibacterial.
- Antitumoral.
- Anti-inflammatory.

• Flavanones

Found in:

- Rutaceae: citrus species (*Chen Pi, Qing Pi*, etc.).

Properties

- Antioxidant.
- Anti-inflammatory.
- Can have an effect on carbohydrate metabolism.
- Immune system modulator.

• Flavones

Found in:

- Polygonaceae: *Rumex* spp. (yellow dock).
- Rutaceae: citrus species (*Chen Pi, Qing Pi*, etc.).
- Leguminoseae: *Glycyrrhizae* spp. (*Gan Cao*).
- Umbelliferae: *Apium graveolens* (celery), *Petroselinum crispum* (parsley).
- Compositae: *Chrysanthemum morifolium* (*Ju Hua*).

Properties

- Anti-inflammatory.
- Anti-allergic.
- Antithrombotic and vasoprotective.
- Tumour inhibitor.

• Flavonol

Found in:

- grapes
- berries
- fruits
- cauliflower
- cabbages.

Properties

- Antioxidant: quercitin has most appropriate configuration as an antioxidant (see Figure 7.6, p. 47).
- Anti-inflammatory.

• Flavan-3-ol (Flavanol)

Found in:

- *Camellia sinensis* (tea): catechin.
- Chocolate.

• Isoflavones

Differ from flavones by the position of the phenyl group (see Figure 21.14). Found in:

- Fabaceae: *Glycine max* (soy bean), *Psoraleae corylifolia* (*Bu Gu Zhi*), *Puerariae* spp. (*Ge Gen*), *Trifolium pratense* (red clover).

Properties of Soy Isoflavones

- Phytoestrogens act like oestrogens in body (see Chapter 38 'Reproductive hormones'. p. 305) working directly on oestrogen receptors.
- Fermentation or digestion of soybeans or soy products results in the release of sugar from the compound to leave the free aglycone (see Chapter 24 'Glycosides', p. 182).

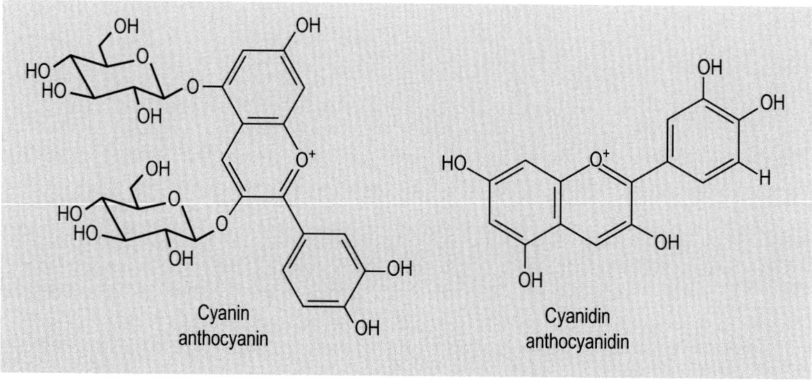

Figure 21.15 Comparison of chemical structures of an anthocyanin and an anthocyanidin.

- The aglycone of genistin is genistein; the aglycone of diadzin is daidzein.
- Modest lowering of low-density lipoproteins.
- Possible linkage with lower breast cancer rates.
- High dietary intake of soy isoflavone might decrease the risk of endometrial cancer.
- Might limit prostate cancer.
- There is some evidence that isoflavone-rich foods are bone sparing; this is not conclusive.
- Soy isoflavone can reduce hot flushes in menopausal symptoms.

● Anthocyanins (Figure 21.15)

- Glycoside (see Chapter 24 'Glycosides', p. 182).
- Water soluble.

● Anthocyanidins (Figure 21.15)

- Aglycone (see Chapter 24 'Glycosides', p. 182).
- **Anthocyanidin** pigments are responsible for the colours such as red, mauve, violet and blue colour in flowers, fruits, and leaves. This can be dictated by the pH of the sap.
- Water soluble.

Both are found in:

- Skins of fruit and in coloured fruit, e.g. grape skins, red apple skins, blackberries, blueberries.

Properties

- Antioxidants.

Tannins

- Polyphenols (made up of more than one unit of phenol).
- They bind and precipitate proteins, but they are not the only plant chemicals to do this. They can bind with proteins, starch, cellulose and minerals.
- Many tannins are glycosides.
- There are two main groups: hydrolysable and condensed (proanthocyanidin).

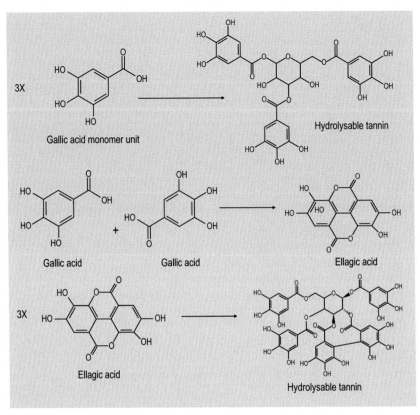

Figure 21.16 The formation of hydrolysable tannins.

- They are soluble in water, with the exception of some high-molecular-weight structures.
- Tannins are produced in two ways: (1) from phenols synthesized via the shikimic acid pathway (hydrolysable tannins); or (2) polymerization (condensation reactions; see Figure 4.7, p. 26) of flavonoids.

Tannins are found in *He Ye* and *Jin Yin Hua*. They are present in plant parts: bark, wood, fruit, fruit pods, leaves, and roots.

Hydrolysable Tannins

- Gallotannins: tannic acid.
- Ellagitannins: ellagic acid (Figure 21.16).

• Properties

- Derivatives of gallic acid.
- Can be hydrolysed by hot water or enzymes. Can also be hydrolysed by mild acids or mild bases to yield carbohydrate and phenolic acids. This will not hydrolyse proanthocyanidins (condensed tannins).

Proanthrocyanidins (Condensed Tannins)

- Do not have glycosides (no sugar attached) (Figure 21.17).
- Related to flavonoid pigment and have polymeric flavan-3-ol (flavanol) as part of structure.
- Catechins (found in green tea) are intermediates in their synthesis.
- Are more common than hydrolysable tannins.

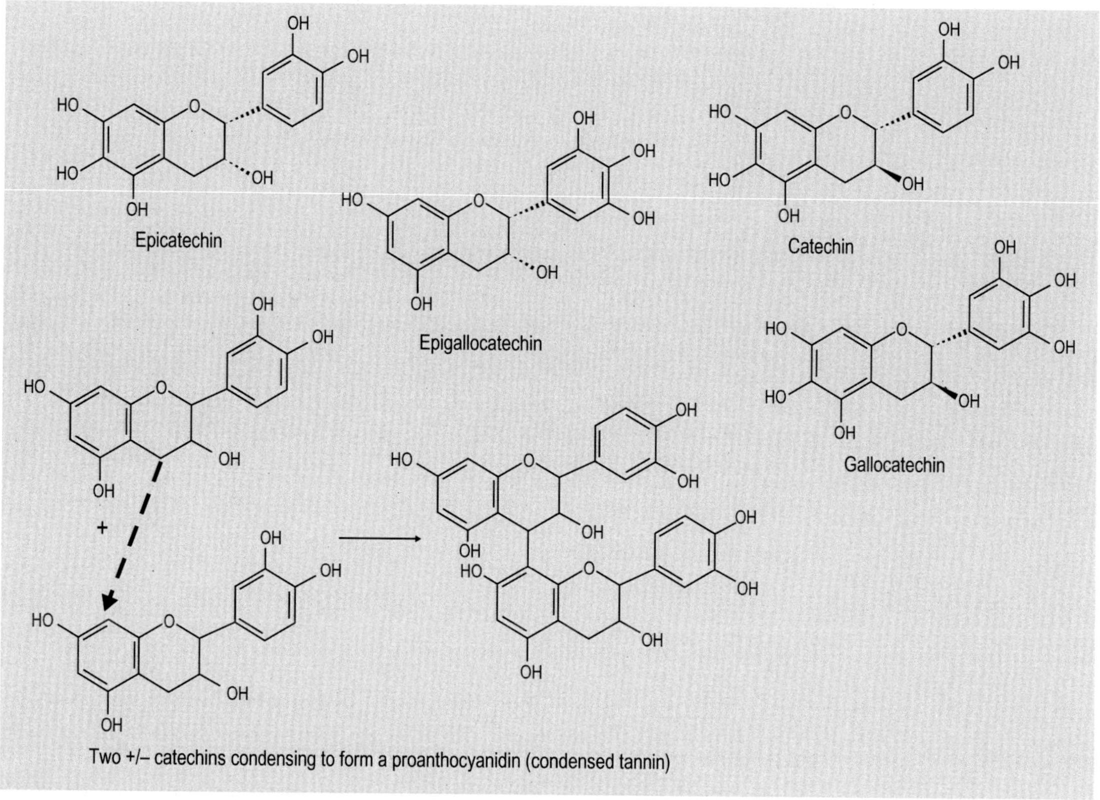

Two +/– catechins condensing to form a proanthocyanidin (condensed tannin)

Figure 21.17 Chemical structures of proanthocyanidin monomers (above) and the condensation reaction to form a proanthocyanidin (condensed tannin) (below).

- Oligomers or polymers of flavonoid units linked by carbon–carbon bonds not susceptible to cleavage by hydrolysis.
- Are called 'condensed tannins' because of their condensed chemical structure.
- **Proanthocyanidins** come from the acid catalysed oxidation reaction that produces red **anthocyanidins** when the proanthocyanidins are heated in acidic alcohol solutions.
- The polymers of proanthocyanidins are variable because the **flavonoid** units can differ.
- Are responsible for the astringent taste of wine.
- Belong to the flavonoid family and can be indicated by the initials OPC (oligomeric procyanidins) or PCO (procyanidolic oligomers).

The Importance of Tannin Interactions

Tannins provide astringent and haemostatic properties to a compound. They interact with:

- carbohydrates
- proteins and therefore enzymes
- polysaccharides
- bacterial cell membranes.

• Reaction with Carbohydrates

- Starch can create cavities in which tannins and other hydrophobic complexes, such as lipid, are embedded.

- Tannins interact directly with cellulose: the tannins seem to react with plant cell walls like lignin. However, this is not clear, as there is a difference in location of tannins and cell wall carbohydrates in living plants, and after digestion by animals.
- The higher the molecular weight of the carbohydrate, the more it interacts with tannins. These carbohydrates are usually not very soluble and mobile in their structure.

Reaction with Proteins

This is a well-recognized interaction; an example is leather tanning. For bonding to take place, the following characteristics have to be present in both the tannins and the proteins. Proteins need:

- large molecular size
- open and flexible structures
- to be rich in proline.

Tannins need:

- high molecular weight
- mobile structures.

How Binding Takes Place: Hydrophobic and Hydrogen Bonding

Hydrolysable tannins and proanthocyanins form tannin–protein complexes in similar ways. These complexes are very stable structures and are very difficult for the gut to break down.

It is possible for proteins to interact with tannins when the amount of protein is in excess of that of the tannin. When this occurs, there is no precipitation and it is difficult to see whether the reaction has taken place.

Insoluble complexes will only form when the amount of tannins exceeds that of protein and a hydrophobic outer layer is formed.

Precipitation is very important and care should be taken when mixing herbs containing tannins; a highly tanninized herb might bind useful constituents. Herbalists can usually see this straight away when they mix tinctures, as they become cloudy. One of the reason that strong black tea is supposed to be good for diarrhoea is that it binds with the proteins in the gut wall and acts as a barrier to prevent water loss.

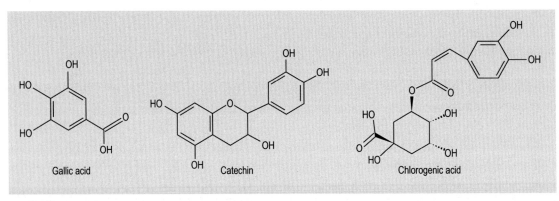

Gallic acid

Catechin

Chlorogenic acid

Figure 21.18 The chemical structures of various pseudotannins.

Pseudotannins

Derived from cinnamic acid, **pseudotannins** (Figure 21.18) are so named because they have some, but not all, the astringent properties of true tannins. For example, they do not react to Goldbeater's skin test (see Chapter 41 'Scientific tests', p. 338).

Lignin

Primary cell walls are soft and their rigidity is maintained by the water inside them, which is why a plant wilts when it is not watered adequately. This does not happen in trees because the primary cell walls contain deposits, which can be much thicker then the primary cell walls, that give the plant a great deal more support.

Lignans and Lignins

Lignans are made up of two units of a phenylpropene derivative joined by C3 side chains or between the aromatic ring and C3 ring (Figure 21.19). They are found in:

- Oleaceae: *Forsythia* spp. (forsythia, *Lian Qiao*).
- Onagraceae: *Oenothera biennis* (evening primose).

Plant lignans are found in foods such as whole grains, legumes, seeds, fruits and vegetables. The best source of plant lignans are flax seeds. Once in the gut, bacteria change the precursors into **mammalian lignans** (enterolactone and enterodiol). These lignans appear to have a weak oestrogenic activity, although the effect does not occur by direct stimulation of the oestrogen receptors.

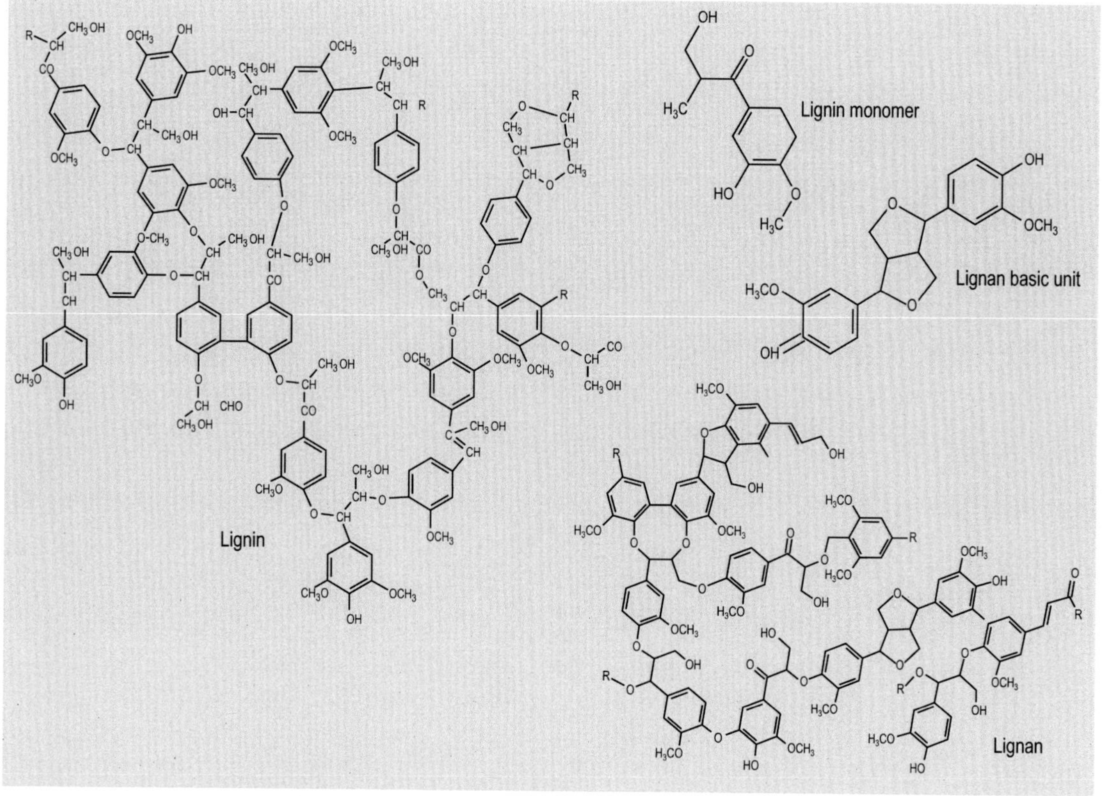

Figure 21.19 Comparison of lignin and lignan chemical structures.

165

Reference

Kim DH, Jung EA, Sohng IS et al. Intestinal bacterial metabolism of flavonoids and its relation to some biological activities. Archives of Pharmacological Research 1998; 21(1):17–23.

Further reading

Kaddu S, Kerl H, Wolf P. Accidental bullous phototoxic reactions to bergamot aromatherapy oil. Journal of the American Journal of Dermatology 2001; 45(3):458–461.

Terpenes

22

Chapter contents

Terpenes are largely found as constituents of essential oils. They are mostly hydrocarbons. The building block is a five-carbon isoprene (CH_2==$C(CH_3)$—CH==CH_2) unit (Figure 22.1). Terpene hydrocarbons have a molecular formula of $(C_5H_8)n$; the n dictates the number of units involved. Terpene hydrocarbons are classified according to the number of isoprene units:

- Monoterpenes: 2 isoprene units, 10 carbon atoms.
- Sesquiterpenes: 3 isoprene units, 15 carbon atoms.
- Diterpenes: 4 isoprene units, 20 carbon atoms.
- Triterpenes: 6 isoprene units, 30 carbon atoms.
- Tetraterpenes: 8 isoprene units, 40 carbon atoms.

Terpenes are found in:

- Lamiaceae (Labiatae): *Melissa officinalis* (lemon balm), *Agastache rugosa* (*Huo Xiang*), *Rosmarinus officinalis* (rosemary), *Lavandula officinalis* (lavender), *Mentha* spp. (mint, *Bo He*).

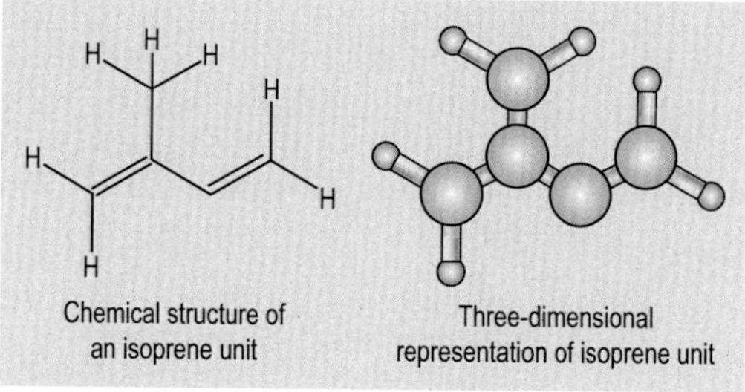

Chemical structure of an isoprene unit

Three-dimensional representation of isoprene unit

Figure 22.1 The chemical structure of the isoprene building block of terpenes and its three-dimensional representation.

- Coniferae: *Thuja occidentalis*.
- Compositae: *Artemisia* spp. (mugwort, *Qing Hao*).
- Leguminoseae: *Glycyrrhizae* spp. (*Gan Cao*).
- Taxaceae: *Taxus* spp. (yew).

Monoterpenes

- Two isoprene units.

General properties of monoterpenes (Figure 22.2):

- Volatile oils: can therefore be administered as inhalations. Have very characteristic odours and are used in perfumes.
- Easily penetrate membranes as non-polar (and therefore lipophilic) compounds. This quality is utilized in aromatherapy.
- Used as flavourings.
- Generally, monoterpenes are antimicrobial (Gram positive and Gram negative; Trombetta et al 2005) and antifungal.
- Antispasmodics.
- Some are glycosides (see Chapter 24 'Glycosides', p. 181) e.g. nerol, citronellol, geraniol.

Menthols

Menthol (Figure 22.3) is a local anaesthetic and reduces irritation.

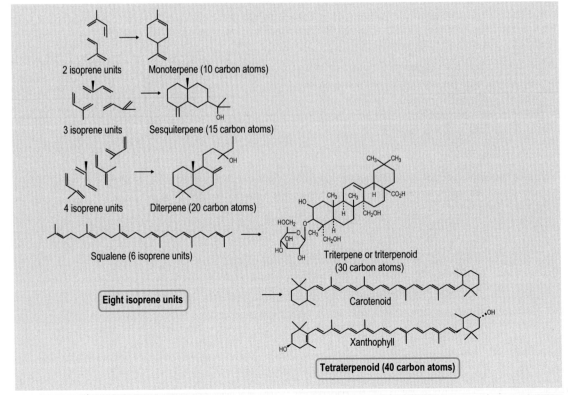

Figure 22.2 The formation of terpenes from isoprene units. This is an oversimplification of the process, but gives a general idea of the components of each type of terpene.

Examples of Actions

- Menthol: found in *Mentha* spp. (mint, *Bo He*) is a carminative.
- Thujone: is the toxic agent found in *Artemisiae annuae* (wormwood, *Qing Hao*).
- The Artemisias are an old remedy in Western herbal medicine for worming.

Iridoids

General properties:

- Derivatives of monoterpenes.
- Most occur as glycosides.
- Have a bitter taste known as 'bitter principles'.
- Cardiovascular, stomachic, choleretic, antihepatotoxic activities and insect attractant and repellant properties.

Examples of Actions

- Aucubin (Figure 22.4) is found in *Eucommiae ulmoides* (*Du Zhong*); harpagoside is found in *Harpagophytum procumbens* (devil's claw). Both have anti-inflammatory properties.

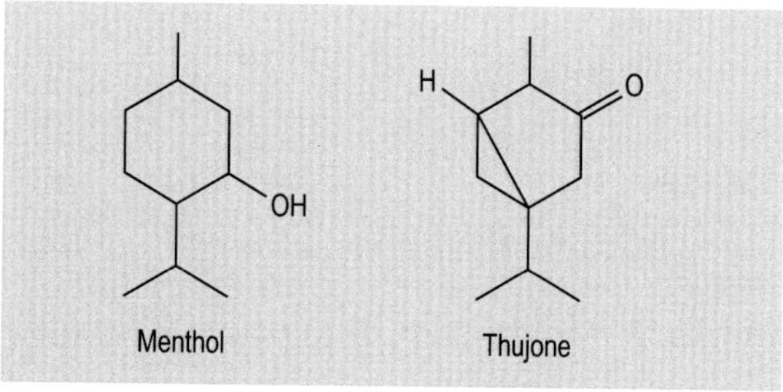

Figure 22.3 Menthol and thujone.

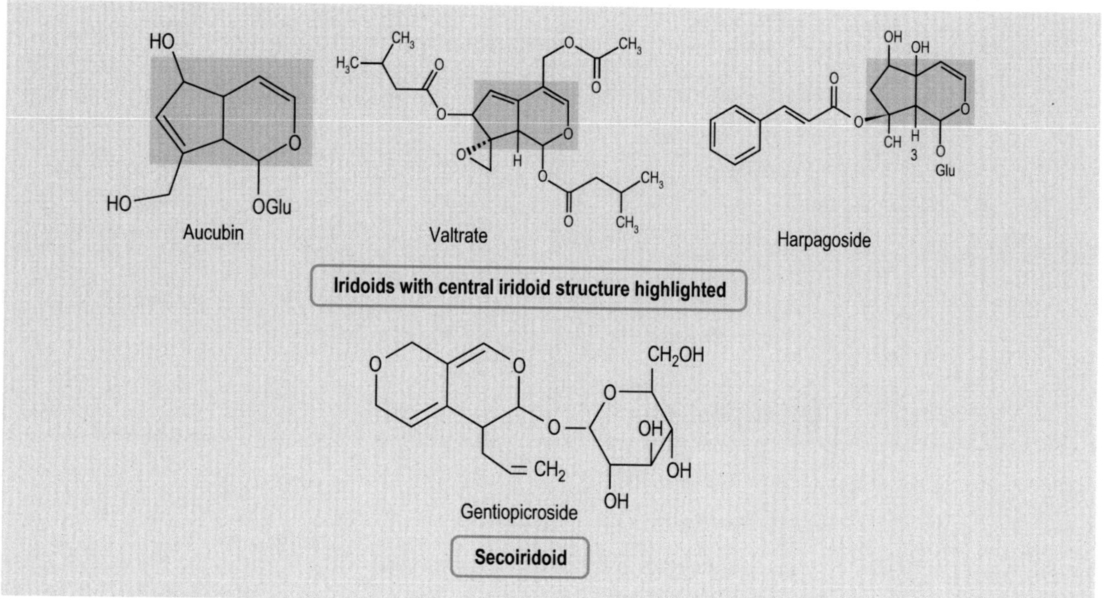

Figure 22.4 Examples of iridoids.

- Valtrate is thought to be one of the compounds responsible for the sedative properties of *Valeriana officinalis* (valerian). It belongs to the class of iridoids associated with valerian and referred to as **valepotriates**.

Iridoids are found in:

- Cornaceae (the dogwood family): *Cornus officinalis* (*Shan Zhu Yu*).
- Gentianaceae: *Gentiana* spp.
- Eucommiaceae: *Eucommiae ulmoides* (*Du Zhong*).
- Antirrhinum (scrophulariaceae): *Rehmanniae glutinosae* (*Shu di Hang* and *Sheng di Huang*).
- Lamiaceae (Labiatae): *Stachys betonica* (wood betony).
- Pedaliaceae (sesame family): *Harpagophytum procumbens* (devil's claw).
- Bigoniaceae: *Kigelia pinnata* (sausage tree).
- Valerianaceae: *Valeriana officinalis* (valerian).
- Verbenaceae: *Verbena officinalis* (verbena).

Secoiridoids

- Often occur as glycosides.
- Gentiopicroside (see Figure 22.4) seems to work on the immune system ultimately affecting the inflammatory system.

The secoiridoids are found in:

- Gentianaceae: *Gentiana* spp. (*Long Dan Cao*).

Sesquiterpenes

- Three isoprene units.
- Not as volatile as monoterpenes.

Sesquiterpenes (Figure 21.5) are found in:

- Cannabaceae: *Humulus* spp. (hops).
- Compositae: *Atractylodes* spp. (*Cang Zhu*, *Bai Zhu*).
- Magnoliaceae: *Magnolia officinalis* (*Hou Po*).
- Cyperaceae: *Cyperus rotundus* (*Xiang Fu*).

General actions of sesquiterpenes:

- antiprotozoal
- antitumour.

Sesquiterpene Lactones

Largely found in:

- Compositae: *Chrysanthemum* spp. (*Ju Hua*), *Taraxacum* spp. (dandelion, *Pu Gong Ying*), *Artemisia* spp. [wormwood (*Qing Hao*), mugwort (*Ai Ye*)].

Diterpenes

- Four isoprene units.

Diterpenes (Figure 22.6) are found in:

- Euphorbaceae: *Croton* spp. (croton, *Ba Dou*)
- Lamiaccae (Labiatac): *Rosmarinus officinalis* (rosemary), *Salvia* spp. (*Dan Shen*).
- Taxaceae: *Taxus* (yew).

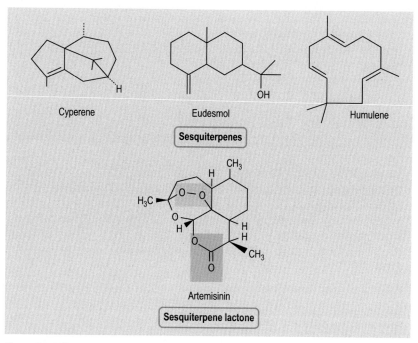

Figure 22.5 Various sesquiterpenes. Artemisinin: green area shows the part of the molecule associated with sequiterpene activity; the purple area shows the part of the molecule that has the antimalarial effect. This is achieved by creating radicals that destroy the malarial parasite. The peroxide group is responsible for this antimalarial effect (Pandey et al 1999).

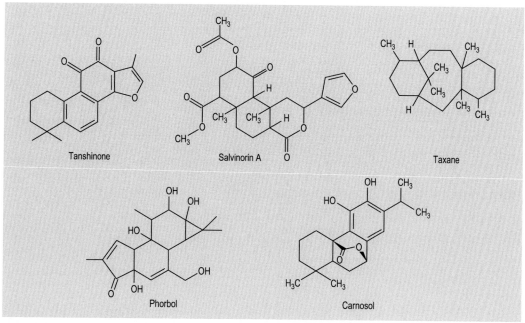

Figure 22.6 Various diterpenes.

Examples of Actions

- Tanshinone found in *Salvia* spp. been of interest in heart conditions.
- Salvinorin A found in *Salvia* spp. is a non-alkaloid kappa opioid receptor agonist (see Chapter 19 'Pharmacodynamics: how drugs elicit a physiological effect', p. 140 and Chapter 32 'Analgesia and the relief of pain', p. 249).

- Taxol is the tradename for taxane, which is used in the treatment of ovarian cancer. Taxane is prepared from *Taxus*.
- Phorbol, from *Croton* spp., has a carcinogenic effect and is used in tumour research.
- Carnosol is found in *Rosmarinus* spp.; it is an antioxidant.

Triterpenes (or Triterpenoids)

- Six isoprene units.
- Very wide distribution including animals.
- Two main types: steroidal (usually tetracyclic triterpenoids, saponins) and the pentacyclic (Figure 22.7).
- When present as glycosides, triterpenes are referred to as saponins (see Chapter 24 'Glycosides', p. 182).
- Squalene is the immediate biological precursor of all triterpenoids (see Figure 22.2).

The triterpene group has a wide range of effects:

- antitumour
- anti-inflammatory
- immunomodulatory

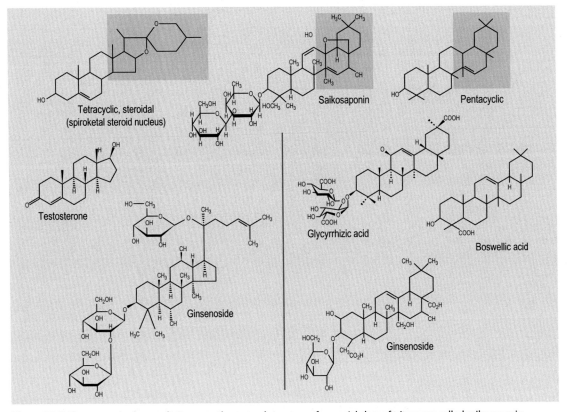

Figure 22.7 The two main classes of triterpene, the general structure of a special class of triterpene called saikosaponin. Boxes highlight differences in structure. Testoterone, a steroidal hormone, is shown for comparison. Note that there are two possible structures of ginsenoside.

- cardiac and antithrombotic
- endocrine.

Steroidal triterpenes are found in:

- Amaryllidaceae: *Agave* spp.
- Araliaceae: *Panax* spp. (ginseng).
- Cucurbitaceae: *Curcurbitae* (bitter melon, *Nan Gua Zi*).
- Dioscoreaceae: *Dioscorea* spp. (wild yam, *Shan Yao*).
- Fabaceae (Leguminosae): *Astragalus* spp. (astragalus, *Huang Qi*), *Trigonella. foenum-graecum* (fenugreek, *Hu Lu Ba*), *Glycine max* (soya).
- Liliaceae: *Trillium* spp. (beth root, wake robin).
- Solanaceae: *Solanum* spp. (these are in the form of steroidal alkaloids).

Pentacyclic triterpenes are found in:

- Apiaceae (Umbelliferae): *Bupleurum* spp. (*Chai Hu*), *Angelica sinensis* (*Dang Gui*) and many others in this group.
- Araliaceae: *Aralia elata*.
- Burseraceae: *Boswellia* spp. (frankincense), *Commiphora* spp. (myrrh, *Guggul*).
- Campanulaceae: *Platycodon grandiflorum* (Chinese bellflower, *Jie Geng*).
- Chenopodiaceae: *Chenopodium* spp. (goosefoot, quinoa).
- Compositae: *Tanacetum* spp. (tansy).
- Fabaceae (Leguminosae): *Glycyrrhiza* spp. (liquorice).
- Myrtaceae: *Myrtus* spp. (myrtle).
- Oleaceae: *Ligustri lucidi* (*Nu Zhen Zi*).
- Phytolaccaceae: *Phytolacca americana* (pokeweed).
- Polygonaceae: *Polygala* spp. (milk wort, *Yuan Zhi*).
- Primulaceae: *Lysimachiae* spp. (*Jin Qiao Cao*).
- Ranunculaceae: *Pulsatilla* spp. (pasqueflower).

Tetraterpenes

- Eight isoprene units.

Carotenoids can be divided into:

- Carotenes.
- Xanthophylls (carotenoids containing oxygen).

General Action

- Antioxidants.

Carotenes

Carotenes (Figure 22.8; see Chapter 13 'Vitamins and minerals', p. 107) are orange, yellow and red pigments found largely in fruit, vegetables and dark green leafy vegetables. They are components of the pigment systems and are involved in the primary light absorption. Two major types of carotene are:

- alpha
- beta: found in carrots.

Beta-carotene is the more common form of the two. **Lycopene** is the red pigment found in red fruit and tomatoes.

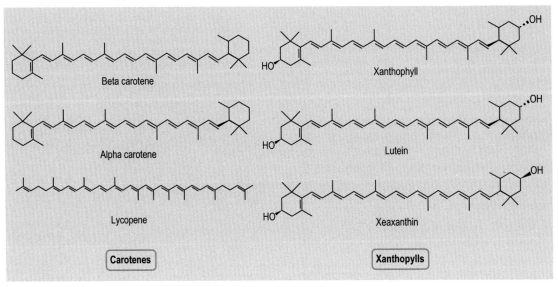

Figure 22.8 Various tetraterpenes.

Xanthophylls

Xanthophyll is yellow pigment found in saffron. **Lutein** and **xeaxanthin** are found in the macula on the retina and are thought to help protect against the potential free radicals produced by the impact of high energy light in that region.

References

Pandey AV, Tekwani BL, Singh RL et al. Artemisinin, an endoperoxide antimalarial, disrupts the hemoglobin catabolism and heme detoxification systems in malarial parasites. Journal of Biological Chemistry 1999; 274(27):19383–19388.

Trombetta D, Francesco C, Sarpietro MG et al. Mechanisms of antibacterial action of three monoterpenes. Antimicrobial Agents Chemotherapy 2005; 49(6):2474–2478.

Amines and alkaloids

23

Chapter contents

This group of pharmacologically active substances is possibly the best known in terms of the effects its members have had on the human population: from Socrates' death by hemlock to the socioeconomic problems caused by heroin and cocaine. This group is now, however, being investigated for cancer treatment.

The distinction between alkaloids and amines is not very clear in some cases, but a general definition of an alkaloid is said to be an amine isolated from a plant.

Amines

- Putrescine (Figure 23.1) is a well-known amine found in decaying material.
- The neurotransmitter, serotonin, is a tryptamine (see Figure 31.6, p. 241).
- Histamine is involved in inflammation and the immune system (see Chapter 30 'Inflammation and the immune system', p. 225 and Chapter 34 'Respiratory diseases', p. 267).

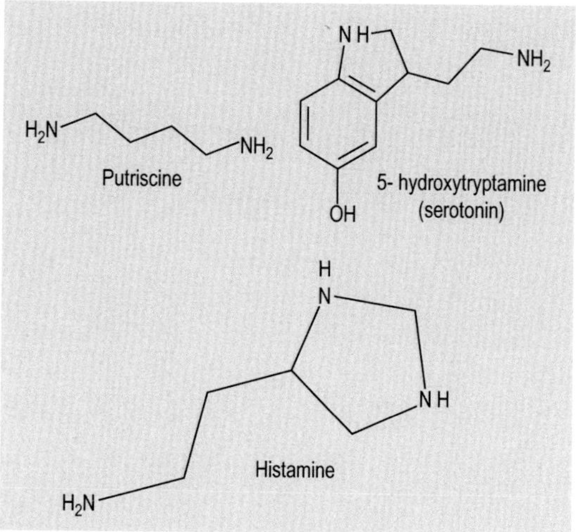

Figure 23.1 Chemical structures of three well-known amines.

Alkaloids

Thousands of different alkaloids have been discovered. They are most commonly found in the following groups:

- Apocynaceae: *Vinca* spp. (periwinkle).
- Berberidaceae: *Berberis* spp. (barberry), *Epimedium* spp. (*Yin Yang Huo*), *Coptis* spp. (*Huang Lian*).
- Fabaceae: *Vicia faba* (fava bean).
- Papaveraceae: *Papaver somniferum* (opium poppy), *Chelidonium majus* (greater celandine), *Cordydalis* spp. (*Yan Hu Suo*).
- Ranunculaceae: *Aconitum* spp. (aconite, *Fu Zi*), *Pulsatilla* spp. (pasqueflower, *Bai Tou Weng*), *Chelidonium majus* (celandine).
- Rubiaceae: *Cephaelis* spp. (ipecacuanha), *Cinchona* spp. (cinchona), *Coffea* spp. (coffee).
- Solanaceae: *Atropa belladonna* (deadly nightshade), *Capsicum* spp. (bell peppers and chilli peppers), *Datura stramonium* (thorn-apple).

Fungi are also well known for their production of alkaloids. The ergot fungus was responsible for the poisoning of thousands of people during the Middle Ages because of its inclusion in rye bread as a result of infected grain. The psychogenic properties of various mushrooms are due to alkaloids.

There are three types of alkaloid (Figure 23.2):

1. True alkaloids:
   - Are always basic in nature (see Chapter 8 'Acids and bases', p. 54).
   - Contain one or more nitrogen atoms in a heterocyclic ring (the ring contains molecules of different elements) (see Chapter 2 'The atom', p. 7).
   - Are synthesized from an amino acid.

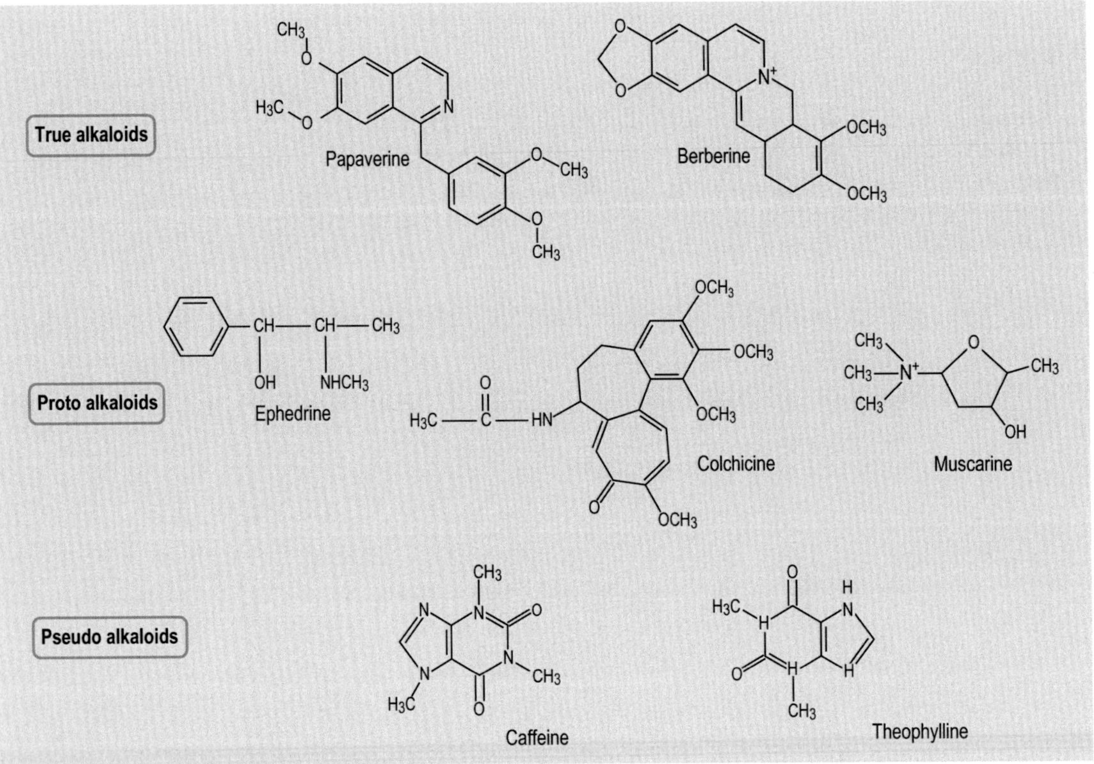

Figure 23.2 The different structures of the three different types of alkaloid.

2. Protoalkaloids:
   - Nitrogen atom is not heterocyclic, e.g. colchicine, ephedrine, muscarine.
   - Are synthesized from an amino acid.
3. Pseudoalkaloids: are not biosynthesized from amino acids, e.g. caffeine and theophylline originate from a purine base (see Figure 12.1, p. 90).

Alkaloids are classified according to:

- The amino acid that provides both the nitrogen atom and the basic structure of the alkaloid skeleton.
- Chemical origins of alkaloids (Figures 23.3 and 23.4):
  - ornithine: trophane, pyrrolidine, pyrrolizidine
  - tryptophan: indole, quinoline
  - tyrosine: benzyl-iso-quinoline, isoquinoline
  - lysine: quinolizidine, piperidine
  - pyridine: pyridine.

There are also variations:

- Amine alkaloids: alkaloids without heterocyclic nitrogen atoms, e.g. muscarine.
- Terpenes: diterpenoids (aconitine), steroids (solanine).
- Betalain alkaloids: pigment alkaloids.

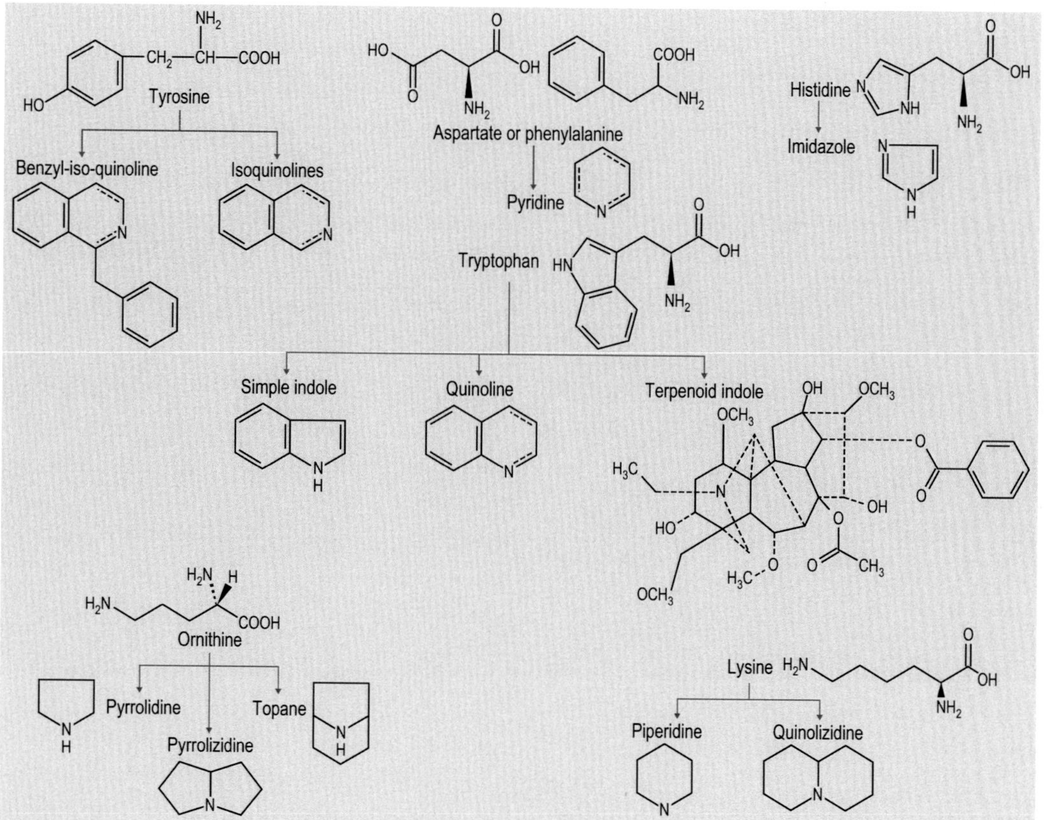

Figure 23.3 The chemical origins of various alkaloids.

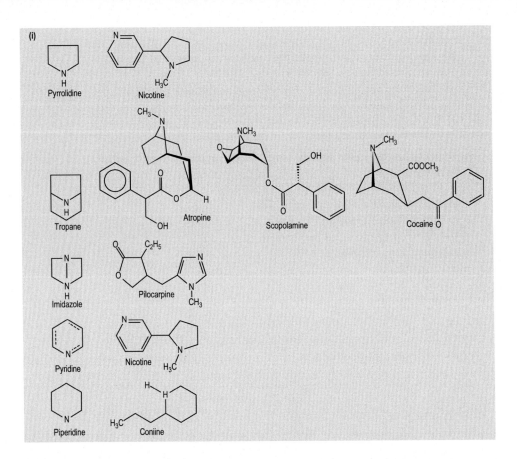

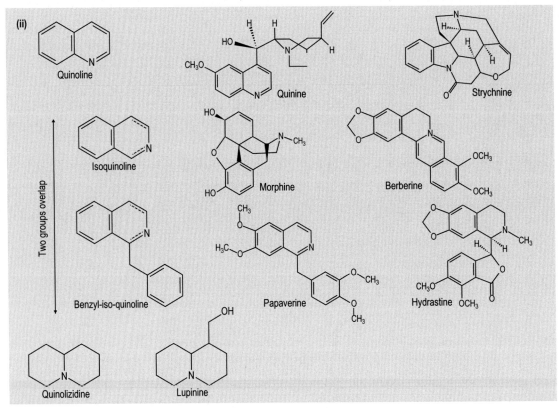

Figure 23.4 The derivation of various groups of alkaloid.

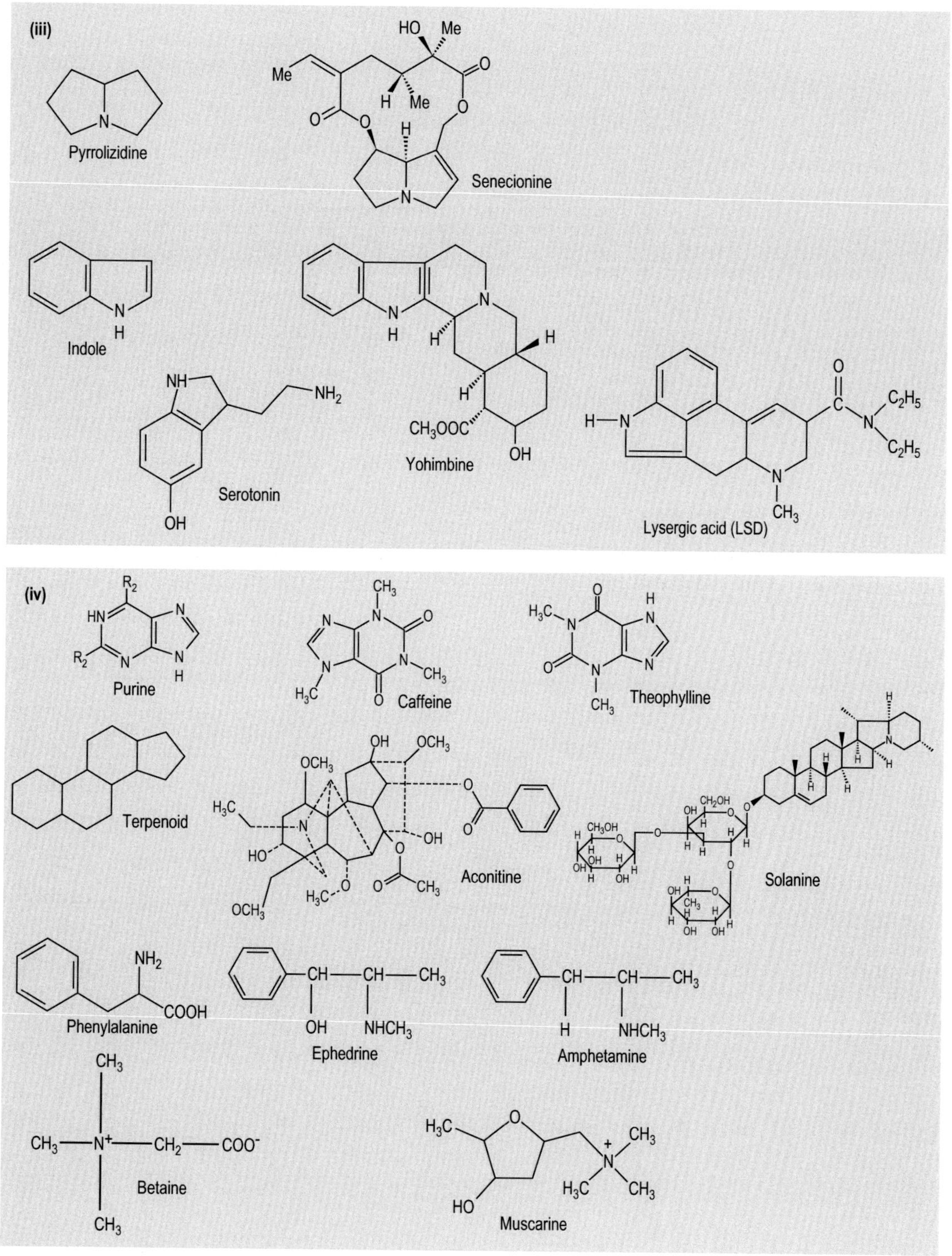

Figure 23.4 (Continued)

Characteristics of Alkaloids

Alkaloids are chemically very active and can produce large effects at small doses, either providing a therapeutic or fatal response. They interfere with:

- Neurotransmitters: see Chapter 31 'The nervous system' (p. 240).
- Active membrane transport: see Chapter 16 'How do drugs get into cells?' (p. 125).
- Protein synthesis: see Figure 11.6 (p. 85).

Therapeutic Use

- Tranquillizers: *Zizyphus spinosa* (sanjoinine, *Suan Zao Ren*), *Papaver* spp. (opium poppy).
- Pain killers: *Papaver* spp. (opium poppy).
- Muscle relaxants: *Chondodendron tomentosum* (tubocurarine).
- Anticancer: vinblastin.

Glycosides

Chapter contents

Many of the plant secondary metabolites are found naturally attached to sugars (glycosides). Mostly, the sugars are monosaccharides (Figure 24.1), such as glucose, but they can be more complicated. The sugars link to a non-sugar part called an aglycone and can be attached by separate bonds or, more commonly, as di-, tri- or tetrasaccharides. This is done by one sugar attaching to the aglycone and the others linking onto that sugar.

The linkage between the sugar and the aglycone (glycosidic linkage) is difficult for human enzymes to break down. This is where having a healthy gut is important, as this job is done by the various microbes in the gut. When the two parts have been separated, the aglycone (the non-sugar part) is small enough to be transported through the gut wall into the bloodstream, where it is sent around the body.

The linkage between the two groups can vary. It can be:

- Phenolic hydroxyl group O-glycoside.
- Carbon group C-glycoside (Figure 24.2), e.g. aloin (which was one of the first glycosides to be isolated).

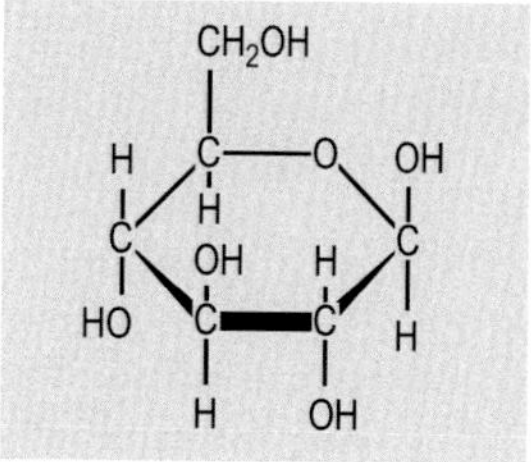

Figure 24.1 The structure of glucose, a common component of glycosides.

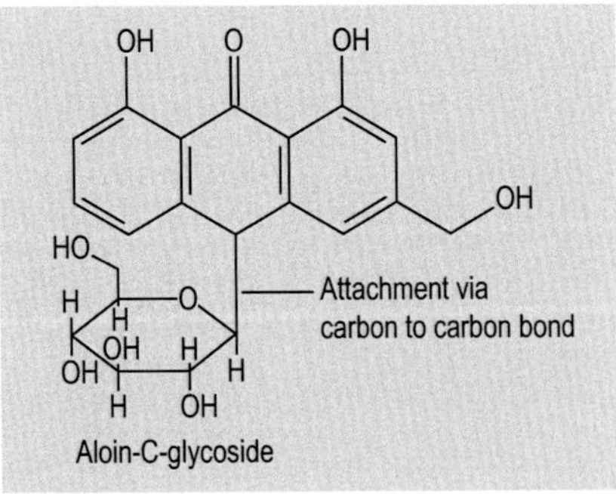

Figure 24.2 The C-glycoside linkage. The sugars attached vary in composition and can consist of one or more sugars.

- Nitrogen-glycoside, *N*-glycoside: this term is falling out of used and is being replaced by glycosylamine.
- Sulphur-glycoside, *S*-glycoside: thioglycoside (glucosinolates; see p. 184).

The well-established naming of glycosides using the termination 'in' (e.g. salicin, aloin) has persisted and results in some confusion, as some substances (e.g. pectin) are not glycosides. Similar examples of this, involving isoflavones, are discussed in Chapter 21 'Phenols' (p. 161). The more modern termination '-oside' can be used (e.g. sennoside) to prevent confusion.

Glycosides are generally inactive and are activated by a process of hydrolysis into:

- a sugar moiety (glycone)
- a non-sugar moiety (aglycone).

This is usually done with the help of specialized bacteria in the colon. Classification of a glycoside is based on the type of aglycone. For example, phenolic glycosides have a phenol attached.

Anthraquinones

It has been shown experimentally that the sugar moiety certainly of sennosides A and B (see Figure 21.9, p. 155) remains unaltered in both the stomach and gut, but is cleaved off in the caecum by the activity of microorganisms, which convert them to dianthrones. The dianthrones that remain in the gut are cleaved again to form an anthrone and anthraquinone (see Figure 21.8, p. 154), which produce the laxative effects.

The activity of the glycosides of anthrones is very high, which is why herbs containing them have to be stored for a while or subjected to heat treatment so that the majority are converted to anthraquinone glycosides.

Saponins

- The glycosides of triterpenes, steroids or steroidal alkaloids found in plants.
- So called because these compounds froth when shaken with water.
- They also cause haemolysis of red bloods cells on direct contact.

Glycyrrhizin (see Figure 24.4) is a saponin.

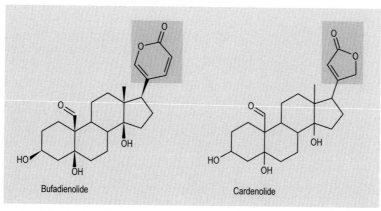

Figure 24.3 Comparison of structures of aglycones of cardiac glycosides. Boxes highlight the difference in structure.

Cardiac Glycosides

- Asclepiadaceae: *Cynanchum* spp. (*Bai Wei, Bai Qian*).
- Lilaceae: *Convallaria majalis* (lily of the valley).
- Ranunculaceae: *Helleborus niger* (black hellebore).
- Scrophulariaceae: *Digitalis purpurea* (foxglove), *Scrophularia* spp. (figwort).

The Heart

Cardiac glycosides exert a positive inotropic effect on the heart in cardiac failure (see Chapter 26 'Cardiovascular disorders', p. 191). Cardiac failure occurs when the heart is unable to pump blood effectively at a rate that meets the needs of the body. The heart muscle can perform only weakly, particularly on ventricular contraction. This reduced pumping capacity results in a reduced heart output. However, as new blood continues to enter the heart, the volume of blood in the heart increases. As the heart is unable to pump this blood out, it becomes congested, hence 'congestive heart failure'. Cardiac glycosides (or the aglycones) increase the capacity of the heart muscle to pump.

The mechanism of action of the cardiac glycosides is still not clear, but the most widely accepted idea is that the cardiac glycosides inhibit the membrane-bound sodium and potassium pumps responsible for the sodium and potassium exchange (see Figure 31.1, p. 235).

There are two types of cardiac glycoside (Figure 24.3):

- bufadienolides: C24 (24 carbon atoms)
- cardenolides: C23 (23 carbon atoms).

Cyanogenic Glycosides

Cyanogenic glycosides (Figure 24.4) yield hydrocyanic acid (HCN) as one of the products of hydrolysis, hence the name 'cyanogenic'. They are capable of producing cyanide when broken down.

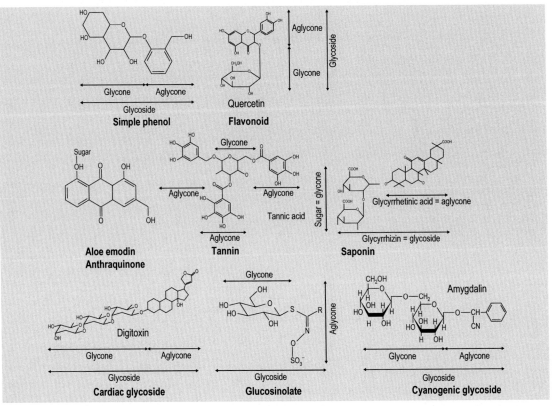

Figure 24.4 Various glycosides, showing position of sugar moiety (glycone) and non-sugar moiety (aglycone) making the whole glycoside.

Amygdalin

The amygadalin in *Pruni armeniacae* (apricot seed, *Xing Ren*) can create toxicity. Even so, the hydrolysis of the glycosides in the gut or liver might be slow enough to allow the body to detoxify the poison. Hence small doses over a short period are not a problem unless the detoxification system is severely impaired.

Isothiocyanates (Glucosinolates)

Found in:

- Liliaceae: *Allium* spp. (onion, garlic).
- Brassicaceae (Cruciferae): *Brassica* spp. (black mustard, cabbage, broccoli, brussel sprouts, etc.), *Sinapis* spp. (white mustard seed, *Bai Jie Zi*), *Amorica rusticana* (horseradish), *Raphani sativi* (radish seed, *Lai fu Zi*).

Properties

- Broken down in cooking and food preparation in the gut to produce isothiocyanates and other products.
- Distinctive hot, pungent flavour caused by breakdown products. This gives brassicas their peppery taste.

- Classed as goitrogens, which are naturally occurring substances that can interfere with the function of the thyroid. Excessive consumption of these foods is inadvisable, particularly in their raw state (many patients are now juicing). Cooking reduces the activity of isothiocyanates.
- Associated with decreased risk of cancer. Research is now being done to examine these glycosides more carefully.

Section 5

Orthodox medication

Orthodox medicine: Introduction

25

This section is designed as an overview of the general orthodox medications that are available. Each chapter has a brief review of anatomy and physiology to make it easier to understand the action of the drugs discussed.

It is possible to learn the actions of each type of medication by rote. On rare occasions, for example with the medication for epilepsy, this will be necessary. For the majority of drugs, however, there is some logic to their use and being able to understand their method of action will allow you to appreciate how they interact with the patient's metabolism.

A deeper understanding of how modern drugs work will enable you, in many cases, to anticipate interactions, not only with orthodox medication but also with herbs and even nutritional supplements. This is a confusing and largely uncharted area; more drugs are developed and made available each year and a practitioner familiar with the principles of basic physiology and pharmacology stands a good chance of identifying problem areas.

Throughout the various chapters in this section, every attempt has been made to cross-reference, both to herbal medicine and nutritional supplementation. The basis of relevant adverse effects is also explained.

The range of orthodox medication is vast and the mechanisms by which they act are equally as numerous and in many cases very complex. For the purposes of this book, the drugs described have been limited to those you are likely to encounter clinically, and descriptions are largely generic. Where appropriate, however, a brief mention will be made of those usually only available under strict medical supervision.

It is impossible to give a complete list of adverse effects; however, these can be accessed in formularies, many of which are available online.

Formularies online

eMIMS: Subscription only. Online. Available: http://www.healthcarerepublic.com/welcome/eMIMS/index.cfm?ctype=OTC-eMIMS/ [accessed 7 March 2008].

Australia: Australian Medicines Handbook. Subscription only. Online. Available: http://www.amh.net.au/ [accessed 7 March 2008].

UK: British National Formulary Home Page, British National Formulary. Online. Available: http://bnf.org/bnf/ [accessed 7 March 2008].

USA: American hospital formulary service online. Online. Available: http://www.ashp.org/ahfs/ [accessed 7 March 2008].

Bibliography

Golan DE, Tashjian AH, Armstrong EJ et al. Principles of pharmacology. The pathophysiologic basis of drug therapy. Baltimore, MD: Lippincott Williams and Wilkins; 2004.

Greenstein B. Trounce's clinical pharmacology for nurses. 17th edn. Churchill Livingstone: Edinburgh; 2004.

Guyton AC, Hall JE. Textbook of medical physiology. 11th edn. Philadelphia: Elsevier Saunders; 2006.

Hardman JG, Limbird LE. Goodman and Gilman's the pharmacological basis of therapeutics. 11th edn. New York: McGraw-Hill; 2005.

Neal MJ. Medical pharmacology at a glance. 5th edn. Oxford: Blackwell Science; 2005.

Rang HP, Dale MM, Ritter JM. Pharmacology. 6th edn. Edinburgh: Churchill Livingstone; 2007.

Reid JL, Rubin PC, Whiting B. Clinical pharmacology. 7th edn. Oxford: Blackwell Science; 2006.

Saeb-Parsy K, Assomull RG, Fakhar ZK et al. Instant pharmacology. Chichester: John Wiley; 1999.

Waller DG, Renwick AG, Hillier K. Medical pharmacology and therapeutics. 2nd edn. Edinburgh: Elsevier Saunders; 2005.

Cardiovascular disorders

26

Cardiovascular disease is an enormous health problem in the Western world and is high in the list of causes of death. Evidence from clinical trials suggests that prevention of hypertension and lipidaemia (see Chapter 27 'Problems with lipid metabolism', p. 203) can significantly reduce cardiovascular disease and deaths.

Physiology of the Heart

The cardiovascular system is effectively a closed system with control mechanisms that normally prevent the pressure becoming too high or too low. The heart is controlled by two main factors:

- hydrostatic pressure
- electrical stimulation.

Hydrostatic Pressure

A constant hydrostatic pressure is maintained in two main ways:

1. **Controlling the amount of fluid in the system**: fluid can be removed from the body if the kidneys are stimulated to extract water, which leaves the body when the patient urinates. Conversely, if it is necessary not to lose fluid, the kidneys will reduce its loss. Two classes of drugs work on this system, **diuretics** and **angiotensin-converting enzyme (ACE) inhibitors** (see p. 195 and p. 200).
2. **Varying the volume of blood pumped out by the heart (inotropic activity)**: after the heart has contracted, there is negative pressure. Because the cardiovascular system is a pressurized system, the blood flows into the heart under pressure and starts to stretch the muscles of the heart wall (Figure 26.1). The amount of stretch created by the venous return of the blood is called **preload**. This elicits a response from the cardiac muscle wall, which encourages the heart stroke. The more stretch, the greater the volume of blood pumped out by the heart. If the heart muscle is stretched too much it becomes dilated and the force of contraction decreases and the heart goes into failure.

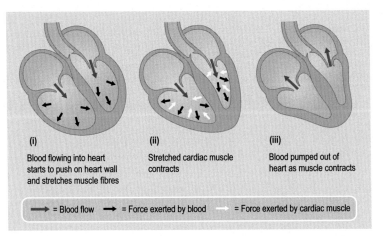

(i)
Blood flowing into heart
starts to push on heart wall
and stretches muscle fibres

(ii)
Stretched cardiac muscle
contracts

(iii)
Blood pumped out of
heart as muscle contracts

➡ = Blood flow   ➡ = Force exerted by blood   ➡ = Force exerted by cardiac muscle

Figure 26.1 Demonstrating the effect volume of blood has on the contraction of the heart.

Cardiac glycosides in **digitalis**, **digoxin** and *Crategus* (hawthorn) increase the force of contraction of the heart (see Chapter 24 'Glycosides', p. 183), which is important in patients with heart failure.

• How the Kidneys can Affect Blood Pressure

The kidneys perform two functions for the cardiovascular system:

1. They regulate water balance.
2. They regulate electrolyte balance.

The two are interlinked.

Stages in the Removal of Water from the Body

Figure 26.2 shows the structure of a nephron, the functional unit of the kidney. The numbers in the figure are explained below.

(i) Filtration

Blood enters the glomerulus of the kidney under pressure. This pressure forces the water and small molecules (e.g. sodium, potassium, glucose) that are present in the blood through the basement membrane of the glomerulus and into the Bowman's capsule (Figure 26.2). At this stage, the filtered fluid is mainly blood plasma minus largely all the plasma proteins (there is some seepage of these, but not much). Factors such as heavy exercise can increase the amount of protein found in the urine, but a large amount of protein in the urine indicates kidney pathology. The fluid flows from the Bowman's capsule into the proximal tubule.

(ii) Active Transport

All the amino acids and glucose, and a large amount of the sodium, potassium and other salts are reabsorbed in the proximal tubule. The active transport of sodium out of the proximal tubule is controlled by angiotensin II. If this is reduced, by medication such as an **ACE inhibitor** (see Figure 26.6), the sodium remains in the tubule, and the water stays with it. As a result, the patient urinates more.

(iii) Loop of Henle

The filtered fluid passes from the proximal tubule into the descending part of the loop of Henle, where the osmotic gradient still encourages water to leave the nephron. The fluid is encouraged to leave the descending part of the loop because, in the ascending part – which is aligned directly opposite – an active transport mechanism

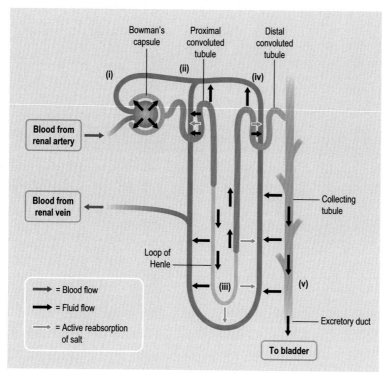

Figure 26.2 The structure of a nephron, showing the flow of fluids and electrolytes.

pulls sodium salts from the loop; water from the descending loop accompanies the salts as the result of osmosis. However, fluid cannot follow the salts from the ascending loop because the wall of the loop is impermeable to water. This is where **loop diuretics** work, by preventing sodium reabsorption.

(iv) Distal Convoluted Tubule

More sodium is removed from the tubules by active transport, with yet more water being pulled out by osmosis. **Thiazides** (Figure 26.5) such as **bendroflumethiazide** act here.

(v) Collecting Tubule

This is where the final balancing of water and electrolytes takes place, before the fluid is removed from the body. **Potassium-sparing diuretics** (Figure 26.5) work here, as well as in the distal convoluted tubules. The collecting tubule is normally impermeable to water, but it can become permeable in the presence of **antidiuretic hormone (ADH)**, which is secreted by the pituitary gland (see Chapter 37 'Metabolic disorders', p. 288). As much as 75% of water in the urine can be reabsorbed as it leaves the collecting duct by osmosis. A failure to produce ADH (due to a fault in the posterior pituitary gland) is seen in the condition known as **diabetes insipidus**, which involves excretion of copious amounts of urine, despite reduced consumption of fluids.

Electrical Stimulation of the Heart

The autonomic nervous system (see Figure 31.5, p. 239) stimulates, and therefore increases, the heart rate through the stimulation of the sympathetic nervous system. This is where the beta-adrenoceptor antagonists (beta-blockers; see below) act (Figure 26.3):

(i)   Stimulation of the heart's electrical system also occurs locally. As the blood flows into the right atrium from the lung circulation, the muscle wall and the

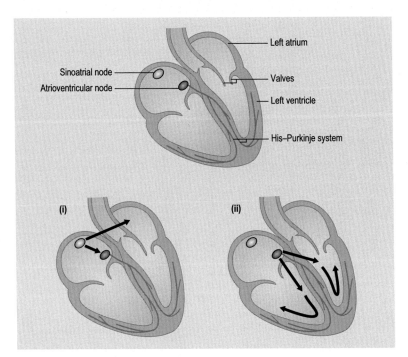

Figure 26.3 Electrical flow around the heart.

     sinoatrial node are stretched. This stimulates an increase in heart rate. The **sinoatrial node** is the heart's natural '**pacemaker**'.

(ii)   The signal is then passed onto the **atrioventricular node**. This node serves as the electrical connection between the atria and the ventricles, which are separated by a membrane. The whole system ensures that the nerve impulse is transmitted in such a way as to make the heart muscle contract in a logical and orderly manner, which ensures that the blood is pumped out and around the body.

The Special Nature of Heart Muscle

Heart muscle is very specialized smooth muscle. Like all smooth muscle it is activated by the autonomic nervous system.

Heart muscle differs from other smooth muscle in that its cell membranes are fused. The connections between the cells are extremely permeable and allow a rapid flow of calcium and sodium ions from one cell to another (**communicating gap junctions**). This partly explains the orderly spread of excitation through the heart.

An **action potential** stimulates the rapid release of sodium ions, followed by the slower release of calcium ions, into the heart muscle. This occurs through voltage-gated ion channels (see Figure 31.2, p. 237). These channels are the site of action of **calcium-channel blockers** and **potassium-channel activators** (see below).

Contraction stops when this flow is shut off and the normal electrolyte balance restored.

The sodium–potassium pump removes sodium and pumps potassium back into the muscle cells against the respective concentration gradients (see Figure 31.1, p. 236). The increased permeability of the membrane to potassium inhibits the generation of the action potential.

Depolarization starts in the sinoatrial (SA) node, spreading over the atria to the atrioventricular (AV) node and on to the conducting fibres in the bundle of His (in the intraventricular septum) and the His–Purkinje system. The ventricular muscle then contracts.

Cardiac Conditions

Hypertension

A blood pressure above 140/85 mmHg is usually the starting point for treatment, although the blood pressure is generally higher when actual medication is given. Family history is taken into account, as this can be significant in preventing heart disease in families.

If blood pressure is high, it is usually tested more than once over a period of time, as emotional situations such as stress or 'white-coat syndrome' can give a false impression of the patient's normal situation.

Treatment

Non-pharmaceutical treatments are preferable as a first option:

- Diet: avoiding convenience foods, sugar, alcohol.
- Exercise: moderate cardiovascular exercise.
- Stopping smoking.

If this does not work, or if patient compliance is poor and the blood pressure continues to increase, then drugs are used.

● Malignant Hypertension

It is unlikely that a complementary healthcare practitioner would see a patient with this condition. The blood pressure is not only very high but there is also swelling of the optic nerve (papilloedema), which is the signature of malignant hypertension. As with ordinary hypertension, the various organs with a high perfusion rate, such as kidneys, brain and lungs, can be damaged, due to the pressure.

Malignant hypertension can be caused if, for example, the patient has a kidney disorder that results in narrowing of the renal arteries of the kidney tissue such as scleroderma, a connective tissue disease that compromises the structure of the kidneys.

Prognosis

Death is commonly within a year unless treated, and is usually due to cerebral haemorrhage or renal failure.

● Pharmacological Treatment of High Blood Pressure

Figure 26.4 illustrates the structures of the different types of cardiovascular medication.

Diuretics

Most diuretics work by inhibiting sodium and water reabsorption at various points in the nephron (Figure 26.5). As the various diuretics increase sodium excretion, water removal occurs by the principle of osmosis (see Chapter 16 'How do drugs get into cells?', p. 123).

Diuretics tend to be used when there is oedema in the legs, which occurs due to gravity. However, they are not given in pregnancy or to nursing mothers (as they can reduce the breast milk). Diuretics with a long half-life are favoured because they do not need to be taken so frequently.

Loop Diuretics

Loop diuretics (e.g. **furosemide**) have a very vigorous action and many patients tend not to go anywhere for a few hours after they have taken them, because they urinate frequently and copiously. Loop diuretics:

- Are the most powerful diuretics.
- Have a short half-life, so the effect is limited to a few hours.

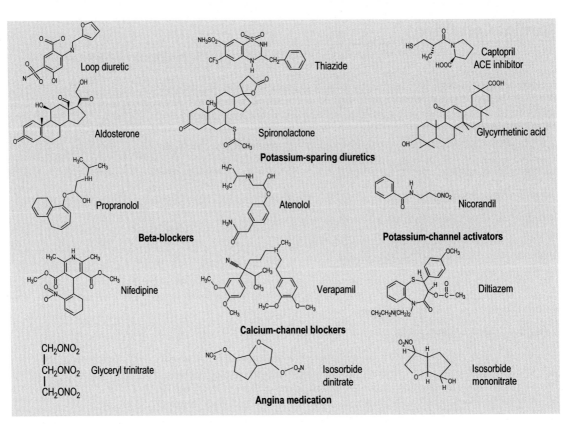

Figure 26.4 Chemical structures of various cardiovascular medications. Note the variations on a similar theme within groups of drugs. Glycyrrhetinic acid is included for comparison with aldosterone.

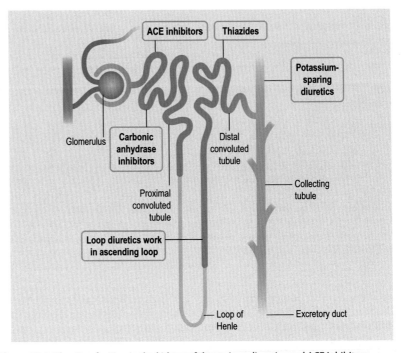

Figure 26.5 The site of action in the kidney of the various diuretics and ACE inhibitors.

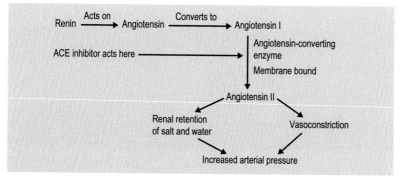

Figure 26.6 The action of the angiotensin-converting enzyme (ACE) inhibitors on the renin–angiotensin system.

- Have a vigorous action that provokes reflex stimulation of the renin–angiotensin system (see Figure 26.6).
- Are potassium depleting.

They are used in:

- congestive heart failure
- acute left ventricular failure
- oedema associated with nephrotic syndrome.

Early Distal Tubule Diuretics

Thiazides e.g. **bendroflumethiazide**:

- Work on the distal tubule (Figure 26.5).
- Are not as powerful as loop diuretics.
- Work on similar principles as the loop diuretics.
- Are potassium depleting.
- Require only a low dosage.

General Adverse Effects of Loop and Early Distal Tubule Diuretics

Hypokalaemia (Low Levels of Potassium)

Levels of potassium are reduced in plasma due to loss of potassium in urine, resulting in:

- muscle weakness
- cramping
- hypotension
- cardiac arrhythmias.

This is why loop diuretics tend to be used for short-term, acute use only. These adverse effects are usually counteracted with potassium supplements or using a combination diuretic with a **thiazide diuretic** and a **potassium-sparing diuretic.**

Hyperglycaemia

Long-term diuretic therapy is associated with an impairment of glucose tolerance and an increased incidence of non-insulin dependent diabetes mellitus. This is due to insulin resistance in peripheral tissues.

Impotence

Reversible on ceasing medication.

Gout

Diuretics compete with uric acid for excretion from the kidney tubules, which can concentrate uric acid in the plasma. Care should be taken if patients suffer from gout.

Other Uncommon Adverse Effects

- **Thrombocytopenia** (low number of platelets) and skin rash.

Potassium-Sparing Diuretics

Potassium-sparing diuretics (Figure 26.5) are the weakest diuretics, but they do reduce sodium loss.

Aldosterone

- Secreted from the outermost part of the adrenal medulla, the zona glomerulosa.
- Main action is to increase sodium reabsorption in the distal tubules of the kidneys, thus maintaining the blood pressure due to maintaining hydrostatic pressure in the blood vessels.
- Also has some potassium-excreting effect, which is inhibited by spironolactone.

Spironolactone

- Is an antagonist of aldosterone and competes for the intracellular aldosterone receptors in the cells of the collecting tubules and, to a lesser extent, in the distal tubules and collecting ducts.
- Is usually given to patients who have not responded to the usual diuretic drugs.

Adverse effects are rare, although spironolactone can upset the gastrointestinal tract and cause rashes.

Glycyrrhitinic Acid

This plant chemical is very similar in structure to aldosterone (Figure 26.4) and is therefore capable of similar pharmacological actions, hence the need to be aware of why *Glycyrrhiza* spp. can increase blood pressure.

• Carbonic Anhydrase Inhibitors

Under normal conditions, the action of carbonic anhydrase retains sodium and bicarbonate in the plasma (see Figure 18.3, p. 135). This mechanism is relevant not only for maintaining blood pressure but also the correct pH of the blood, which must be kept within very narrow limits (see Chapter 8 'Acids and bases', p. 58).

Carbonic anhydrase inhibitors prevent sodium being reabsorbed and increase the volume of water being lost by the kidneys due to the increased osmotic pressure in the tubules. Although carbonic anhydrase inhibitors can be used for high blood pressure, they are currently more commonly used for such conditions as **glaucoma**.

Adverse Effects

Most commonly unusual tiredness or weakness.

• Beta-Blockers

Beta-blockers attach themselves to the **beta-adrenoreceptors** of the sympathetic nervous system, thus making the receptors unavailable to the usual messengers. There are two types of **beta-adrenoreceptor:**

- beta 1: predominantly in the heart.
- beta 2: predominantly associated with lung, peripheral blood vessels and skeletal muscles.

The beta-adrenoreceptors are found in three main areas of the body:

- **Heart**: beta-blockers result in a decrease in the heart rate and in the volume of blood pumped out of the heart, which decreases cardiac output.
- **Kidney**: beta-blockers cause a decrease in sodium and water retention. Inhibition of the sympathetic nervous system inhibits renin release.
- **Central and peripheral nervous system**: inhibition of the beta-receptors in the brainstem and periphery decreases sympathetic nervous system activity, resulting in general vasodilatation of blood vessels.

Propranolol is lipid soluble, and therefore depends on the liver for clearance. Drugs cleared by the liver usually have a short half-life, and several doses a day of propranolol might be needed for it to be effective.

Atenolol is water soluble and depends on the good function of the kidney for clearance. It has a longer half-life the propranolol and can be used once a day at a high dose.

Side Effects

- Bradycardia: slowing of the heart rate.
- Difficulty with heart contraction: decreased ionotropic effect (see p. 191).
- Cold hands and feet, or Raynaud's phenomenon: there is a loss of beta-receptor vasodilatation in cutaneous vessels.
- A sense of 'being under the weather': beta-blockers slow the heart rate, which can make patients feel unwell.
- Bronchospasm: inhibiting the action of the sympathetic nervous system causes constriction of the bronchi. **Beta-blockers cannot be used on patients with asthma.**
- Tiredness and fatigue: cardiac output is reduced and there is reduced muscle perfusion in exercise.
- Masking of hypoglycaemia: glucose is normally released in response to adrenaline surges. Beta-blockers reduce this response.
- Metabolic disturbances: small increase in triglycerides and reduced levels of high-density lipoprotein.

199

• Calcium Antagonists (Calcium-Entry Blockers, Calcium-Channel Blockers)

Calcium antagonists affect the cellular entry of calcium, rather than its action on the cell.

Muscle contraction is calcium dependent (see Chapter 31 'The nervous system', p. 237). There are muscles in the peripheral blood vessel walls and the heart is predominantly muscle. If the calcium channels are blocked then vasodilatation of the blood vessels takes place and the contractility of the heart muscle is reduced. There are three classes of calcium antagonist:

1. **Dihydropyridine derivatives**, e.g. nifedipine, amlodipine: directly relax the vascular smooth muscle and therefore have pronounced peripheral vasodilator properties. Drugs in this class can produce a transient reflex tachycardia; the other two classes do not.
2. **Phenylalkylamines**, e.g. verapamil: act directly on the heart. Their short half-life is due to an extensive first-pass metabolism. If used for a long time they will inhibit hepatic drug metabolism and therefore last longer.
3. **Benzothiazepines**, e.g. diltiazem: have an action between the dihydropyridines and the phenylalkalamines.

All the calcium antagonists are subject to the first-pass metabolism to a great degree.

Side Effects

Dihydropyridines

- Headache and facial flushing.
- Cardioacceleration and palpitations.
- Swelling of ankles and occasionally hands: due to drug-related disturbance of the haemodynamics of the microcirculation of the periphery and effects of gravity.

Phenylalkylamines

- Bradycardia or atrioventricular conduction delay.
- Constipation as the muscles of the gut wall do not contract as well.
- **Drug interactions with autoimmune drugs.**

Benzothiazepines

- Bradycardia and atrioventricular conduction effects.
- Occasional skin rash.
- **Drug interactions with autoimmune drugs.**

• Angiotensin-Converting Enzyme Inhibitors

Angiotensin-converting enzyme (ACE) inhibitors inhibit the activity of angiotensin-converting enzyme (Figure 26.6). Angiotensin makes the kidneys retain salt and water. ACE inhibitors:

- **Act directly on the kidneys** to cause salt and water retention.
- **Cause the adrenal glands to reduce secretion of aldosterone**: angiotensin is an aldosterone agonist (see Chapter 19 'Pharmacodynamics: how drugs elicit a physiological effect', p. 140). Aldosterone increases salt and water reabsorption by the kidney tubules. This action is blocked by ACE inhibitors, leading to loss of salt and water.

Side Effects

- Profound hypotension (the blood pressure can become dangerously low). This might occur with the first dose of the drug.
- Impairment of renal function.
- **Dry unproductive cough**: the enzyme kininase II is the same as angiotensin-converting enzyme and so is inhibited by ACE inhibitors. This results in bradykinin not being metabolized. Bradykinin is spasmogenic and affects bronchial muscles to produce the cough.
- Taste disturbances, and skin rash.

Medication for high blood pressure starts with one drug but patients might find themselves taking up to three drugs: a diuretic, a beta-blocker and an ACE inhibitor.

Angina

In angina, the coronary circulation is unable to meet the demands placed on it. If the blood supply around the heart muscle is increased by dilating the blood vessels then heart function improves. Dilating the coronary artery relieves anginal pain. There are two types of angina:

1. **Stable**: due to coronary artery disease. Occurs with excitement or exertion and diminishes when both are reduced. Treatment aims to increase the oxygen supply to the tissues of the heart or to reduce the amount of oxygen required by the heart.
2. **Unstable**: occurs at rest or with a little exertion.

Treatment is directed towards clearing the coronary arteries. An antithrombotic (see Chapter 28 'Blood disorders', p. 212) is used as the primary treatment. Surgery might be necessary in severe cases (bypass surgery or coronary angioplasty).

• Pharmacological Treatment of Angina

Glyceryl Nitrate

- Powerful, short-acting smooth muscle relaxant with non-specific vasodilator activity.
- Results in a marked dilatation of large veins, leading to a reduction in the central venous pressure. Providing there is no heart failure, **this reduces the cardiac output by reducing the preload on the heart**.

Remember:

- As the blood volume returning to the heart increases, preload increases and there is enhanced filling with ventricular dilation (see Figure 26.1).
- Increased ventricular stretch usually leads to increased contractility.
- Increased preload and increased contractility leads to increased stroke volume and ultimately an increase in arterial pressure.
- Reducing the preload reduces the arterial pressure.

Glyceryl trinitrate is metabolized virtually 100% in the first-pass metabolism, so it is given sublingually or transdermally to initially bypass the liver. It has a **half-life of 2 minutes so is quickly broken down**. Glyceryl trinitrate is taken only in emergencies or when the patient has to do something that will induce the angina.

Adverse Effects

- Headache.
- Flushing and postural dizziness: these arise because the vasodilatation is non-specific and occurs throughout the body. However, they do not usually last long because of the short duration of action of the drug.

Isosorbide Dinitrite and Isosorbide Mononitrate

- The action of these drugs is similar to glyceryl trinitrate, but the half-life is 40 minutes or more.
- There is usually a 6- to 8-hour break in medication every 24 hours to prevent drug tolerance.
- Care has to be taken in this period that no unusual activity takes place, to prevent an angina attack.

Potassium-Channel Activators

These have a similar action to nitrates and relax the walls of the coronary arteries, improving blood flow. Smooth muscle relaxation occurs by selectively increasing the membrane permeability to potassium, which flows out of the cell quickly after the muscle cell has been activated. The resulting charge across the membrane makes it more difficult to generate another action potential, leaving the muscle in a state of rest for longer (see Figure 31.2, p. 237).

Beta-Blockers

These help angina by:

- Keeping the heart rate down, even with exercise.
- Reducing the force of contraction of the heart.
- Increasing the length of diastole, which is the period during which coronary blood flows.

Adverse Effects

Rebound worsening of angina, myocardial infarction or tachycardia can occur if beta-blockers are suddenly withdrawn. The dose has to be lowered over a 24- to 48-hour period.

Calcium Antagonists

Calcium antagonists inhibit the action of the calcium channels by:

- Decreasing the tone of the vascular smooth muscle.
- Decreasing the ability of the heart muscles to contract.
- Reducing the electrical conduction around the heart: **verapamil** and **diltiazem** also help to act as antiarrhythmic agents.

All the **dihydropyridines** have pronounced peripheral vasodilator properties. **Verapamil** and **diltiazem** limit heart rate.

Side Effects

- Headaches.
- Nausea.
- Flushing.
- Swollen ankles.
- Can interact with beta-blockers.

Homocysteine

See Chapter 37 'Metabolic disorders' (p. 296).

Problems with lipid metabolism

27

Fatty acids are an important source of energy: potentially, triglycerides can release as much energy per kilogram as carbohydrates or proteins. Lipids are components of membranes in the form of phospholipids (see Chapter 10 'Lipids', p. 73).

Ultimately, the carbohydrates that are not utilized by the body end up as fatty acids, which are stored as triglycerides. This fact is conveniently side-stepped by food manufacturers, who produce low-fat products that often have a very high sugar content.

Fatty acids are usually eaten as triglycerides, which are broken down into free fatty acids and monoglycerides by lipases in the small intestine. This process is assisted by bile salts, which emulsify the fats and increase the efficiency of the enzymes (see Chapter 4 'Bonds continued', p. 25).

Lipids are absorbed largely as fatty acids (although some are absorbed as free glycerol and diglycerides). After absorption, they are packed with protein to create a lipoprotein, which acts as a carrier for the lipid in the bloodstream.

There are four main classes of lipoprotein:

1. **Chylomicrons**: carry triglycerides from the gut to the liver and **adipose (lipid storage) tissue**.
2. **Very-low-density lipoproteins (VLDL)**: carry triglycerides made in the liver from the liver to the adipose tissue.
3. **Low-density lipoproteins (LDL)**: carry cholesterol from the liver to the rest of the body. **Large amounts of LDLs are undesirable**.
4. **High-density lipoproteins (HDL)**: gather cholesterol from the body returning it to the liver. **High amounts of HDLs are desirable.**

What Happens to Lipids after Absorption?

Figure 27.1 outlines the fate of lipids after absorption. The numbers below correspond to those in the illustration:

(i) Most lipids are absorbed as fatty acids and a small amount as free glycerol and diglycerides.

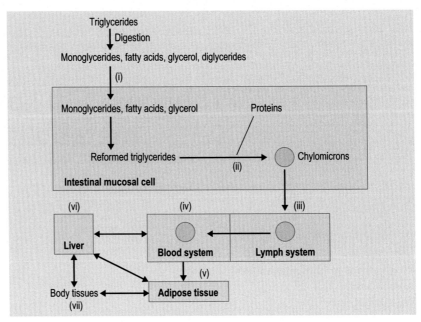

Figure 27.1 General metabolism of lipids.

(ii) In the cells of the gut wall (**enterocytes**) they reform into triglycerides, and are packaged into **chylomicrons** along with lipoproteins and other lipids.

(iii) The chylomicrons are then released in the lymph system (**sugars and amino acids are absorbed directly into the bloodstream**).

(iv) At the thoracic duct, the chylomicrons are released into the sublclavian vein, where they bind to the membranes of adipose cells (v) or pass to the liver (vi) or to the tissues of body to be broken down by lipoprotein lipase in the cell membranes and the resulting fatty acids used as an energy source (vii).

If the lipids are unused, they are stored.

The liver is the key organ for lipid metabolism.

Atherosclerosis

Thrombus Formation

Figure 27.2 illustrates the formation of a thrombus, which is the basis of atherosclerosis. The numbers below relate to those in the illustration:

(i) Lipids are present in the bloodstream under normal conditions.

(ii) High levels of cholesterol in the blood can damage the lining of an artery, causing an inflammatory reaction, which then enables cholesterol and other fats to gather in that area.

(iii) The injury to the lining of the arteries (endothelial cells) encourages the attachment of monocytes; the endothelial cells also bind LDL independently. This situation is exacerbated in hyperlipidaemia.

(iv) The attached monocytes generate free radicals (see Chapter 7 'Free radicals', p. 42), which oxidize the attached LDL, resulting in lipid peroxidation.

(v) The modified LDL is taken up by the macrophages via their 'scavenger receptors'.

(vi) These macrophages (now called **foam cells**) migrate into the blood-vessel wall. These and T lymphocytes form fatty streaks.

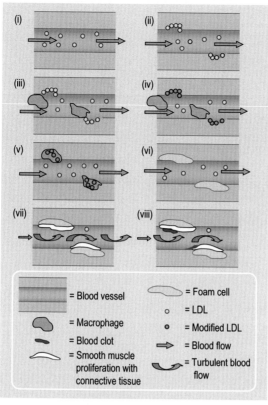

Figure 27.2 The formation of fat deposits in the blood vessels and thrombus formation.

(vii) Proliferation of the smooth muscle and connective tissue occurs, and creates an atherosclerotic plaque. This structure is very inflexible and not only reduces the blood flow but can also cut off flow entirely.

(viii) The combination of this foreign formation and the turbulence caused by its presence creates a thrombus (blood clot).

Facts about Atheroslerosis

- Atherosclerosis is largely found in the large and intermediate-sized arteries.
- Calcium salts are included in the atheroma, which creates 'hardening of the arteries'. This can make the blood vessel more liable to rupture due to its inflexibility.
- HDLs are preferable to LDLs.
- Cholesterol is present in cell membranes and in the membranes of the internal organelles of all cells. It is an important starting material for sex hormones, hydrocortisone, aldosterone (water metabolism) and therefore has a far ranging effect in the body. Thus some cholesterol in the body is necessary.
- Cholesterol will be produced by the body as required.

Why HDLs are 'Good' and LDLs 'Bad'?

Small lipoproteins, i.e. the LDLs, cause the most damage because their small size allows them to pass easily into the blood-vessel walls. This means that they can transport cholesterol from the liver to the walls of the blood vessels. This cholesterol can form the basis of an atheroma. Thus, LDLs are considered 'bad'.

HDLs take in excess cholesterol from the tissue and return it to the liver (i.e. taking it away from the artery wall). This beneficial function is considered 'good'.

Hyperlipidaemia

Hyperlipidaemia is one of the most common metabolic disorders. It occurs when lipids in the plasma in the form of lipoproteins are abnormally high. There are several categories of this disease, some of which can be inherited. High levels of LDLs are associated with, and increase the risk of, atheromas and coronary thrombosis.

• Causes: Lifestyle Factors

- Diabetes mellitus.
- Hypothyroidism.
- Smoking.

Treatment

• Conservative

- Diets that encourage lower blood cholesterol, such as eating a diet low in fat and sugar.
- Taking antioxidants.
- Exercise.
- Quitting smoking.

• Orthodox

Lipid-Lowering Medication

Figure 27.3 shows the location of action of lipid reduction drugs.

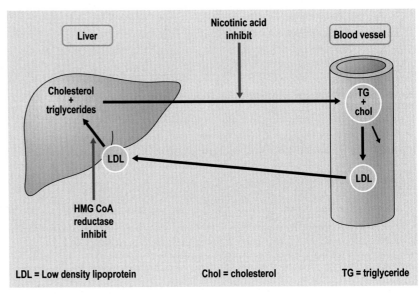

Figure 27.3 Location of action of lipid reduction drugs.

LDL receptors are present on the cell membranes of liver cells (hepatocytes) and other cells throughout the body. They enable cholesterol to enter normal body cells. Once attached to LDL receptors on the hepatocytes, LDLs release their cholesterol and triglycerides. The cholesterol is stored or oxidized to bile salts or secreted into the bile unchanged.

Excess cholesterol in the cells suppresses the formation of new LDL receptors, so the intake of cholesterol in the form of LDL into the cells decreases. Cholesterol synthesis is also suppressed. This system is utilized by the designers of drugs that lower cholesterol.

HMG CoA Reductase Inhibitors (Statins)

- Interfere with the production of cholesterol in the liver, reducing the hepatic synthesis of cholesterol.
- The liver compensates by making more LDL receptors, which results in an increase in the uptake of LDLs and so effectively feeds more lipids into cholesterol production.
- This reduces the LDL concentration in the blood as more LDL is ultimately taken out of the circulation by the liver.

Other facts:

- Cholesterol is largely synthesized during sleep, so the drugs are usually administered at night.
- The statins are derived from fungal metabolites.
- Liver function tests have to be performed every so often as the drugs can affect liver enzyme function Chapter 41 'Scientific tests', p. 335).

Fibrates

- Reduce the amount of cholesterol and triglycerides made in the body, which is why they are **used in mixed hyperlipidaemia** (elevated cholesterol and triglycerides) as well as in other types of lipidaemia.
- Activate peroxisome-proliferator-activated receptors (PPARs), which are intracellular receptors that alter carbohydrate and fat metabolism.
- Increase LDL uptake in the liver.
- Reduce plasma fibrinogen and improve insulin resistance (hence their use in patients with syndrome X; see Chapter 37 'Metabolic disorders', p. 294).
- Secrete the fats that are still produced by the body more actively with fibrates.

Adverse Effects

- Gastrointestinal irritation.
- Nausea.
- Headache.
- Skin rash.

Nicotinic Acid

- Reduces the release of VLDLs and therefore lowers plasma triglycerides.
- Lowers levels of cholesterol and increases HDLs.
- Increases the tissue plasminogen activator (which is involved in the clot-dissolving mechanism) and decreases plasma fibrinogen, decreasing the risk of thrombosis.

Adverse Effects

- Flushing.
- Palpitations.
- Gastrointestinal disturbances.

Antiobesity Medication

Orlistat inhibits the enzyme pancreatic lipase, which breaks down triglycerides in the intestine. As a result, free fatty acids are not absorbed and the triglycerides are removed from the gut undigested. Vitamin D supplementation is recommended if there is concern about the level of fat-soluble vitamins.

Adverse Effects

- Flatulence and general gastrointestinal disturbance (reduced by lowering fat intake).
- Diarrhoea.
- Tooth and gingival problems.
- Headache.
- Menstrual irregularities.
- Hypoglycaemia.
- Anxiety.
- Fatigue.
- Respiratory infection.
- Urinary tract infection.

Blood disorders

28

Red blood cells (erythrocytes) perform two functions:

- They transport oxygen from the lungs to the tissues of the body: they are able to perform this task because of the haem-based structure they contain (haemoglobin; see Chapter 13 'Vitamins and minerals', p. 96).
- They catalyse the reversible reaction between carbon dioxide and water, thus enabling the removal of large amounts of carbon dioxide from the body tissues: erythrocytes contain the enzyme carbonic anhydrase, which makes it possible for the blood to transport carbon dioxide in the form of bicarbonate ions (HCO_3^-) (see Figure 18.3, p. 135).

Red blood cells are so constructed as to be able to deform to squeeze through capillary walls without rupturing. Their life span is relatively short (around 120 days); mature erythrocytes have no nucleus.

Erythropoietin

Around 90% of the hormone erythropoietin is produced by the kidneys; the rest is produced by the liver. As erythropoietin controls the rate of red blood cell production, it follows that patients are likely to become anaemic in cases of severe kidney disease (or their removal). This is worth bearing in mind if you have an anaemic patient with a chronic kidney condition.

Anaemias

Iron-Deficiency Anaemia (Microcytic Anaemia)

- Usually discovered with a full blood count (Chapter 41 'Scientific tests', p. 331) and is one of the most common types of anaemia.

- There is not enough iron in the body to form haemoglobin.
- Blood cells are of normal size and content, but are fewer in number than normal.
- Can vary from mild, with no signs or symptoms, to severe, in which the patient experiences extreme fatigue and weakness.

For reasons for iron deficiency, see Chapter 13 'Vitamins and minerals' (p. 97).

• Treatment

- Iron supplementation.

Pernicious Anaemia

- Macrocytic, normochromic anaemia: blood cells are large, with a normal amount of haem.
- Autoimmune type of anaemia: due to the patient producing antibodies against the intrinsic factor needed for efficient absorption of vitamin B_{12}.
- Pernicious anaemia can also refer to the anaemia caused by a deficiency of vitamin B_{12} due to other causes (see Chapter 13 'Vitamins and minerals', p. 105).

• Treatment

- Lifelong injections of vitamin B_{12}.

Megaloblastic Anaemia

Generalized description of a type of anaemia that is usually the result of vitamin B_{12} and folate deficiency. The red blood cells are larger than normal and there is an accompanying reduction in the numbers of white blood cells and platelets.

• Treatment

Vitamin B_{12} and folate supplementation (see Chapter 13 'Vitamins and minerals', p. 105).

Aplastic Anaemia

The bone marrow stops making an adequate number of blood cells so there is a noticeable reduction of blood cells, including red blood cells.

• Treatment

- Nearly all patients require transfusions.
- Ultimately, treatment will be directed at the cause of anaemia, e.g. the patient might have leukaemia and will therefore require the appropriate treatment for that condition.

Sickle-Cell Anaemia

- The body makes abnormal-shaped red blood cells.
- Genetic: commonly found in people of sub-Saharan African descent.

• Treatment

- Transfusions.
- Oral antibiotics from 2 months to 5 years to prevent pneumonia: it is therefore important to consider health of the gastrointestinal tract of such patients (see Chapter 17 'Metabolism', p. 132).

Thalassaemia

- Similar to sickle-cell anaemia.
- Genetic: very often of Mediterranean descent.

Treatment

Transfusions.

Note: with both sickle-cell anaemia and thalassaemia, avoid supplementation with omega 3 oils.

Leukaemia

Abnormal growth of the cells in the bone marrow that develop into white blood cells.

Treatment

● Underlying Cause Leucopenia

- Decreased white blood cells: most commonly neutrophils (neutropenia; see Chapter 30 'Inflammation and the immune system', p. 224).
- Increased risk of infection (see Chapter 30 'Inflammation and the immune system', p. 225).
- Might be due to leukaemia, autoimmune disease or vitamin B_{12} or folate deficiency (see Chapter 13 'Vitamins and minerals', p. 105).

Treatment

● Underlying Cause Thrombocytopenia

- Reduction in platelet count.
- Increased clotting time.
- Caused by leukaemia, lymphoma, aplastic anaemia, vitamin B_{12} or folate deficiency anaemias, an enlarged spleen, AIDS.

Treatment

● Underlying Cause Porphyria

- Any iron in the body that is not associated can create free radicals (see Chapter 7 'Free radicals', p. 41) because it attaches itself to any protein it comes into contact with. Liver cirrhosis is a result of this. Iron must therefore be carefully controlled.
- Excess iron usually not a problem in a healthy individual because iron that is absorbed from the duodenum binds immediately to a carrier molecule called transferrin, which transports the iron to storage as ferritin. The transferring molecule binds very strongly with the cell membranes of erythroblasts (precursors to red blood cells) in bone marrow, ensuring that at no time is free iron released.
- About 15% of iron is stored.
- The body has no means of actively excreting iron (although about 0.6 mg is lost in the faeces every day and approximately 1.3 mg per day in menstruation). Regulation of the amount in the body is done by regulating uptake.
- Too much iron in the gastrointestinal tract can damage the cells lining the lumen, which are responsible for regulating the entry of iron into the bloodstream. The large amount of iron will lead to free iron entering the body.
- Treatment is by chelation. This binds up the iron, thus neutralizing its activity.

Haemostasis

Haemostasis (the arrest of bleeding) occurs because of the creation of an abnormal environment in the blood vessels.

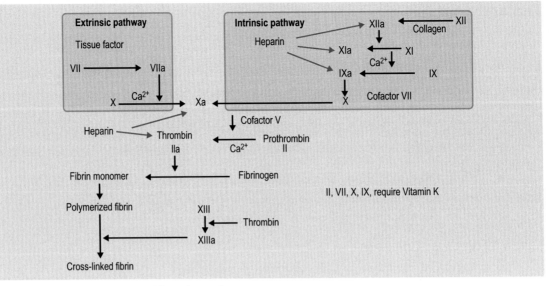

Figure 28.1 The blood coagulation (clotting) cascade.

Normal Events in Haemostasis

- The process of repairing a blood vessel starts with vasoconstriction and the formation of a platelet plug at the site of an injury.
- This is then stabilized by the formation of a fibrin network, which is the end result of the coagulation cascade (Figure 28.1).
- The fibrin is removed during healing as fibrinolytic enzymes digest it.

● The Different Pathways Involved in Clotting

Two different pathways are involved in the clotting cascade (Figure 28.1):

- The **extrinsic pathway**: activated by tissue factor (a protein, released from damaged tissue, that triggers the clotting cascade), which is expressed by cells during injury.
- The **intrinsic pathway**: activated when blood comes into contact with a foreign surface, e.g. an atheroma

● Formation of a Thrombosis

A **thrombosis is a blood clot in the wrong place**. A thrombosis forms due to:

- Abnormalities of the vessel wall: an atheromatous plaque in an artery wall (see Figure 27.2, p. 205).
- Abnormalities of flow in a blood vessel: blood stasis in veins, e.g. deep vein thrombosis (DVT) as a result of a long period of immobility (e.g. on a long-haul flight).
- Abnormalities of blood constituents: e.g. uterine material with tissue factor activity gains access to the maternal circulation. Certain bacterial endotoxins also cause generation of tissue factor.

Antiplatelet Drugs

Antiplatelet drugs are preferred to anticoagulants as they are less likely to cause excess bleeding.

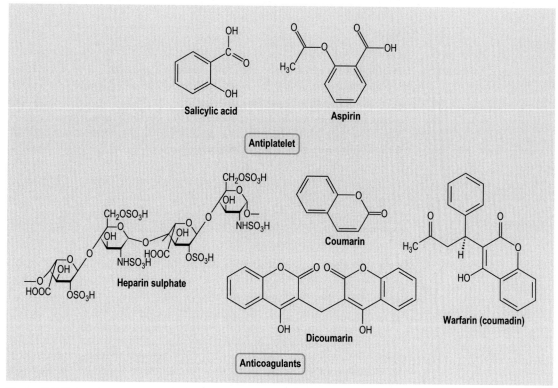

Figure 28.2 Various haemostatic medications, demonstrating the natural derivatives of modern medications.

Aspirin

- Originally derived from salicylic acid (Figure 28.2 and see Figure 21.4 on p. 151).
- Aspirin is commonly used, as it is cost effective and easy to administer. A loading dose is initially required.
- Aspirin inactivates a key enzyme involved in the platelet synthesis pathway. This is an irreversible reaction as the platelets have no nucleus. Recovery from taking aspirin for an antiplatelet effect is 10 days, the time it takes to produce more platelets.
- Aspirin is used in transient ischaemic attacks (TIAs) and myocardial infarction.

Note: cerebral haemorrhages have to be considered in the differential diagnosis as the symptoms can be similar. Aspirin in this case is *not* administered, as it would make the situation worse. A brain scan usually differentiates between the two.

• Adverse Efects

- Bleeding of the gut wall.
- Allergy reaction to aspirin. Not given to some one with a known allergy to aspirin.

Note: this applies to herbs and foods containing salicylates.

- **Aggravates asthma.**
- Possibility of renal failure in patients with renal artery stenosis and patients taking ACE inhibitors.
- Cerebral haemorrhage.

Note: it is not a good idea to give aspirin to some one with a disease such as haemophilia or any type of sickle-cell anaemia. Omega 3 fish oils are also considered a problem in these cases.

Anticoagulants

• Heparin

- Heparin (see Figures 28.1 and 28.2) is injected into a vein or under the skin.
- It is used in the first instance in DVT or pulmonary embolism.
- It is also used in renal dialysis circuits and cardiopulmonary bypasses.
- **It is usually bovine or porcine in origin**.
- Heparin is a large, highly charged molecule with very little ability to cross the blood–placenta barrier. As warfarin can cross the placenta, patients on warfarin treatment have to use heparin when pregnant.

Adverse Effects

- Bleeding.
- Heparin-induced thrombocytopenia: the heparin forms a heparin–antibody complex that binds to the platelet surface membrane forming platelet clumps, which can cause vessel obstruction.

Five days of heparin treatment is usually all that is required to treat a venous thrombosis. By this time patients will be taking oral anticoagulants at the same time as the heparin, and so heparin treatment can be safely stopped.

• Warfarin

- Is modelled on dicoumarol the natural anticoagulant derived from coumarin (see Figure 28.2 and Chapter 21 'Phenols', p. 157). Acts as a vitamin K antagonist.
- When the vitamin K acts on a cofactor it is recycled by reductase reactions. If this processes is inhibited the active vitamin K is not able to act on the factors in the cascade pattern.
- Warfarin therapy is monitored very carefully because it can sometimes prove difficult to balance. Much of the warfarin administered to a patient binds to plasma proteins, but can be easily displaced, releasing higher levels of free, unbound warfarin into the bloodstream than desirable (see Chapter 16 'How do drugs get into cells', p. 125). The converse is true when too little warfarin is administered.

Note: consumption of large amounts of spirits has been documented to increase clotting time. Chronic consumption of large amounts of alcohol by warfarinized patients appears to potentiate the effects of warfarin.

Adverse Effects

- Bleeding.
- Skin rashes.

Contraindications

- Lack of patient compliance.
- Do not use in first trimester of pregnancy.

Interactions

As warfarin is so easily displaced, there is an almost endless list of interactions and a formulary needs to be consulted. Herbalists who wish to treat patients would be advised to ensure that a regular check is done on the warfarin levels in the patient's blood. In terms of Chinese medicine, this means avoiding any blood-moving herbs, such as *Rhizoma Sparganii stolonifera* (*San Leng*), *Rhizoma Curcumae ezhu* (*Er Zhu*).

Even simple herbs like **garlic** and **gingko** can interfere with the function of warfarin. Herbs such as **St John's wort** can **upregulate the P450 enzyme** in the liver, clearing the drug too fast through the system and thus making it less effective.

Vitamin K

Vitamin K (see Chapter 'Vitamins and minerals', p. 108) is essential for normal haemostatic and antithrombotic function.

Haemophilia

- Characterized by a decrease in clotting factor (see Figure 28.1) and therefore increased clotting time.
- The skin is easily bruised and bleeding into joints or hollow internal organs can occur.
- Genetic.

Treatment

Injection of clotting factor VII or IX.

Note: omega 3 is associated with decreased platelet activation and aggregation and so might cause prolonged bleeding in patient with blood disorders such as haemophilia.

Antimicrobials

Bacterial Structure

The cell wall of a bacterium is unique. Although not present in every bacterial species, it is usually a very important part of maintaining the integrity of the bacterium.

Animal and plant cells exist in a relatively constant chemical environment, but bacterial cells mostly live in an unfavourable environment. The cell wall is therefore a very important part of maintaining the integrity of the bacterium. Bacteria do not have a nucleus, but instead the genetic material exists in the form of a single chromosome that holds all the genetic information of the cell lying free in the cells. Bacteria have no mitchondria.

The function of the cell wall of a bacterium is to:

- Maintain the cell's characteristic shape: to prevent the phosphoplipid membrane of the cell wall from adopting a spherical shape.
- Withstand considerable changes in osmolarity.
- Provide a rigid platform for structures such as flagellae.

The structure of the bacterial cell wall varies considerably between species, and classification is largely on the reaction of the bacterial cell wall to the Gram stain (named after the Danish bacteriologist Hans Christian Gram). **Gram-positive bacteria** retain more of the stain than **Gram-negative bacteria**, due to the different constituents of the cell walls.

Most of the work on wall structure has been done with Gram-positive cocci and bacilli, and with enteric bacteria (found in the intestine) and other Gram-negative rods.

Gram-Negative Bacteria

- Exhibit some flexibility in their nutritional needs, using inorganic nitrogen compounds, mineral salts and a simple carbon source for synthesis of their whole structure.
- Have a low internal osmotic pressure (see Figure 16.1, p. 124).

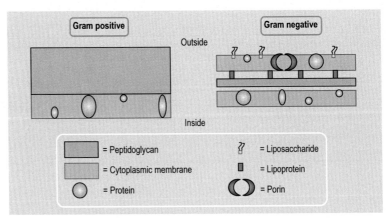

Figure 29.1 The structure of the bacterial cell wall.

Gram-Positive Bacteria

- Gram-positive cocci or bacilli have more specific nutritional requirements. Several bacteria lack some synthetic abilities and require various amino acids, vitamins and accessory factors for growth
- These have a high internal osmotic pressure.

However, these characteristics do not always hold true:

- Some cocci, rickettsias, the Chlamydias and spirochaetes are Gram-negative and have exacting growth requirements.
- Mycoplasmas lack a rigid wall structure; although technically Gram-negative, they are a separate group.

Finding medication that is effective against these microorganisms is anything but straightforward.

The Bacterial Cell Wall

- ### Gram-Positive Bacteria
  - Relatively simple wall.
  - 90% of the Gram-positive cell wall comprises peptidoglycans (a polymer of sugars and amino acids) (Figure 29.1).

- ### Gram-Negative Bacteria
  - The cell wall is much more complex, consisting of layers of membranes.
  - The cell wall is much thinner than the Gram-positive wall.
  - Only 20% is peptidoglycans.
  - The cell wall has protein components, which penetrate the layer partly or completely and form the membrane 'mosaic'.
  - The cell wall contains porins (membrane proteins that allow the passage of small molecules through the membrane).

Antimicrobial Medication

Actions

- **Bactericidal**: e.g. penicillins – lethal to bacteria.
- **Bacteriostatic**: not lethal but inhibit the ability of bacterial cells to reproduce. The body's immune system therefore has to be efficient enough to destroy the microbe itself.

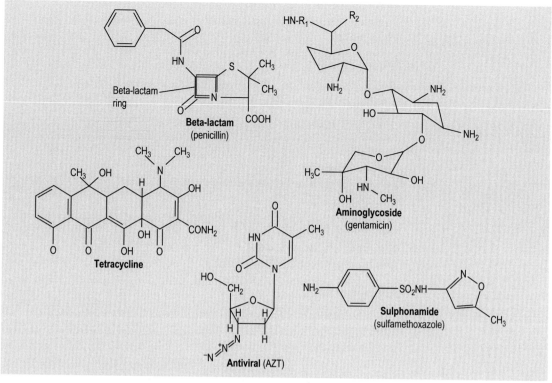

Figure 29.2 The main antibiotic groups and azidothymidine (AZT).

Main Antibiotic Groups

- Beta-lactams.
- Aminoglycosides.
- Tetracyclines.
- Sulphonamides.

Beta-Lactams

- Penicillins (Figure 29.2), cephalosporins.
- Have a beta-lactam ring, which is the active part of the molecule.
- Inhibit cell wall synthesis by preventing cross-linking of peptidoglycans.
- Act on Gram-positive anaerobic bacteria, e.g. streptococci and meningococci.
- Absorbed by most tissues, except the central nervous system (CNS).
- Some patients have an allergy to penicillin.
- Low toxicity.
- Removed largely unchanged in urine.

Aminoglycosides

- Gentamicin (see Figure 29.2): note the carbohydrate structure.
- Inhibit protein synthesis.
- Act on Gram-negative facultative bacteria (they can metabolize both with and without oxygen), e.g. staphylococci, *Listeria* and *Corynebacterium* spp.
- Poorly absorbed, therefore injected.
- Concentrate in renal cortex, not easily accessible to CNS and eye.

- Removed by kidney, therefore renal function must be good.
- Problems with nephrotoxicity, ototoxicity (can damage eighth cranial nerve, leading to deafness or vertigo).

• Tetracyclines

- Act on Gram-negative and Gram-positive bacteria (i.e. are **broad spectrum**).
- Inhibit protein synthesis (see Figure 11.6, p. 85).
- Absorption varies depending on the tetracycline.
- Bind to calcium (can therefore be incorporated into teeth and bone structure, causing discoloration of teeth and impairment of bone formation). **Avoid taking with milk.**
- **Secreted in milk by breast-feeding women.**
- Distributed to almost all tissues.
- Some are removed unchanged in the urine; others are metabolized in the liver and removed in the bile.
- Used for *Chlamydia* infections.
- Can cause gastrointestinal disturbances.

• Sulphonamides

- Act on Gram-negative and Gram-positive bacteria (i.e. broad spectrum).
- Work by resembling a bacterial metabolite: the sulphonamide effective blocks the metabolic process by depriving the bacteria of folic acid, which it needs for purine synthesis (see Chapter 12 'Purines and pyrimidines', p. 89). DNA synthesis is therefore inhibited.
- **Bacteriostatic.**
- Good distribution to all tissues.
- May be partly removed unchanged by the kidneys and or metabolized in the liver.

Facts Associated with Antibiotics

- Age and health are important factors in dosage and response to the drug (see Chapter 19 'Pharmacodynamics: how drugs elicit a physiological effect' p. 143).
- The kidneys eliminate most antimicrobials (very few are processed by the liver), so good renal function is vital.
- A complete course of antibiotics has to be taken to ensure that all the bacteria have been eliminated. Not taking a complete course might result in another upsurge of the bacteria and a return of the disease.

Pregnancy

This is a very important consideration in the use of antibiotics.

Treatment with Antimicrobials

Broad-spectrum drugs can be given initially but if the disease persists then a sample is taken, usually a throat swab in the case of a throat infection, or a mid-stream urine sample. Cultures are then made and tested against the appropriate antibiotic, so that a more effective antibiotic can be used.

• Main adverse reactions

Hypersensitivity

- Immediate: if extreme anaphylactic shock.
- Delayed: usually a skin rash.

Ototoxicity

Damage to the sensory cells in the cochlea and vestibular organ of the ear can lead to vertigo, ataxia and auditory disturbances, including deafness.

Prophylaxis

Although it is not advisable to give antibiotics prophylactically, this is sometimes necessary, for example when an individual has been exposed to a bacterial form of meningitis, or when an individual might be susceptible to infection after surgery to prevent septicaemia, e.g. open heart surgery.

Bacterial Resistance

Methicillin-resistant*Staphylococcus aureus* (MRSA) has become a big problem in hospitals due to the overuse of antibiotics. The more powerful antibiotics are saved for such infections. Very careful personal hygiene is hugely important in this situation.

Antiviral Drugs

The major problem with viruses is that they integrate themselves into the host cell's biochemistry. This intertwining of virus and host cell makes them difficult to attack.

Azidothymidine

The structure of azidothymidine (AZT; see Figure 29.2) is similar to that of nucleosides (see Figure 12.2, p. 90):

- AZT is an antiproliferative immunosuppressant.
- The AZT is changed – in infected and non-infected cells – to a substance that is a chain terminator of DNA. This makes it fairly toxic, as DNA synthesis in all the body's cells is affected.

Adverse Effects

- Increased susceptibility to infection.
- Nausea and vomiting.
- Alopecia.
- Bone marrow suppression.
- Small risk of carcinogenicity, particularly lymphomas.
- Great risk of potential drug, herb, or supplement interactions.

Inflammation and the immune system

30

It is difficult to separate the immune system from the anti-inflammatory system; the two are interrelated and any defect in the immune system has far-reaching effects on a patient's health.

To properly understand the immune system it is necessary to have a reasonable understanding of its working components. The explanation here is very simplified but is more than adequate for the scope of the book and for a basic understanding of the underlying principles of the complicated processes of the immune and anti-inflammatory systems.

Origins of the Immune System

Communication in early evolution was cell to cell. This means of communication survived as we evolved to become the immune system and the inflammatory response.

The Function of the Immune System

The immune system is the body's defence system against bacteria, fungi, parasites, viruses and other pathogens entering the body. It is also a means of eliminating these pathogens before they cause serious harm.

The construction of the immune system allows it to adapt so as to mount a more rapid and vigorous attack each time it encounters a particular pathogen.

Why is An Anti-Inflammatory Response Necessary?

The anti-inflammatory response is a defensive response to tissue injury or damage. It is designed to remove the irritant and repair damaged tissue.

Components of the Immune System

Leucocytes

Leucocytes – white blood cells – are part of the body's mobile defence system. There are five types of white blood cell:

- Neutrophils
- Eosinophils } Granulocytes produced in bone marrow; 6-day supply in the
- Basophils marrow.
- Lymphocytes: continually in the circulatory and lymph systems. Produced mainly in the lymph system (lymph glands, spleen, thymus tonsils, etc.).
- Monocytes: change to macrophages after entering the tissues.

• Neutrophils

- Respond to the chemicals released by bacteria and dead tissue cells, moving to the area of highest concentration.
- Phagocytose the foreign cells and destroy them.
- Die soon after phagocytosis, as the process uses up their glycogen reserves. The dead neutrophils accumulate, with tissue fluid, to create pus.

• Eosinophils

- Increase in allergic reactions.
- Increase in most parasitic infections.
- Have surface receptors for immunoglobulin E (IgE).

• Basophils

- Similar to mast cells but mobile.
- Highly specific receptors to IgE (see mast cells, below).

• Lymphocytes

- Increase in viral infections.
- Two major types: B and T lymphocytes.

• Monocytes

- **Leave the bloodstream to become tissue macrophages**, which remove dead cell debris. Also attack some bacteria and fungi (neutrophils do not deal with these effectively).
- Have a longer life than neutrophils as they are able to replace their digestive enzymes.

Other Components

• Mast Cells

- Found in connective tissue and contains granules of **histamine** (p. 175) and **heparin** (see Figure 28.2, p. 213).
- Involved in wound healing and defence against pathogens.

- Involved in allergic (Chapter 34 'Respiratory diseases', p. 267) and anaphylactic reactions.
- Highly specific receptors to IgE.

How Does the Immune System Work?

Pathogens that invade the body stimulate the immune system, which has three main stages of response:

1. To neutralize the pathogen by:
   - secreting cytotoxic proteins: proteins lethal to pathogens
   - phagocytosis: engulfing the pathogen and effectively digesting it.
2. To fragment the pathogen by phagocytosis: the fragments are presented on the surface of **antigen-presenting cells (APCs)** in the lymph tissue and provide a marker that enables the cells of the immune system to recognize that type of pathogen. The APCs also release a cytokine (interleukin-1; see below), which encourages the proliferation of B and T cells.
3. To secrete interleukins: the above stimulates the cells of the immune system to secrete interleukins, which further stimulate the immune system. The **B and T lymphocytes** are cloned in the lymph nodes. Some cells produce a pool of **memory cells (M)** specific to a particular antigen, which will enable the body to respond much faster with another exposure. This takes place in the lymph node and is known as the **induction phase**. The other cells go on to the **effector phase**.

The **effector** phase is one of the following:

- **Humoral-mediated phase**: involves antibodies, which act in the fluid of the blood and tissues to **involve the B cells**. There is also some added stimulation from interaction between the B cells and T helper cells.
- **Cell-mediated phase**: this works where the antibodies cannot reach, deals with pathogens in cells and **involves the T cells**.

Humoral Response

A humoral-mediated response (Figure 30.1):

- Is an **immediate** reaction. Hence the speed of anaphylactic shock, hay fever, asthma and some food allergies. It is a **type 1 reaction**.
- The **T helper cells** not only activate **B cells** but also release **interleukins** (signalling molecules and part of a group classed as **cytokines**). These **interleukins** stimulate **eosinophils**, **mast cell production** and the generation of IgE, which are the **mediators** in **chronic inflammation.**
- **IgE** has a strong tendency to attach to **mast cells** and **basophils**, changing the composition of their cell membranes so that they release their contents. People with **atopic allergies** have high levels of IgE in their blood.
- Some of the components are histamine, protease, platelet-activating factors, etc., which open-up the local blood vessels, attracting the **eosinophils** and **neutrophils** to the site. The eosinophils and neutrophils attack and destroy bacteria. The site is also damaged by the contents such as the proteases. There is loss of fluid into the tissues and contraction of the local smooth muscles.

Antibodies or **immunoglobulins** (hence the shorthand Ig) have two main functions:

1. To recognize and interact specifically with particular antigens (Figure 30.2): this can provide some damage limitation.
2. To activate the immune system: the tails act as a tag to activate the complement sequence (see below).

There are five classes of antibody: IgA, IgD, IgE, IgG and IgM.

225

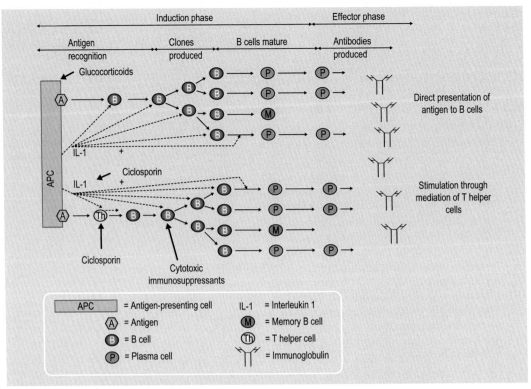

Figure 30.1 Humoral (antibody)-mediated response showing points of immunosuppressant intervention.

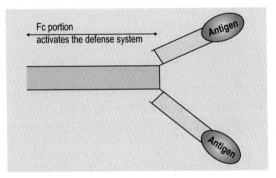

Figure 30.2 Structure of an antibody showing its attachment to antigens.

• The Complement System

This is similar in mechanism to the coagulation cascade (see Figure 28.1, p. 212). It is activated by interaction in several ways:

- Antigen–antibody complex (classical pathway)
- the antigen (alternative pathway)
- complex carbohydrates (see Chapter 9 'Carbohydrates' p. 71).

The final part of complement activation produces a **membrane attack complex**, which creates holes in the outer membrane of Gram-negative bacteria (see Figure 29.1, p. 218).

The complement cascade has a feedback mechanism, which in theory should limit its action. However, several of the products of the complement cascade are

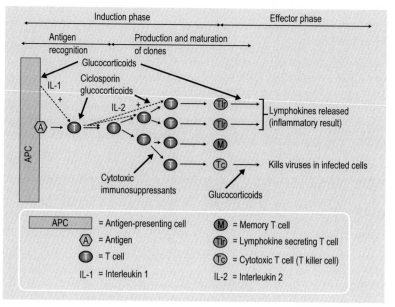

Figure 30.3 Diagram demonstrating the cell-mediated response showing points of immunosuppressant interventions.

powerful inflammatory stimulants, so it is possible for the inflammatory response to get out of hand.

Cell-Mediated Response (Figure 30.3)

- T cells move to an inflammatory area.
- Two types of T cell are involved: cytotoxic T cells, which ensure the death of a cell displaying a foreign antigen, and T helper cells, which assist the immune response.
- This response is not as well understood as the humoral response and is considerably more complex.
- This is a **delayed reaction** (possibly a few days).
- The absence of T helper cells means that the immune system is virtually unable to function.
- **Type IV hypersensitivity: e.g. the tuberculin reaction – this is one example of a delayed response.**
- Rheumatoid arthritis (RA), multiple sclerosis and insulin-dependent diabetes are all examples of cell-mediated response conditions.

The Inflammatory System

The Inflammatory Response

The inflammatory response occurs in the following way:

- Vasodilatation of the local blood vessels increases the local blood flow.
- Increased permeability of the capillaries allows leakage of large amounts of fluid into the interstitial spaces.
- Clotting of the fluid in the interstitial spaces due to excessive amounts of fibrinogen and other proteins leaking from the capillaries.

- Migration of large numbers of neutrophils, basophils, monocytes and eosinophils into the tissues.
- Swelling of the tissue cells.

An inappropriate **cell-mediated immune response** is stimulated and there is infiltration of mononuclear (cells with one nucleus, e.g. lymphocytes, as opposed to polymorphonuclear cells, e.g. neutrophils) cells and release of various cytokines.

Inflammation can continue after it is needed if the pathogen or antigen persists. Hence, a practitioner can see this lingering for weeks, months or years. Chronic inflammation is the result of the type IV cell-mediated immune response and chronic autoimmune diseases are therefore thought to be due to the reaction initially set off by a pathogen.

Inappropriate T-cell activity underlies all types of hypersensitivity.

Components Involved in Inflammation

• Eicosanoids

The name implies molecules derived from 20-carbon essential fatty acids. These are usually omega 3 and omega 6 essential fatty acids. The main source of eicosanoids is arachidonic acid. There are four types of eicosanoid (Figure 30.4):

- prostaglandins PG) ⎫
- prostacyclins ⎬ Prostanoids.
- thromboxanes ⎭
- leukotrienes: found in inflammatory exudates. Present in rheumatoid athritis, psoriasis and ulcerative colitis. Potent spasmogens causing contraction of the bronchioles.

Prostaglandins

- Prostaglandins (PG) are active in very low hormone level concentrations.
- Can regulate blood pressure, smooth muscle contraction, gastric secretions and platelet aggregation.

228

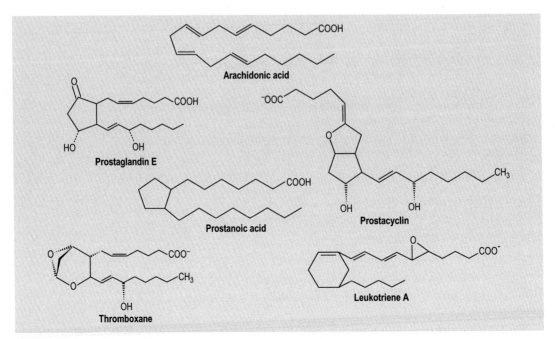

Figure 30.4 Various eicosanoids.

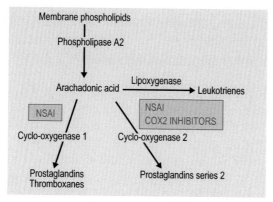

- Generated from phospholipids. Very important in the anti-inflammatory system.
- Are produced by cyclo-oxygenase (COX) enzymes. There are two pathways: COX-1 and COX-2.

Prostaglandin PGE1

- Causes vasodilatation.
- Prevents platelet aggregation.
- Anti-inflammatory effect.
- Increased synthesis useful.
- Formed from a precursor of arachidonic acid.

Prostaglandin PGE2

- **Biphasic action**: although largely thought of as a vasoconstrictor, PGE2 is also a **powerful vasodilator**, therefore encouraging a greater blood supply to that area and more histamines and inflammatory components. The histamines then increase the inflammatory problem.
- Proinflammatory.
- Formed from arachidonic acid.

Prostaglandin PGE3

- Prevents platelet aggregation.
- Anti-inflammatory effect.
- Formed from eicosapentoic acid (EPA).

Prostacyclins

- Inhibit platelet aggregation.
- Inhibit vasoconstriction.

Thromboxanes

- Vasoconstrictors, therefore hypertensive agents (see Chapter 26 'Cardiovascular disorders', p. 195).
- Facilitate aggregation of platelets: aspirin works by inhibiting the COX enzyme responsible for producing thromboxanes (see Figure 30.5), thus preventing platelet aggregation.

Figure 30.5 The prostaglandin and leukotriene production pathway, demonstrating points of intervention.

Leukotrienes

- Leukotrienes are synthesized from arachidonic acid, by a lipoxygenase found in leucocytes and macrophages.
- Leukotrienes act on G protein receptors (see Figure 19.5, p. 141).
- Involved in asthmatic and allergic reactions.
- Sustain inflammatory reactions.
- Increase vascular permeability.
- Encourage leucocyte chemotaxis (i.e. the movement of leucocytes towards an area of inflammation).

Proteins Involved in the Inflammatory and Immune Systems

Cytokines

- Regulate inflammatory and immune reactions.
- Interleukins are a form of cytokine.
- Interferons are a form of cytokine that has antiviral activity.

● Tumour Necrosis Factor Alpha (TNF-Alpha)

- TNF-alpha is a cytokine that is important in the inflammatory response.
- Induces the synthesis of interleukins.
- Macrophages, mast cells and activated T cells secrete TNF-alpha.
- Stimulates macrophages to produce cytotoxic metabolites thus increasing the activity of phagocytes.
- TNF-alpha been implicated in rheumatoid arthritis and Crohn's disease.

Anti-Inflammatory Medication

- Glucocorticoids.
- Non-steroidal anti-inflammatories.

Glucocorticoids (Corticosteroids)

- Steroids are normally produced by the adrenal glands and are made and released as required.
- Cholesterol is the framework from which steroids are made. Steroids produced by the body will have an anti-inflammatory action and immunosuppressive effects.
- Used in serious cases of inflammation, e.g. rheumatoid arthritis, ulcerative colitis or chronic active hepatitis.

    Prednisolone is a commonly used oral steroid.

● Adverse Effects

The adverse effects of corticosteroids are tied up with the hormonal system, which in its natural state is a delicate balance of hormonal interactions with the various glands in the body.

- Metabolic effects: rounded, 'moon face'; deposits of fat creating a buffalo hump; obesity of the trunk leaving thin arms and legs; a tendency to bruising; possible diabetes; muscular weakness.
- Fluid retention and possible hypertension.
- Osteoporosis (see Chapter 37 'Metabolic disorders', p. 290).

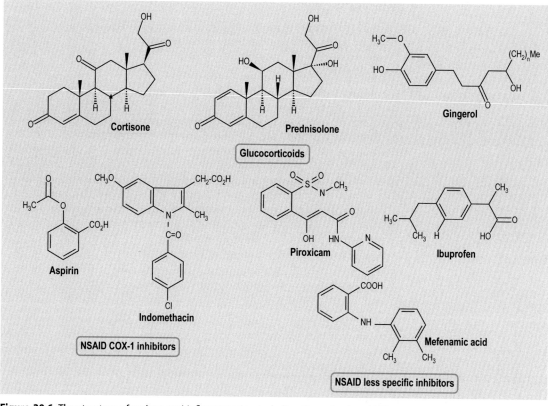

Figure 30.6 The structure of various anti-inflammatories, including the natural anti-inflammatory agent gingerol (note the similarity in structure to ibuprofen and aspirin). NSAI = non-steroidal anti-inflammatories.

- Might get a sense of euphoria, but might also get mood swings; the steroids can also precipitate a depressive illness.
- Cataracts: rare.
- Dyspepsia.
- Suppression of immune system leading to repeated infections.

Non-Steroidal Anti-Inflammatory Drugs (NSAIDs)

The anti-inflammatory effect of non-steroidal anti-inflammatories (NSAIDs) is due to inhibition of the COX enzyme (Figure 30.5). These drugs have three major effects:

- anti-inflammatory
- analgesic
- antipyretic.

• Anti-Inflammatory Effect

Different NSAIDs work on different COX enzymes (Figure 30.6):

- Indometacin, aspirin: COX-1.
- Diclofenac, naproxen: equal effect on COX-1 and COX-2.
- Piroxicam, ibuprofen, mefenamic acid: less selective.

Although the NSAIDs reduce inflammation, the mechanism is still not well understood.

• Analgesic Effect

PGE1 and PGE2 sensitize pain fibres to bradykinin or 5-hydroxytryptamine. Blocking their production will reduce this effect.

• Antipyretic Effect

NSAIs reset the internal thermostat when there is a fever. This is thought to be the result of prostaglandin production by the hypothalamus.

• Adverse Effects

- Gastrointestinal effects (diarrhoea, nausea, vomiting, dyspepsia): due to direct mucosal irritation or because of inhibition of the synthesis of the prostaglandins that normally inhibit acid secretion, as well as protecting the gut layer. This problem was thought to have been overcome with the development of COX-2 inhibitors, which, because they were more specific for the COX-2 pathway, allowed the COX-1 pathway to function, thus reducing the incidence of mucosal irritation. However, widespread usage found a link with increased myocardial infarction when COX-2 inhibitors were taken continuously for 18 months. This is thought to be the result of an **imbalance in the thromboxane and prostacyclin** levels, which might lead to an increase in platelet aggregation, one of the factors involved in blood haemodynamics.
- Skin: mild rashes, urticaria and photosensitivity.
- Lungs: can cause difficulties in breathing with asthmatics.
- Kidneys: can cause renal insufficiency. PGE2 involved in renin–angiotensin system.

• Aspirin

Aspirin is a derivation of salicylates, which are found naturally occurring in willow bark, meadowsweet, etc. Salicylic acid and acetyl salicylic acid (aspirin) were among the earliest drugs synthesized.

Adverse Effects

- Aspirin can irritate the lining of the gut and cause bleeding (*Note*: willow bark, meadowsweet and other salicylate-containing herbs are used by Western herbalists to help heal stomach ulcers).
- Some patients are allergic to salicylates.
- Can bring on or make asthma worse.
- Can cause serious imbalance in warfarin levels as aspirin is more favourably bound to plasma proteins than warfarin (see Chapter 16 'How do drugs get into cells?', p. 126), thus releasing more free warfarin into the blood.

Immunosuppressants

- Prevent tissue rejection in organ transplants.
- Used in autoimmune diseases, e.g. rheumatoid arthritis, systemic lupus erythematosus.
- Used in certain types of cancer.

In a normal person, the T cells are largely responsible for killing the cells of an organ transplant or graft (e.g. following bone marrow transplantation), so their suppression – far more than the plasma antibodies – is a priority in treatment.

There is an overlap between pure immunosuppressant drugs and chemotherapy (see Chapter 39 'Chemotherapy', p. 309). Immunosuppressant drugs are used at much lower doses than for chemotherapy. **They require lifelong use**.

Approaches to Suppression of the Immune System

- Suppression of growth of lymphatic tissue due to inhibition of gene expression: glucocorticoids.
- **Use of cytotoxic agents** to deplete expanding lymphocyte populations: **antimetabolites** (azathioprine), methotrexate (see Figure 39.2, p. 311) and **alkylating** agents (cyclophosphamide) to suppress the formation of antibodies and T cells.

- Inhibition of lymphocyte signalling to block activation and production of lymphocytes: ciclosporin (specific for T cells and does not affect other parts of the immune system).
- Inhibition of cytokines (interleukins and TNF) essential for mediating the immune response: TNF-alpha inhibitor.
- Use of antibodies to deplete the immune system of specific cells: used for prevention and treatment of organ transplant rejection.

Glucocorticoids

- Suppress the growth of lymphoid tissue and, as a result, decrease the formation of both antibodies and T cells.
- Inhibit the production of inflammatory mediators, including platelet-activating factor, leukotrienes, prostaglandins, histamine and bradykinin.
- Work both as immunosuppressives and anti-inflammatories, therefore useful for conditions such as rheumatoid arthritis.

Adverse Effects

See p. 230.

Cytotoxic Agents

- Alkylating agents: used to treat some types of glomerulonephritis caused by a systemic inflammatory condition, e.g. systemic lupus erythematosus.
- Antimetabolics (antiproliferative): azathioprine suppresses the formation of antibodies and T cells by mimicking a purine.

Inhibition of Lymphocyte Signalling

Ciclosporin

- Fat-soluble antibiotic of fungal origin.
- Impairs production and release of interleukins, which activate T-cell growth, and so prevents T-cell activation. Specificity to T cells means that other parts of the immune system are left intact.

Adverse Effects

- Nephrotoxicity.
- Hypertension: might require medication to lower blood pressure.
- Possible convulsions.
- Tremor.
- Possible nausea, vomiting or anorexia.
- Hyperglycaemia.
- Hyperlipidaemia.
- Liver dysfunction.
- Hirsutism.
- **Potential for serious drug, herb and supplement interactions.**

Inhibition of Cytokines

TNF-Alpha Inhibitors

- Bind to TNF-alpha blocking its action.
- Have been used in the treatment of rheumatoid arthritis.

Adverse Effects

- Possibility of increased infection and malignancy.
- Injection-site reactions.

233

• Interleukin Inhibitors

- Have been used in rheumatoid anthritis.
- Possibility of increased infection and malignancy.
- Injection-site reactions.

As TNF-alpha and interleukins are very close in action, therapy using the combination of the two is being investigated.

• Use of Antibodies to Deplete the Immune System of Specific Cells

- Used for prevention and treatment of organ transplant rejection.
- Batches vary in efficacy and toxicity.

Adverse Effects

- Fevers and chills.
- Possible hypotension.
- Glomerulonephritis.

A combination of immunosuppressant drugs might be used.

Immunostimulants

Used in immunodeficiency and some cancers.

Interferons

- Immune-enhancing properties.
- Increase antigen presentation.
- Macrophage, natural killer cell and cytotoxic T lymphocyte activation.
- Used mainly as therapeutic agents with melanoma, renal cell carcinoma and chronic myelogenous leukaemia.

Adverse Effects

- Fever, chills and general malaise.
- Myalgias.
- Myelosuppression.
- Headache.
- Depression.

The nervous system

31

How an Electrical Impulse is Generated

As previously discussed (see Chapter 19 'Pharmacodynamics: how drugs elicit a physiological effect', p. 139), proteins span the cell membrane and can affect the rate of flow or direction of ions. These proteins are of two main types:

- Ion pumps: energy dependent and physically move ions against a concentration gradient.
- Ion channels: open or close according to the voltage (**voltage gating**) across the membrane or by activation from the attachment of a molecule.

Both play in important role in conduction of a nerve impulse and muscle contraction.

Production of an Action Potential

Normally:

- The **potassium concentration inside** a cell is **higher** than the potassium concentration outside the cell.
- The **sodium concentration outside** the cell is **higher** than the sodium concentration inside the cell.

The sodium–potassium pump (Figure 31.1) is a form of active transport as both the sodium and potassium are moving against a gradient. It is responsible for maintaining an electrical balance across a cell membrane. The sodium–potassium pump actively pushes sodium molecules out of the cell and pumps potassium molecules in against a gradient. With each cycle, **three Na$^+$ ions are pumped out** and **two K$^+$ ions are pumped in**. The net result, as there are also negative ions such as Cl$^-$ (chlorine) present both inside and outside the cell, is a net negative charge inside the cell and a positive charge outside the cell. This means that there

235

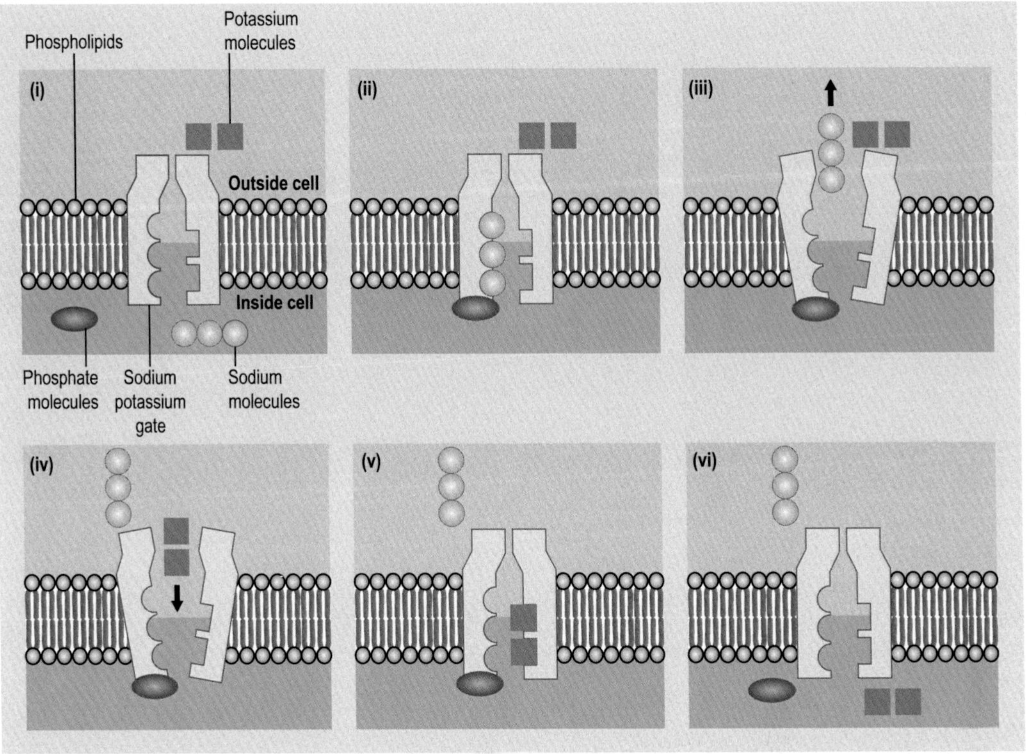
Phospholipids
Potassium molecules
(i)
(ii)
(iii)
Outside cell
Inside cell
Phosphate molecules
Sodium potassium gate
Sodium molecules
(iv)
(v)
(vi)

Figure 31.1 The sodium–potassium pump mechanism. (i) Sodium pump before phosphorylation. (ii) Sodium pump after phosphorylation (which provides the energy for the pump); sodium moves into the gate. (iii) The gate opens and sodium moves out. (iv) Potassium moves in. (v) The gate closes. (vi) The concentrations of potassium and sodium are reversed temporarily until (i) is restored by normal movement down the concentration gradient.

is a **potential difference across the cell membrane**, known as the **resting potential**. To produce an action potential (Figure 31.2):

(i) The normal resting potential of a cell membrane is −60 to −70 mV, which means the inside of the cell is 60 to 70 mV less than the outside. If the membrane of the cell suddenly becomes more permeable to the ions then this situation will change. Permeability to ions is selective and occurs through ion channels, which will only permit certain ions to pass through them. Once the channel is open, the ion will pass either in or out of the cell down the concentration gradient. This dramatically changes the potential across the cell membrane.

(ii) In a nerve or muscle cell, if the ion channel for sodium is opened the sodium floods into the cell down the concentration gradient, taking its positive charge with it. The potential difference across the membrane now becomes positive. In other words, the inside of the cell becomes more positive than the outside. This is the **depolarization phase**. When the membrane reaches a certain **threshold level**, the nerve cell fires or the muscle cell contracts; if this threshold level is not reached, the nerve cell will not fire and the muscle cell will not contract. The size of the action potential (the spike in Figure 31.2) that is produced when the threshold level is reached is fixed; the action potential always fires at this size. This is **the all-or-none principle**.

(iii) When the action potential has been produced, the sodium gates start to close and the potential difference across the membrane opens the potassium gates, which allow potassium to flood out of the cell. This is the **repolarization phase**.

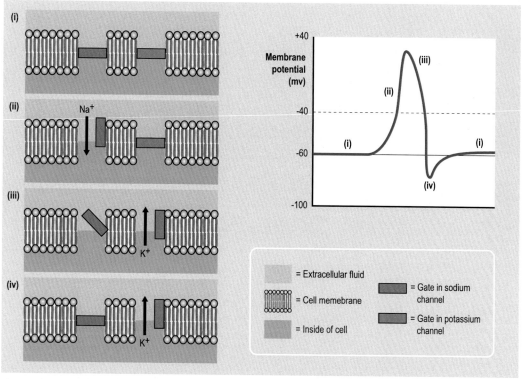

Figure 31.2 The function of ion channels due to membrane potential (see text for explanation).

(iv) There is an overshoot, until the voltage across the membrane closes the potassium gate allowing the sodium–potassium pump to restore the balance once again (i). Blockage of these channels can be achieved by local anaesthetics (see Chapter 32 'Analgesia and relief of pain', p. 254) and some anticonvulsant medication (Chapter 33 'Neurological disease', p. 255).

Muscle Contraction

The action potential activates the voltage-gated calcium ion channels (channels opened by change in voltage across them) on the end of the axon at the synapse. The principle is very much the same as that for the sodium–potassium channel. Calcium enters the axon membranes, stimulating the release of the neurotransmitter acetylcholine into the neuromuscular synapse. This is taken up by the **nicotinic receptors** (see below) on the motor endplate. The sodium and potassium ion channels then open, allowing the sodium into the endplate and the potassium out. As the membrane is more permeable to sodium, the amount of sodium entering the cell is greater than the potassium leaving it, making the overall charge on the inside of the cell more positive. This action potential then spreads through the T-tubule network of the muscle fibres, ultimately releasing calcium ions from the endoplasmic reticulum in the muscle cells.

The actin filaments in the muscle cells are composed of three protein components:

- Actin strands: which are wrapped around one another.
- Tropomyosin.
- Troponin: which is actually three loosely bound protein subunits that normally block the actin myosin-binding sites.

Figure 31.3 illustrates the process of muscle contraction. In (i) and (ii), the released calcium ions interact with the troponin units, making them change shape and allowing the tropomyosin to slide out of its groove to expose the actin myosin-binding

237

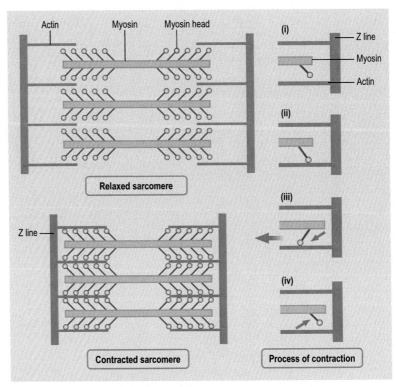

Figure 31.3 The process of muscle contraction.

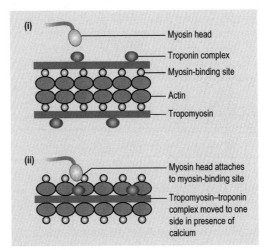

Figure 31.4 The action of the tropomyosin–troponin complex: the myosin head to attaches to myosin binding sites on the actin filament.

sites and allow the cross-bridge components of the myosin to interact with the actin (Figure 31.4). Figure 31.3(iii) shows how this interaction results in the head of the myosin tilting towards the arm and dragging the actin filament with it (the **power stroke**). At the end of this power stroke (iv) the myosin head is cocked back. Adenosine triphosphate (ATP) is released and binds to the myosin head, releasing it from the actin filament. The myosin head swings back ready to attach again and take another power stroke. In this way, the filaments are walked past one another, or 'ratcheted'. The cross-bridges are reputed to work independently, each one attaching, pulling along and detaching in a continuous cycle.

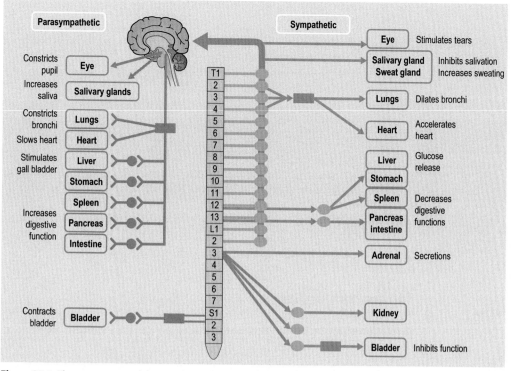

Figure 31.5 The components of the autonomic nervous system.

As the action potential passes, the calcium ions are pumped back into the sarcoplasmic reticulum and, **as the calcium is removed from the muscle fibres, the muscle relaxes**. The theory is that, the greater number of cross-bridges that are attached at one time, the greater the force of contraction. All this is very energy dependent; the power source is ATP (see Figure 12.3, p. 91).

Rigor Mortis

When the energy source is depleted and the calcium is pumped back into the endoplasmic reticulum to be stored once more, the muscle fibres change configuration, blocking the binding sites and the contraction ceases.

In **rigor mortis**, the calcium levels inside the muscle cells rise and the body's ATP levels drop. At high levels of calcium, the myosin cross-bridges bind to the actin, contracting the muscles. As there is no ATP to reset the cross-bridges, the muscles remain contracted.

The Autonomic Nervous System

The sympathetic and parasympathetic nervous systems comprise the autonomic nervous system. The physical and chemical arrangement of each differs (Figure 31.5). Both systems use neurotransmitters.

Sympathetic Nervous System

This is arranged in two parts:

- The cell bodies of the **preganglionic neuron** originate in the thoracic and lumbar areas of the spinal cord.
- After the synapse, the next group of neurons, the **postganglionic neurons**, are located near to the spinal cord. It is this set of neurons that goes on to the 'target organ', e.g. lungs, heart.

The sympathetic nervous system therefore involves two synapses, each with a different transmitter:

- Between the preganglionic and postganglionic neurons (near the spinal cord): acetylcholine is the neurotransmitter.
- Between the postganglionic neuron and the target organ: noradrenaline (norepinephrine) is the neurotransmitter.

Parasympathetic Nervous System

Is also arranged in two parts:

- The cell bodies of the parasympathetic nervous system are located in the spinal cord at the sacral region and in the medulla. The cranial nerves III, VIII, IX and X form the preganglionic neurons. These go a long way, almost to the target organ, before they form a synapse.
- The postganglionic neuron is therefore very short before it embeds itself into the target organ.

Both synapses in the parasympathetic nervous system use acetylcholine.

Neurotransmitters

Neurotransmitters are chemicals that enable neurons to pass signals to each other. There are three main groups:

- **Amino acids**: the two main amino acid neurotransmitters are glutamate (excitatory) and gamma amino butyric acid (GABA) (inhibitory) (Figures 31.6 and 31.7). GABA is produced from glutamate. These transmitters are involved in epilepsy and brain damage due to ischaemia.
- **Peptides**:
  - **Endorphins**: chemicals produced by the body and which resemble opiate drugs both in structure and in effects, which enables them to contribute to pain relief and perhaps to some pleasurable emotions (hence 'runner's high').
  - **Substance P**: works on sensory C-type nerve fibres and is responsible for mediating pain transmission from the peripheral nerves to the spinal cord. Depletion of substance P does not occur immediately but requires a topical preparation to be applied 4–5 times a day for a period of 4 weeks.
  - **Capsaicin**: the pungent principal of *Capsicum* (chilli pepper) is traditionally applied topically to arthritic joints. It works by causing a depletion of substance P from the local sensory C-type fibres.
- **Monoamines**: noradrenaline (norepinephrine), dopamine, serotonin and acetylcholine. **Catecholamines** are derived from phenylalanine. Tyrosine is a subdivision of the monoamines that encompasses any compounds whose structure usually contains a catechol nucleus (see Chapter 7 'Free radicals', p. 47) and an amine group. Noradrenaline (norepinephrine), adrenaline (epinephrine) and dopamine are examples.

Phytochemistry note: alkaloids, such as atropine and **scopolamine (hyoscine)** and **ephedrine**, bind to the **muscarinic receptors** in the nervous system, where they compete with acetylcholine.

Pharmacology in the Central Nervous System

The function of the peripheral nervous system (PNS) is a great deal less complicated than that of the brain. The PNS utilizes acetylcholine and noradrenaline (norepinephrine) as its neurotransmitters; the brain has many more neurotransmitters

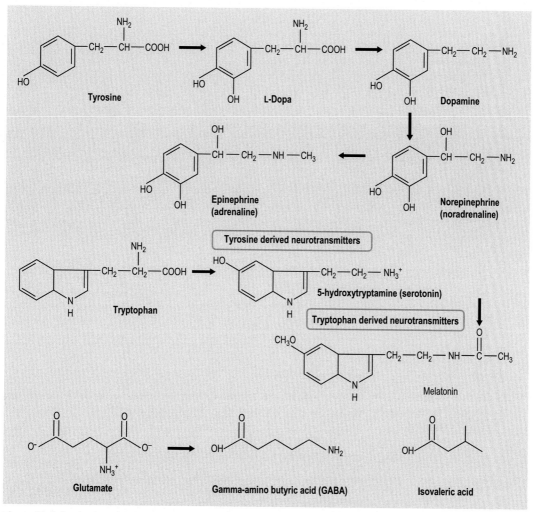

Figure 31.6 Production of various neurotransmitters and isovaleric acid found in valerian, which is structurally similar to gamma-amino butyric acid (GABA).

because it is required to manage some very complicated functions, such as emotion. Not only are the transmitters in the central nervous system more diverse, but so are their actions:

- Some neurotransmitters excite (glutamic acid) whereas others inhibit (GABA).
- Some neurotransmitters have different functions depending on the area of the brain they are working on; dopamine is a prime example.
- The type of receptor can affect the speed of the transmission: acetylcholine acts on two different types of receptor, **nicotinic** and **muscarinic**. Each produces different pharmacological and physiological responses. **Nicotinic receptors work very quickly** whereas the **muscarinic receptors** act through an intermediary system, and therefore **work more slowly.**

Amino Acids

• Glutamate

- A major excitatory neurotransmitter that is associated with learning and memory.
- Thought to be associated with Alzheimer's disease, the first symptoms of which include memory malfunctions.

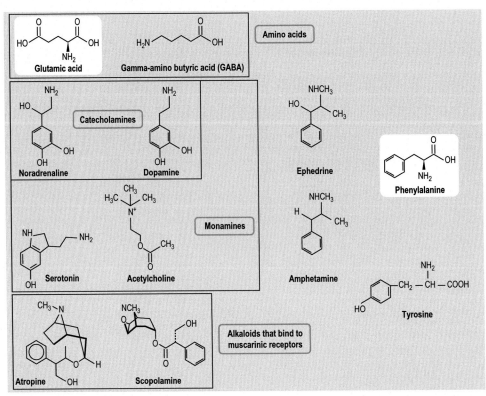

Figure 31.7 Neurotransmitters, including ephedrine (from *Ephedra* spp.) and amphetamine, which interact with noradrenaline (norepinephrine) receptors and two phytochemicals (atropine and scopolamine) that interact with acetylcholine receptors.

• Gamma-Amino Butyric Acid (GABA)

- An inhibitory neurotransmitter that is very widely distributed in the neurons of the cortex and which contributes to motor control, vision and many other functions of the cortex. In other words, it acts as a 'brake' on the nervous system.
- Varying levels can affect the degree of anxiety of an individual: drugs for epilepsy and patients suffering from Huntington's disease increase the level of GABA in the brain.

Peptides

- The opioids bind to the postsynaptic receptors activated by opium. This and its derivatives are very useful in analgesia.
- Opioid peptides are widely distributed throughout the brain and are often located with other small-molecule neurotransmitters such as GABA and serotonin (5-hydroxytryptamine; 5-HT). These opioid peptides tend to be depressants.
- Endogenous of opioids are also involved in complex behaviours such as sexual attraction and aggressive/submissive behaviours. They might also be involved in psychiatric disorders such as schizophrenia and autism, although this is still a topic of heated debate.
- Constant stimulation of the opioid receptors can lead to addiction.
- The opioid system is still not properly understood.

Monoamines

• Dopamine

The **basal ganglia** (Figure 31.8) are a collection of nuclei embedded deep in the white matter of the cerebral cortex. The substantia nigra is a part of the basal ganglia. The

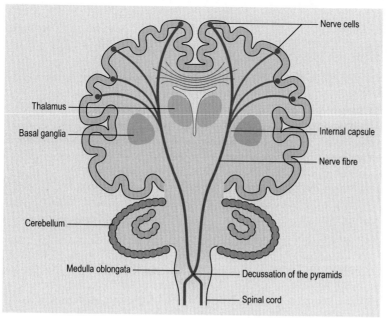

Figure 31.8 Location of the basal ganglia.

ganglia are responsible, with the cerebellum, for organizing movement on a moment-to-moment basis (hence the problems associated with Parkinson's disease).

Dopamine (DA) is concentrated in the basal ganglia. If levels of dopamine are not optimal, movements are jerky, clumsy and uncoordinated. Dopaminergic neurons are widespread in the brain and distribute in three dopamine pathways. The main dopamine-containing area of the brain is the substantia nigra, which is important in body movements.

Dopamine is synthesized in neurons in the substantia nigra from L-dopa (**levodopa**), which is used for treating Parkinson's disease. **Dopa decarboxylase inhibitor** has to be given to prevent metabolism of L-dopa before it can have a therapeutic effect.

Drugs Enhancing Dopamine Activity

Used for:

- Parkinson's disease: decreased levels of dopamine are present in Parkinson's disease.
- Chorea.
- Dystonia.
- Hallucinations and delusions.
- Antiemetic activity.

Drugs Reducing Dopamine Activity

Used in:

- Schizophrenia; overactivity at dopamine synapses is associated with schizophrenia.
- Delusion.
- Chorea.
- Parkinsonism.
- Tics.
- Nausea.
- Vertigo.

Cocaine and amphetamines increase activity at dopamine synapses.

Dopamine is a contributor to voluntary movement and pleasurable emotions, depending on which receptor it acts on.

Serotonin (5-hydroxytryptamine (5-HT))

Serotonin is synthesized from the amino acid **tryptophan**. There are several types of serotonin receptor, and drugs act on these receptors in several different ways:

- **Agonists**: lithium, sumatriptan.
- **Partial agonists**: buspirone, LSD (lysergic acid).
- **Antagonists**: e.g. clozapine, the antagonists have different degrees of ability to occupy sites.
- **Re-uptake** inhibitors: fluoxetine, sertraline, venlafaxine, MDMA (methylenedioxy methamphetamine; ecstasy).

Actions of Serotonin

The CNS contains less than 2% of the total serotonin in the body. It is mainly localized in the neurons emerging from a group of nuclei at the centre in the midbrain, pons and medulla. The pathways then branch out over much of the CNS. Serotonin is thought to be involved in many brain disorders. Serotonin is also involved in the regulation of sleep and wakefulness, eating and aggression, pain perception, body temperature, blood pressure and hormonal activity.

Low serotonin levels are thought to create insomnia and depression. Abnormal levels are thought to contribute to depression and obsessive–compulsive disorder.

Histamine

This potent agent is believed to be involved in the regulation of sleeping and waking states.

Noradrenaline (Norepinephrine) and Adrenaline (Epinephrine)

There are four types of adrenoreceptor, alpha-1, alpha-2, beta-1 and beta-2:

- Alpha receptor stimulation: leads to vasoconstriction of the arterioles and pupillary dilation.
- Beta-1 receptor stimulation: leads to an increase in pulse and contractility of the heart.
- Beta-2 receptor stimulation: leads to bronchodilatation, uterine relaxation and arteriolar vasodilatation.

Drugs enhancing adrenergic activity are used in asthma (adrenaline administrated in emergency) and heart failure. Interestingly monoamine oxidase inhibitors (MAOIs) and tricyclic antidepressants (TCAs; see Chapter 33 'Neurological disease', p. 262) are thought to act by increasing synaptic noradrenaline (norepinephrine) in the CNS.

Drugs that reduce adrenergic activity are used in angina, hypertension, arrhythmias, thyrotoxicosis anxiety. Cocaine and amphetamines increase the activity at nerve-ending synapses.

Action of Noradrenaline (Norepinephrine)

Noradrenaline (norepinephrine) is found in cell bodies in the pons and medulla. These bodies project neurons to the hypothalamus, thalamus, limbic system and cerebral cortex. It comes as no great surprise, therefore, to discover that noradrenaline contributes to control of mood and arousal and can affect sleep patterns.

Depletion of noradrenaline (norepinephrine) in the brain has been shown to cause a decrease in drive and motivation and might be linked to depression. It is part of the 'fight or flight' response, which increases heart rate, etc.

Ephedra spp. (Ma Huang)

Ephedrine:

- Displaces noradrenaline (norepinephrine) from storage vesicles in presynaptic neurons.
- The displaced noradrenaline (norepinephrine) is released in large quantities into the synapse, where it activates the adrenergic receptors.

Amphetamine (Figure 31.7) works in a similar way, to cause:

- Increased heart rate.
- Bronchodilation by acting as a bronchial muscle relaxant, hence its use in asthma.
- Vasoconstriction of the blood vessels leading to raised blood pressure.

Ephedrine has moderately potent bronchial muscle relaxant properties and is therefore used for symptomatic relief in milder cases of asthmatic attacks. It is also used to reduce the risk of acute attacks in the treatment of chronic asthma.

High doses of *Ephedra* (*Ma Huang*) can cause:

- restlessness and anxiety
- dizziness
- insomnia
- tremor
- rapid pulse
- sweating
- respiratory difficulties
- confusion
- hallucinations
- delirium
- convulsions.

Points to note:

- High blood pressure and rapid irregular heart rate are very dangerous symptoms.
- This can be brought about by only two or three times the therapeutic dose.
- The elderly are particularly sensitive to overdose.
- There have been instances of psychosis similar to amphetamine psychosis.

Drug interactions include:

- digoxin
- antihypertensives such as beta-blockers.
- monoamine oxidase inhibitors (MAOI)
- other neurotransmitter-related drugs.

• Acetylcholine (Muscarinic and Nicotinic Receptors)

There are two types of acetylcholine receptor, which are named for the substances that block them:

- muscarinic
- nicotinic.

Although acetylcholine sets off each response, the different types of receptor are responsible for a different physiological effect:

Nicotinic

- Fast onset (voltage-gated receptor, therefore fast acting).

- Short duration.
- Excitatory.
- Blocked by the alkaloid nicotine.

Muscarinic

- G protein, therefore slower (see Chapter 19 'Pharmacodynamics: how drugs elicit a physiological response', p. 141).
- Excitation or inhibition.
- Blocked by the alkaloid muscarine.

The cholinergic pathways in the specific regions of the brainstem are thought to be involved in cognitive function, particularly memory. Alzheimer's disease is thought to be due to advanced damaged of these pathways.

Peripherally, acetylcholine is the main neurotransmitter of the parasympathetic nervous system. This is why some of the antidepressants that block cholinergic receptors have the side effect of a dry mouth: the salivary glands are not stimulated to produce saliva.

- **Centrally acting anticholinergic drugs used in**: parkinsonism, dystonias, motion sickness.
- **Peripheral antimuscarinic drugs used in**: asthma, incontinence, pupil dilation (so that the interior of the eye can be more easily examined).
- **Peripheral cholinergic agonist used in**: glaucoma (pilocarpine from the *Pilocarpus* spp.; see also carbonic anhydrase inhibitors, Figure 26.5, p. 198 for different approach), myasthenias.
- **Atropine**, a tropane alkaloid (see Figure 23.4, p. 178) extracted from *Atropa belladonna* (deadly nightshade) is used to open the iris for examination or surgical procedures.

Analgesia and relief of pain

32

Pain is a very necessary sensation as its purpose is to signal harm to an organism. It allows the organism to adapt to its surroundings so that it can remove itself from the sensation or in the case of humans actively resolve the problem by treatment.

All pain receptors are free nerve endings and are called **nociceptors.** These are part of the process that transmits the pain to the brain (the process of **nociception**). Various sensory receptors found throughout the body react to a variety of stimuli, such as hot, cold, pressure and chemical, all of which can give the patient the subjective experience of pain. Different types of neuron carry the pain signal to the central nervous system (CNS):

- **First-order neurons**: transmit pain impulses. There are two subtypes:
  - rapidly conducting (12–30 m/s), myelinated A fibres
  - slow conducting (0.5–2 m/s) non-myelinated C fibres.
  These terminate in the dorsal (posterior) columns of the spinal cord (Figure 32.1).
- **Second-order neurons**: carry the pain stimuli to the **thalamus** (Figure 32.2) via the **lateral spinothalamic tracts.**

Synapses are formed by both A and C fibres in the dorsal horns (dorsal or posterior columns) of the spinal cord. There is also regulation of the transmission between the nociceptive neurons and those in the spinothalamic tract. Descending fibres from the higher centres can inhibit transmission.

- **Third-order neurons** go from the thalamus to the cerebral cortex. The thalamus plays a large role in the integration of pain input, whereas the cortical area deals with the meaningful subjective interpretation of pain and can in some cases override the sensation of pain.

The various pain stimuli are:

- Mechanical.
- Thermal.
- Chemical: can be triggered chemically at the free nerve ending by changes in the concentration of hydrogen ions (H^+), serotonin (5-hydroxytryptamine (5-HT)), histamine, bradykinin and eicosanoids (see Figure 32.3, p. 249).

247

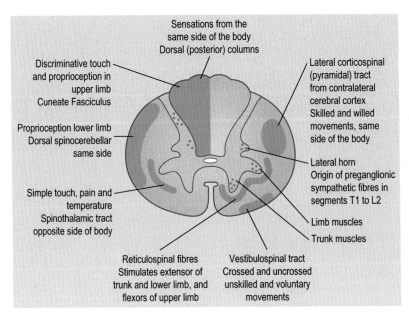

Figure 32.1 Anatomy of the spinal cord, showing related sensory and motor areas.

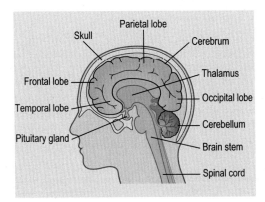

Figure 32.2 Cross-section of the brain and upper spinal cord.

Bradykinin (Figure 32.3) is released when tissue is damaged and so is found in inflammatory processes, e.g. joint inflammation. It stimulates and sensitizes nerve endings, which leads to the stimulus that registers pain with the body. Anti-inflammatories and aspirin inhibit prostaglandin synthesis and therefore the release of mediators that create pain (see Chapter 30 'Inflammation and the immune system', p. 228).

Analgesics

Sites of Action

- At the site of injury, by decreasing the pain caused by an inflammatory reaction: **aspirin, non-steroidal anti-inflammatories.**
- In neurons, to alter the way the nerve conducts: **local anaesthetics.**
- In synapses in the dorsal horn: **opioids and antidepressants.**
- At the level of the brain by affecting the perception of pain: **opioids and antidepressants.**

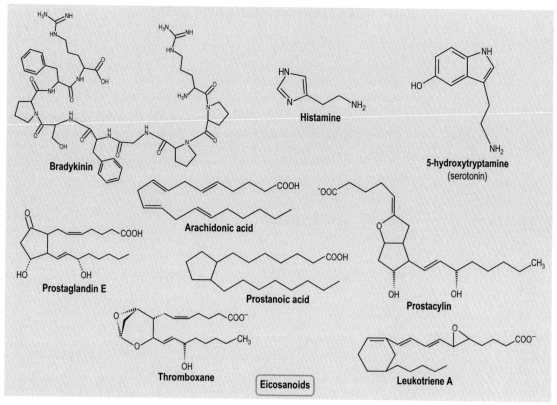

Figure 32.3 Pain stimulants.

Terminology

- **Analgesia**: refers to the specific blocking of the pain receptors, leaving the function of other receptors, such as touch and temperature, intact.
- **Anaesthesia**: the blocking of all sensations.

Opioid Receptors

• Location

- Substantia gelatinosa (in the dorsal or posterior column) and central grey matter of the brainstem.

• Subgroups

- **Mu and kappa receptors**: these are responsible for analgesia and respiratory depression.
- **Delta receptors**: bind endogenous opiates such as enkephalins, endorphins and dynorphins. These are released as neurotransmitters from specific opiate-containing neurons and modify pain sensation. This quality is exploited by morphine-like drugs.

Pain Pathway Transmitters

- Substance P: see Chapter 31 'The nervous system' (p. 235).
- Other opioid peptides: see Chapter 31 'The nervous system' (p. 235).
- 5-HT (serotonin): see Chapter 31 'The nervous system' (p. 235).
- Excitatory amino acids: see Chapter 31 'The nervous system' (p. 241).

Principles Behind Analgesic Drugs

There are two types of pain:

- **Visceral**: dull, poorly localized pain, e.g. abdominal pain arising from the peritoneum.
- **Somatic:** sharply defined, e.g. from a cut on the skin, or a broken bone.

Pain is useful, to a point, because it makes us aware of a diseased organ or damage to the body. **Congenital analgesia (congenital insensitivity to pain)** is a rare condition in which sufferers do not feel any pain, which makes it life threatening. This is because it is difficult for them to register that they have damaged themselves or have a visceral disease such as peritonitis.

Specific Analgesics

Paracetamol

Paracetamol (Figure 32.4) acts largely as a painkiller and has very little effect on inflammation.

- ## Side Effects

  - Allergic skin reactions.
  - Paracetamol in large doses can be lethal (see Chapter 7 'Free radicals', p. 49).

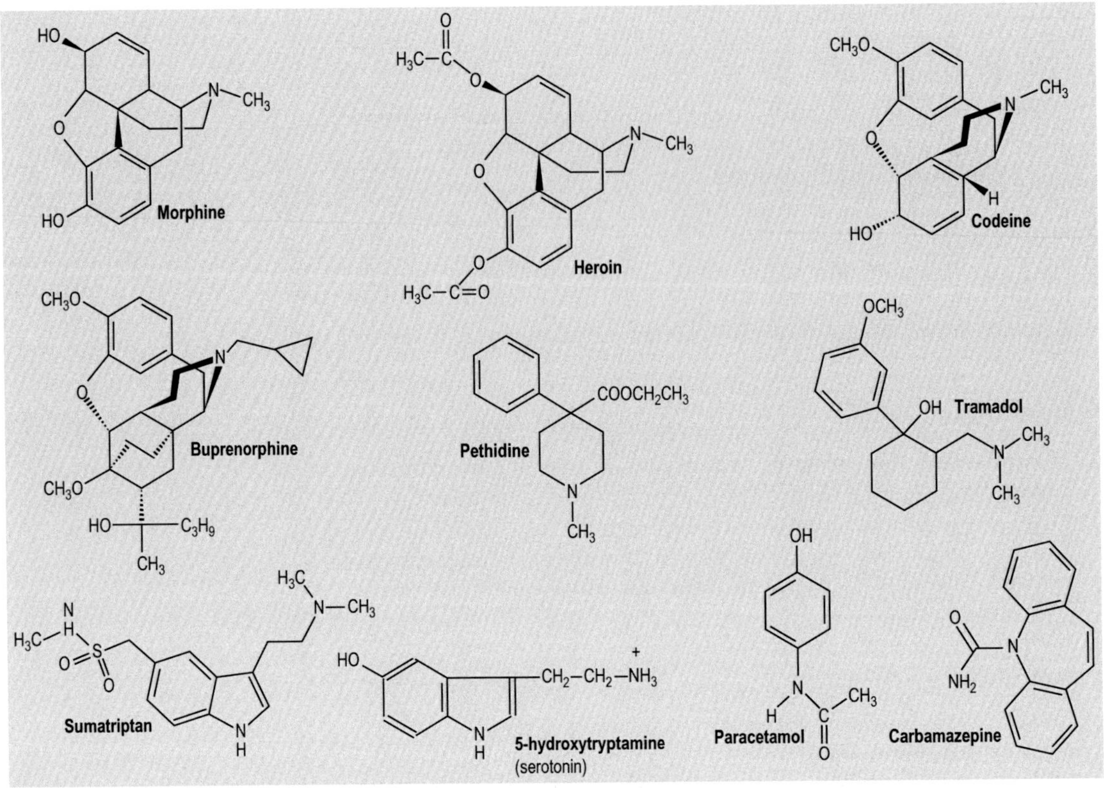

Figure 32.4 Chemical structures of painkillers.

Opioid Analgesics

The opiate-based drugs alter the perception and response to pain.

• Morphine

Morphine has a depressant effect on the body by acting centrally on the mu opiate receptors in the CNS and peripheral tissues. CNS effects (general opioid action including derivatives to a lesser degree) are:

- Analgesia: including euphoria and sedation. Particularly useful if a patient is terminal or in a great amount of pain.
- Depression of the vasomotor centre: leading to hypotension.
- Depression of respiration and cough suppression: very dangerous, particularly in the critically ill and the elderly.
- Release of antidiuretic hormone: decreases the urination of the patient leading to urinary retention.
- Miosis (constriction of the pupil of the eye).
- Peripheral effects: smooth muscle contraction as opposed to striated, which is the voluntary muscles.
- Reduced motility of the gastrointestinal tract with accompanying reduced secretion: for this reason, many morphine-derived preparations cause constipation.
- Biliary spasm.
- Constriction of the bronchi partly as a result of histamine release: this adds to the problem of the breathing induced by morphine's action on the CNS.
- Vasodilatation: a flushing on the skin and itching.
- Nausea and vomiting.

A slow-release oral form is usually used because morphine has a high first-pass metabolism. About 90% of the dose leaves the body within 24 hours.

Adverse Effects

These are usually an extension of the pharmacological effects:

- problems breathing
- hypotension
- nausea and vomiting
- constipation
- tremor
- skin reaction and itching
- addiction to the drug and tolerance if used over a long period of time.

Types of Morphine Administration

Oral

Not the most effective way to give lasting relief because morphine is subject to a high first-pass metabolism (see Chapter 17 'Metabolism', p. 129). Manufacturers have, however, produced a slow-release oral preparation.

Intravenous

This is **the usual route of administration**. In terminal cases, use is made of a pump system that patients can operate independently when pain relief is required. Otherwise morphine can be given intramuscularly or subcutaneously. Very little of the administered drug crosses the well-protected blood–brain barrier. What medication does get there peaks between 30 and 45 minutes after administration.

Drug Interactions

- Morphine delays the absorption of other orally administered drugs.
- Its depressant effects are potentiated by phenothiazines such as chlorpromazine, which are used as antiemetics, and migraine medication and tricyclic antidepressants such as dosulepin.
- Morphine potentiates most hypnotics, e.g. diazepam and some anaesthetics.

Uses

- Pain relievers: visceral and traumatic.
- Cough suppressants: codeine derivatives are used in some cough mixtures, hence it is possible to get addicted to the cough mixtures.
- Antidiarrhoeal agents: not used so much now. Kaolin and morphine used to be used. Kaolin is a clay, which was used to line the gut, acting as a physical barrier to prevent more water loss; the morphine slowed down gut contractions.

• Other Opioid Derivatives

Heroin

- Is more lipid soluble than morphine. As a result, it is absorbed much more easily by phospholipid membranes of cells.
- Is ultimately metabolized in the body to morphine.
- Its abuse is well documented.

Codeine

- Its properties are similar to morphine, but it is a less powerful analgesic.
- Is used as a cough suppressant in cough mixtures.
- Can control diarrhoea.
- Is combined with aspirin or paracetamol as an analgesic.
- Metabolized to morphine in the body.

Pethidine

- Pethidine is a type of opioid.
- Often used as a short-acting pain reliever, particularly in childbirth or biliary and ureteric colic.

Opiate Partial Agonists and Opiate Antagonists

• Buprenorphine

- A partial agonist of mu opiate receptors but acts as an antagonist on kappa receptors (see Chapter 19 'Pharmacodynamics: how drugs elicit a physiological effect', p. 140 and Chapter 32 'Analgesia and pain relief', p. 249).
- Has such a high affinity for the receptors that it is difficult to antidote in the case of an overdose.
- It is a potent and long-lasting analgesic.
- Used as a substitute for management of heroin addicts.

Adverse Effects

Similar to opioids.

• Tramadol

- Acts as a partial agonist, which creates only a partial physiological response (see Chapter 19 'Pharmacodynamics: how drugs elicit a physiological effect', p. 140) at the mu receptors and by activating 5-HT and noradrenaline (norepinephrine) pathways. Pain is therefore inhibited at a spinal level.

- Low occurrence of respiratory depression and low potential for abuse make this a useful drug for pain relief.
- Can have side effects of nausea and vomiting.

Carbamazepine (Tegretol)

- Maintains the sodium channels in a closed position, meaning that neurons in the brain become less excitable, thus calming the nervous system and the patient.
- Also used for schizophrenia and bipolar disorders, but at much higher doses.

Adverse Effects

- Drowsiness.
- Fatigue.
- Headache.
- Diplopia (double vision).
- Ataxia.
- Vertigo.
- Dizziness.
- Nausea and vomiting.
- Dry mouth.
- Allergic skin reactions.
- Effects on the formation of blood cells.
- Oedema and fluid retention.

Drug Interactions

- Various antibiotics.
- Drugs working on the nervous system.
- Steroids.
- Cardiac medication.
- Potential for interactions with a wide variety of herbs and supplements.

Migraine Medication

Migraine is a debilitating condition characterized by severe headaches and various other symptoms such as vomiting. It affects about 10% of the population in the UK. The majority of sufferers are women and there appears to be a relationship between the menstrual cycle and migraine attacks. The current theory is that there is a sudden vasodilatation of cranial blood vessels, but the overall cause is not well understood.

Treatment

NSAIDs and opiate-based painkillers can be used in some cases; otherwise specialized migraine medication has to be used.

Triptans

- The best known is sumatriptan (Imigran; see Figure 32.4), used in the acute stage of the attacks. They are not useful as prophylactics.
- **Selective 5-HT (serotonin) agonists**: 5-HT is thought to act as a mediator for migraine headache. The triptans either cause constriction of the intracranial blood vessels, leading to a reduction of pressure, or they block the release of proinflammatory neuropeptides from presynaptic nerve terminals.

- Triptans such as sumitriptan can be sprayed up the nose; this is useful in patients who are prone to vomiting.
- Antiemetics can also be used if vomiting is severe.

Adverse Effects

- Drowsiness.
- Transient increase in blood pressure.
- Hypotension.
- Bradycardia or tachycardia.
- Visual disturbances.

Local Anaesthetics

Lidocaine and novocaine are sodium-channel blockers (see Figure 19.6, p. 141 and Figure 31.2, p. 237). When sodium is not allowed to move through the channels, depolarization in the neurons is no longer possible. This means that the neuron will be unable to transmit an action potential; it is this that creates the anaesthesia.

Neurological disease

33

Chapter contents

Epilepsy

- Occurs because of abnormal discharges by the cortical neurons.
- Patients may experience recurrent seizures for which there is no apparent cause.

The different epileptic syndromes are divided into two main types:

- Partial seizures.
- Generalized seizures: tonic–clonic (grand mal) and absence (petit mal) seizures are the most commonly known.

The highest rates of epilepsy are in children and elderly people.

The neurotransmitters involved in epilepsy are largely amines. Drugs associated with neurological disease tend to be a type of amine, which is why plant alkaloids can have a similar effect (see Chapter 23 'Amines and alkaloids', p. 175).

Aetiology

- Cerebrovascular disease.
- Cerebral tumours.
- Genetic.
- Congenital.
- Alcohol.
- Drugs.
- Toxins.

- Head trauma.
- Encephalitis.
- Meningitis.

Diagnosis

- Blood tests: might indicate an underlying metabolic disorder.
- Magnetic resonance imaging: looks for lesions on the brain.
- Electroencephalography: looks for abnormalities in electrical activity of the brain and can be used to support the diagnosis.

Treatment

The drug is matched to the individual patient and the type of epileptic seizures. Between 70 and 80% of epileptic patients will become seizure free with the appropriate medication.

General Discussion of Medication

The aim is to treat the patient without causing side effects and using a single drug. **Sodium valproate** is usually the drug of choice. **Carbamazepine** (Tegretol or Carbatrol; see Figure 33.5) and **phenytoin** (Dilantin or Phenytek) can be used in its place, but are considered alternatives.

Lamotrigine is now rapidly becoming a drug of choice, as it does not need constant monitoring and has relatively few side-effects.

Carbamazepine is the drug of choice for partial seizures. It is a **tricyclic antidepressant derivative** and is thought to work by blocking the calcium and sodium channels on the neurons (see Chapter 31 'The nervous system', p. 237). Because of this, it has been used in neuralgias and certain types of dystonia. Because it induces its own metabolism (it is an enzyme inducer) its half-life can fall dramatically during chronic administration. It is therefore started at a low dose, which is gradually increased.

Ethosuximide is used instead of **sodium valproate** for absence (petit mal) seizures.

Phenobarbital is now only used when other treatments fail; it is an inexpensive medication.

Pharmacokinetics of Anticonvulsants

Anticonvulsants tend to have interactions with a wide range of drugs, but particularly those that bind to the plasma proteins (see Chapter 16 'How do drugs get into cells?', p. 126) or those metabolized by the liver (see Chapter 17 'Metabolism', p. 129).

One of the problems is that they can increase the chances of toxicity without increasing the antiepileptic effect. Supplements or herbal treatment do, therefore, have the potential to interact with these powerful drugs. Valproate and newer antiepileptic drugs do not require such careful monitoring of the plasma levels, but the newer drugs are expensive and tend to be used not in isolation but with other drugs that have reached their optimum dosage and are not having the required effect.

A third of patients will need more than one drug to keep the condition under control.

• Adverse Effects

These vary greatly with each type of medication. Adverse effects of the two most common treatments are outlined below:

Carbamazepine

- Measles-like rash.
- Rare idiosyncratic risk of bone marrow supression (leukopenia and thrombocytopenia; see Chapter 28 'Blood disorders', p. 211).

- Liver disorders.
- Vestibulocerebellar symptoms in acute toxicity (usually result in dizziness).
- Cognitive and behavioural effects.
- Paradoxic seizures as a symptom of toxicity.

Valproate

Valproate is well absorbed, readily bound to protein and is metabolized by the liver; it is therefore contraindicated in active liver disease and porphyria. Regular liver function tests have to be performed in the first 6 months of therapy.

Parkinson's Disease

- A progressive, chronic, age-related disease.
- Affects movement, cognitive function, emotion and autonomic function.
- Develops predominantly in the elderly.
- A genetic factor might be involved in those who develop it at or before the age of 50 years.
- There is difficulty in walking, accompanied by rigidity and tremor.
- The diagnosis is made clinically and is often difficult.
- Characterized by the classic triad of bradykinesia, rigidity and tremor due to lesions in the pyramidal tract (see Figure 32.1, p. 248).

Aetiology

The substantia nigra deteriorates. This is the area of the brain that sends signals down the spinal cord to control the muscles of the body. Dopamine, the main neurotransmitter, is made by the cells of the substantia nigra.

The basal ganglia, the red nucleus, the substantia nigra, the reticular formation and the cerebellum are all part of the extrapyramidal system, which controls gross autonomic motor movement (Figure 33.1). The basal ganglia inhibit the rapid firing of the motor neurons. This control is reduced when the inhibitory function of dopamine is lessened; hence the increase in tremors through lack of inhibition.

Treatment

Dopamine cannot cross the blood–brain barrier and therefore cannot be used as therapy. However, its precursor, **levodopa**, can cross the barrier and enter the brain. Once in the brain, it is converted to dopamine (Figure 33.2), thereby increasing the levels and helping to reduce symptoms. **Dopamine agonists** are used largely in an effort to maintain the dopamine levels in the body.

Adverse Effects

These are extensive:

- anorexia
- nausea and vomiting
- taste disturbance
- postural hypotension (rarely labile hypertension) and dizziness
- tachycardia and arrhythmias
- reddish discoloration of urine and other body fluids
- abnormal involuntary movements
- depression
- drowsiness
- agitation

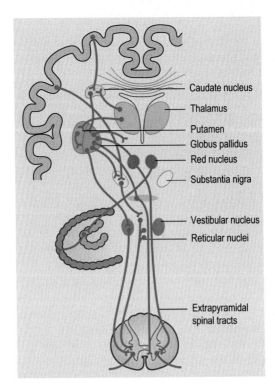

Figure 33.1 The basal nuclei and their linkage to motor tracts.

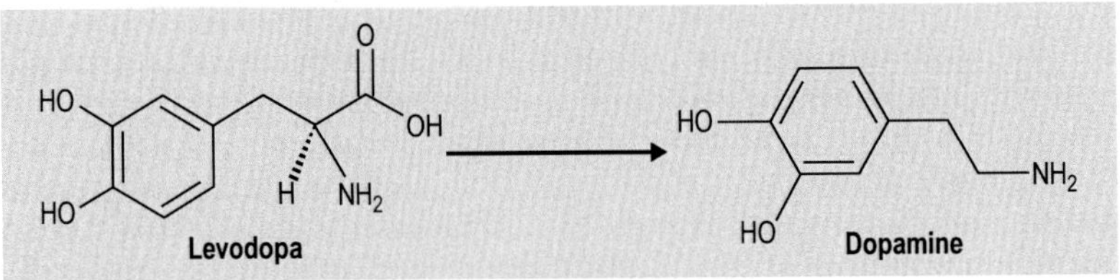

Levodopa — Dopamine

Figure 33.2 The conversion of levodopa to dopamine.

- headache
- insomnia
- flushing and sweating
- gastrointestinal bleeding
- peripheral neuropathy
- pruritus and rash.

Antimuscarinic Drugs

These are used in patients in whom Parkinson's has been induced by antipsychotic drugs or recreational drugs. They reduce the effects of the cholinergic excess in the CNS, which occurs as a result of dopamine deficiency (Figure 33.3).

Tardive dyskinesia (involuntary, jerky movements of the body, limbs and face) is not improved by antimuscarinic drugs, which might even make the condition worse.

Multiple Sclerosis

The exact cause is unknown but it is thought to be due to an autoimmune attack that creates patches of inflammation on the myelin sheath, thus damaging the sheath and impairing the transmission of the signals passing down it.

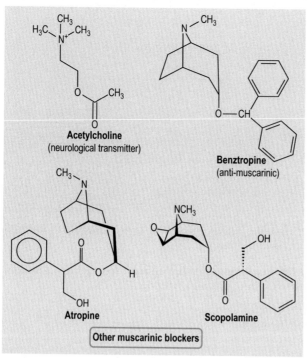

Figure 33.3 Chemical structures of the neurotransmitter acetylcholine, benztropine (an antimuscarinic used to counteract cholinergic symptoms) and other types of muscarinic blocker, demonstrating the similarities between the structures.

As well as corticosteroids and immunomodulatory therapy with interferon, other more unusual methods, such as cannabis sublingual spray, have been used (tetrahyrocannabinol – the active compound – seems to have an effect on various neurotransmitter systems, particularly with the treatment of the spasticity of the muscles in mind).

Myasthenia Gravis

This disease is characterized by episodes of muscle weakness caused by loss or dysfunction of acetylcholine receptors. This is due to an autoimmune attack that destroys or impairs the function of the acetylcholine receptors at the postsynaptic neuromuscular junctions, thus interfering with neuromuscular transmission.

Treatment

- **Anticholinesterases** (Figure 33.4): are reversible, non-competitive or competitive inhibitors of the enzyme that removes acetylcholine from the synapse, thus allowing what receptors there are the greatest possible opportunity to function.
- **Plasmapheresis**: relieves the symptoms. During this process the plasma is removed from blood cells by a cell separator. The separator works either by spinning the blood at high speed to separate the cells from the fluid or by passing the blood through a membrane with pores so small that only the fluid part of the blood can pass through. The cells are returned to the person undergoing treatment; the plasma, which contains the antibodies, is discarded and replaced with other fluids. Medication to keep the blood from clotting (an anticoagulant) is given through a vein during the procedure. This procedure is not used very often.

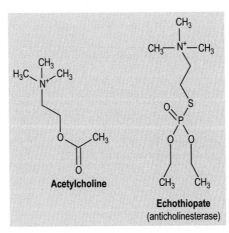

Figure 33.4 Comparison of chemical structures of acetylcholine and an anticholinesterase to demonstrate similarity in structure.

- **Corticosteroids**, **iummunosuppressant** drugs and **thymectomy**: can be used to interfere with the autoimmune pathogenesis.

The Psychoses

The exact mechanism of psychoses is not clear and the mechanism of drug action is still not understood. Overactivity of dopamine is one hypothesis, as increased dopamine concentrations have been found in the brains of treated and untreated patients. But drugs such as clozapine (Figure 33.5), which are classed as atypical and have additional effects, work when the other 'typical' neuroleptics (major tranquillizers) do not. So the dopamine hypothesis is only part of the explanation.

Uses of Neuroleptic Drugs (Antipsychotics, Major Tranquillizers)

The main aim of these drugs is to inhibit extreme behavioural disturbances of psychosis to enable the patient to function as normally as possible in society.

● Schizophrenia

In this case, the drugs are used to try and help the emotional disturbance created by delusional thinking, hallucinations, inappropriate behaviour and anxiety. In chronic cases medication is continuous to prevent a relapse.

● Bipolar Disorders

Neuroleptics in this case control the manic phase and the delusions and anxiety in the depressive phase.

● Drug-Related Disorders

The use of recreational drugs may create psychoses.

Conventional Neuroleptics

● Chlorpromazine

- Can be taken orally.
- Once in the liver it is metabolized into several compounds, some active and some inactive. It has a half-life of over 16 hours. However, as the first pass accounts for 80% of the drug, intramuscular injection is frequently used.

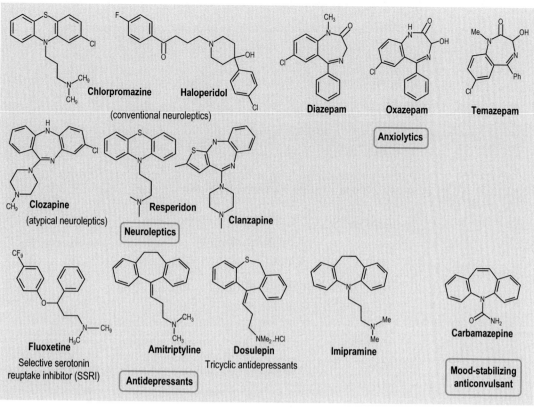

Figure 33.5 Various neurological drugs. Note the similarities in structure.

- Can be used in lower doses to treat nausea and vomiting and some labyrinthine disturbances and during drug-withdrawal reactions.

Adverse Effects

- Dose related:
  - dystonia (slow movement or extended spasm in a group of muscles)
  - parkinsonism
  - **tardive dyskinesia**: due to the effect it has on the extrapryamidal tracts.
  - increased prolactin leading to galactorrhoea, infertility and impotence.
- Hypersensitivity reactions (not related to dose):
  - cholestatic jaundice
  - postural hypotension: due to inhibition of alpha-1 receptors
  - blurred vision, constipation, urinary hesitancy, dry mouth, tachycardia or arrhythmias: due to anticholinergic effects
  - sedation: histamine-1 receptor inhibition
  - hypothermia in the elderly
  - potentially fatal hyperthermia, muscle rigidity and autonomic dysfunction
  - various adverse effects such as confusion, nightmares, insomnia and weight gain.

• Haloperidol

- Fifty times more potent than chlorpromazine.

Adverse Effects

- Similar to chlorpromazine.

New (Atypical) Neuroleptics

Atypical means that the drug produces fewer extrapyramidal symptoms.

• Clozapine

- Best-known drug in this group.
- Has an affinity for 5-HT and D4 receptors (a type of dopamine receptor).
- Tends to be the drug of choice because it can treat patients who do not respond to the conventional neuroleptics.

Adverse Effects

- Along with similar drugs in this group it has a tendency to cause extrapyramidal side effects, particularly **tardive dyskinesia**.
- Weight gain.
- Sedation.

Clozapine tends to be initially restricted to hospitalized patients who can be monitored on a weekly basis.

• Risperidone and Olanzapine

- Similar effects to clozapine.
- These are drugs of preference in patients with a dual diagnosis of drug abuse and psychosis.

• Adverse Effects

Similar to clozapine.

Depression

Clinical depression is characterized by the following:

- despair
- lack of appetite
- insomnia or broken sleep
- weight loss
- delusional behaviour: this is not common, but can occur.

The underlying problem is thought to be a chemical, at the neurotransmitter level, where the actions of noradrenaline (norepinephrine) or 5-HT have an effect. For more detail on neurotransmitters, see Chapter 31 'The nervous system' (p. 240). Antidepressants are used to relieve the symptoms of depression.

Monoamine Oxidase Inhibitors (MAOIs)

- Non-competitive irreversible antagonists (see Chapter 19 'Pharmacodynamics: how drugs elicit a physiological effect', p. 138) of monoamine oxidase type. They break down noradrenaline (norepinephrine) and serotonin, leading to an increase in transmitter activity.
- The enzyme (monoamine oxidase) is inhibited not only in the brain, but also in the peripheral neurons, enterocytes and platelets.
- Inhibition of the enzyme leads to increases in serotonin, noradrenaline (norepinephrine) and dopamine (see Chapter 31 'The nervous system', p. 242) in the brain.
- Because of this widespread inhibition, MAOIs are now used only under tight supervision, for example in patients who are institutionalized and whose diets can be controlled. Other antidepressants tend to be favoured because they have fewer severe side effects.

- It can take 2–3 weeks before enough of the drug accumulates for the effects to be felt, and the same amount again to recover because these are irreversible antagonists and it takes time for the enzyme to be remanufactured.

Adverse Effects

- Postural hypotension.
- Headache.
- Anticholinergic side effects: dry mouth, constipation, sexual dysfunction.
- Drug-induced liver damage.
- Hypertensive crisis: this is noteworthy because it occurs following foods, drinks or drugs containing the amine tyramine (cheese, meat, yeast extract, soy, beer, some wines and many processed foods). Inhibition of the monoamine oxidase enzyme in the gut wall makes it easier to absorb tyramine and other sympathomimetic substances (i.e. simulating an apparent release of noradrenaline-like substances; see Chapter 31 'The nervous system', p. 244) from food.

Herbal remedies, particularly those containing alkaloids, can be detrimental to a patient's health. Amines can displace the normal noradrenaline from the storage sites, which leads to hypertension, tachycardia and headaches. If the rise in blood pressure is severe enough then there is the possibility of a cerebrovascular accident.

Tricyclic Antidepressants

- Amitriptyline, imipramine and dosulepin (dothiepin): have a three-ring structure, hence the name 'tricyclic'.
- Block the reuptake of noradrenaline (norepinephrine) and/or 5-HT by the synapses; therefore, in the short term, they increase the levels of transmitter in the synapse. Long term, this leads to an adaptation by a reduction of the numbers of the pre- and postsynaptic adrenoreceptors and 5-HT receptors in the brain.
- The therapeutic response to the tricyclics develops over 3–4 weeks, so anyone prone to suicidal tendencies has to be carefully monitored in this time.
- Readily metabolized by the liver, but metabolites of the medication can further extend the duration of the drug. Once a day is usually sufficient for tricyclics.
- There is a wide difference in the plasma levels of tricyclics from one person to another: dosage is carefully considered on an individual basis.

Adverse Effects

- Sedation.
- Confused emotional state.
- Anticholinergic effects: e.g. dry mouth, constipation, sexual dysfunction.
- Postural hypotension.
- Cardiac tachyarrhythmia with an overdose.
- Poisoning: tricyclic overdose is common.
- Seizures on withdrawal.

Selective Serotonin Reuptake Inhibitors (SSRIs)

- Inhibit the reuptake of 5-HT in the CNS.
- Have long half-lives (2 days), so need to be given only once a day.
- Less sedative than the tricyclics.

Drug Interactions

Have a synergistic effect on carbamazepine, phenytoin (anticonvulsants), monoamine oxidase inhibitors, benzodiazepines (for anxiety), lithium and probably warfarin.

- ● **Adverse Effects**
  - Nausea.
  - Diarrhoea.
  - Headache.
  - Insomnia.
  - Agitation.

Mania and Hypomania

Patients with mania or hypomania usually have a pathologically elevated mood and lack of inhibitions. This behaviour usually occurs as part of a bipolar disorder.

Mania

Expansive mood with general restlessness and overactivity, non-stop chatter, grandiose ideas and a loss of grip on reality. The manic phase is treated with a heavy-duty tranquillizer. Lithium salts are used both as an acute treatment and prophylactically (because it takes a while to build up).

Anticonvulsive agents such as carbamazepine and sodium valproate are also used as prophylactic agents in bipolar disorders.

- ● **Lithium Carbonate**
  - The mechanism is not clear, but it seems to act as a substitute for sodium and potassium cations (positively charged ions) in cellular transport.
  - Affects the release of monoamine neurotransmitters and alters intra- and extracellular ion concentrations.
  - Rapidly and easily absorbed after being taken orally. It takes 5 days to reach a steady dosage.
  - Not metabolized by the body, being excreted – unchanged – by the kidneys, which means the dosage will have be adjusted for patients with impairment of renal function and also in the elderly. Its therapeutic range is very narrow. The drug is very carefully monitored for optimal control.
  - Dehydration, salt depletion or diuretic therapy increase the concentration of the drug in the blood. Diuretics are an issue because they can make the lithium levels rise.
  - Steroid and angiotensin-converting enzyme (ACE) inhibitors also alter the sodium balance.
  - Large number of drug interactions.

Not used if the patient has:

- severe cardiovascular disease
- renal disease
- severe debilitation
- dehydration
- sodium depletion
- brain damage
- conditions requiring low sodium intake.

Adverse Effects

- Thirst.
- Gastrointestinal discomfort and diarrhoea.
- Nausea and vomiting.
- Anaemia.

- Vertigo.
- Muscle weakness, psychomotor retardation, changes in muscle tone or tension, fine tremor of the hands, loss of muscular coordination.
- Dazed feeling.
- Stupor.
- Acne.
- Increase in amount of urine.
- Fatigue, drowsiness.
- Ringing and/or buzzing of the ears.
- Blurred vision.
- Loss of appetite.
- Restlessness.
- Anaesthesia of the skin.
- Slurred speech.
- Blackout spells.
- Headache.
- Seizures.
- Coma.

Interacts with:

- Medication for asthma, bronchitis, cystic fibrosis, emphysema and sinusitis.
- MAO inhibitors (within 14 days)
- Lithium: can cause serious, even fatal, interactions.
- Antithyroid pills or diuretics (such as furosemide and spironolactone) and drugs such as methyldopa, indometacin, phenylbutazone and piroxicam can all increase lithium concentrations.
- Acetazolamide, sodium bicarbonate, sodium chloride, theophylline and mannitol can decrease lithium concentrations.
- Phenothiazines, carbamazepine or phenytoin taken with lithium can increase neurotoxicity.
- ACE inhibitors such as captopril can increase lithium levels.

Interactions with herbs and supplements are therefore extremely likely.

• Carbamazepine

This is used in acute mania and as bipolar disorder prophylaxis. It is not as effective as lithium but can be used instead if lithium is contraindicated. For mechanism of action, see Chapter 32 'Analgesia and relief of pain' (p. 253).

Anxiety

Anxiolytics are medication used for treating anxiety (see Figure 33.5):

- Used to control symptoms of anxiety without serious impairment of normal physical or mental function.
- Potentiate gamma-aminobutyric acid (GABA) transmission and therefore calm the patient.
- Act on the limbic system, cerebral cortex and ascending amine systems, which govern arousal.

Benzodiazepines

- Are in widespread use, quite often as premeds for minor procedures such as endoscopy or patients with extreme anxiety in the close confines of an MRI scanner.

- **Temazepam can also be used as a hypnotic** (see below).
- **Diazepam** is rapidly absorbed from the gastrointestinal tract and metabolized by the liver to form several active metabolites including oxazepam. The plasma half-life is 24 hours and its effect last even longer as each of the active metabolites have half-lives of several days (this can be longer in the elderly).

• Adverse Effects

Patients can acquire a dependency problem with these drugs. A patient who has been taking a benzodiazepine over a period of time should have the dosage reduced gradually. Prescriptions are supposed to be limited to 6 weeks; these drugs should be given only if the anxiety is debilitating.

Beta-Blockers

- **Propranolol** (see Chapter 26 'Cardiovascular disorders', p. 198) is normally used; this is a non-selective beta-blocker.
- The use is limited but patients with performance anxiety can find it helpful.

Tricyclic Antidepressants and SSRIs

- Used at a low dosage.
- Imipramine and SSRIs are used in the treatment of recurrent panic attacks.

Insomnia

Hypnotic Drugs

- Short-term use only to prevent addiction.
- They provide normal restful sleep by allowing the patient to go to sleep.
- Tend to be the **benzodiazepines.**

Respiratory diseases

The respiratory passages from the nose to the terminal bronchioles in the lungs are moistened by a layer of mucus over the epithelial lining. This is secreted by special cells called goblet cells, and partly by small submucosal glands. The passages are also lined with cilia, which beat continually in the direction of the pharynx, enabling trapped particles to be swallowed or coughed to the exterior (cigarette smoke reduces this capability).

Sinuses

As discussed in Chapter 15 'Methods of administration' (p. 120), the thin, highly vascular lining of the sinuses makes it easy to reach with soluble orthodox medication (in the form of sprays) and vapourized aromatic oils. This, combined with their fat solubility, ensures rapid absorption into the body and also the brain.

Because of this feature, it is usually one of the first areas in a patient to be affected by allergens.

Allergies

An allergic reaction is the body's response to an antigen (see Chapter 30 'Inflammation and the immune system', p. 225). This reaction can range from allergic rhinitis, hay fever and urticaria to drug hypersensitivities. The respiratory system plays a significant role in allowing allergens to enter the body.

The initial allergic reaction occurs in the following way:

- The antigen is phagocytosed by macrophages.
- B lymphocytes produce immunoglobulin E (IgE) in response to the antigen (see Figure 30.1, p. 226).
- IgE fixes to mast cells and basophils; the IgE cells become sensitized.

A second exposure to the antigen activates a much greater response from the immune system, as the mast cells break open releasing histamines that react on mucosal membranes, smooth muscle, skin or other organs. The mast cells are concentrated at sites that are likely to incur most injury, e.g. mouth, nose, feet, blood vessels, skin, lungs and gut mucosa. This can create a problem if the mast cell activity gets out of hand and tissues from a variety of areas – from skin and joints to internal organs – are affected.

Allergic Rhinitis and Hay Fever

Airborne allergens react with IgE-sensitized mast cells in the nasal mucosa and the mucous membranes around the eyes. This is treated by oral antihistamines or nasal spray.

• Antihistamines

Histamine

- Found in most of the tissues of the body, but is in higher concentrations in the lungs, skin and the gut.
- Usually found in basophils and mast cells.
- Released from mast cells during inflammatory or allergic reactions.
- H2 histamine receptors are found in the acid-secreting cells in the stomach.

There are two types of antihistamine drug: H1-receptor antagonists, the classic antihistamine drugs, and H2-receptor antagonists, which affect gastric secretion:

- Cimetidine (Figure 34.1), an H2 antagonist, is used to treat stomach ulcers.
- Ceterizine, an H1 antagonist, is used to treat allergies.

H1-Receptor Antagonists (H1 Antihistamines)

Ceterizine

- Blocks the classical histamine H1 receptors and interferes with the actions of histamine released in type 1 immune reactions.
- Used in hay fever, allergic rhinitis, urticaria and other acute allergic reactions.
- Used to settle down itching and skin reactions such as wheals and hot allergic lumps.
- Potential for drowsiness but not as sedative as effects of the older antihistamines as it is more specific for peripheral H1 receptors.

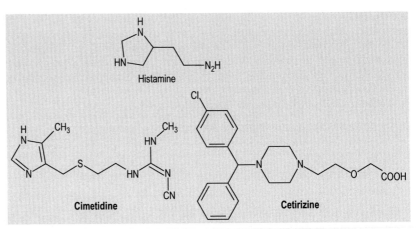

Figure 34.1 The structure of histamine and two different types of antihistamine.

Respiratory Diseases

Asthma

Asthma occurs as a result of a restriction of airflow caused by the contraction of the smooth muscles of the bronchioles and mucosal oedema. It is due to an increased responsiveness of the trachea and bronchi to various stimuli. This reaction is reversible, but in some cases a severe asthma attack can be fatal if not treated quickly. Triggers can be:

- **Specific** such as allergens, chemicals or drugs, e.g. non-steroidal anti-inflammatories.
- **Non-specific**, e.g. exercise, irritants or cold air.

Childhood asthma or **extrinsic asthma** is associated with increased levels of IgE antibodies. In adult or **intrinsic asthma** the symptoms appear in middle age and tend to be persistent.

The **initial response** occurs suddenly and is due to spasm of the smooth muscles of the bronchioles. The antibodies attach to the mast cell, which reacts to the allergen by releasing **histamine**, **leukotrienes**, **eosinophils**, **macrophages**, **platelets** and **bradykinins**. Leucocytes are attracted into the area, which leads to the second or **delayed response**.

The **delayed response** does not occur immediately and is a progressive inflammatory reaction. The usual inflammatory cells are found at the site, with cytokine-releasing T cells and eosinophils, the contents of which damage the epithelium. The products of these cells stimulate the nerve cells to constrict the bronchioles. A thickening of the mucosal walls along with copious amounts of mucus, which accumulate over a period of time, decrease the lumen of the bronchioles further. There is often a family history of hay fever or eczema.

Blood Tests

- Serum eosinophil levels might be raised.
- The levels of IgE might be normal.

Beta-2 Adrenoceptor Agonists

Beta-2 adrenoceptor agonists (see Chapter 31 'The nervous system', p. 244) are used; these:

- act on the smooth muscles
- inhibit the release of contents from the mast cells
- inhibit the action of the vagus nerve
- increase the action of the cilia to improve mucus clearance.

Usually, different types of medication are given:

- Short-acting drugs: **salbutamol** (Figure 34.2) is a beta-2 agonist that works within 30 minutes, the effects of which last 4–6 hours.
- Longer-acting drugs: **salmeterol** is a beta-2 agonist, its effects last 12 hours. It should therefore not be used more than twice a day.

Doses are given by inhalation.

Adverse Effects

- Tremor: due to the beta receptors being stimulated.

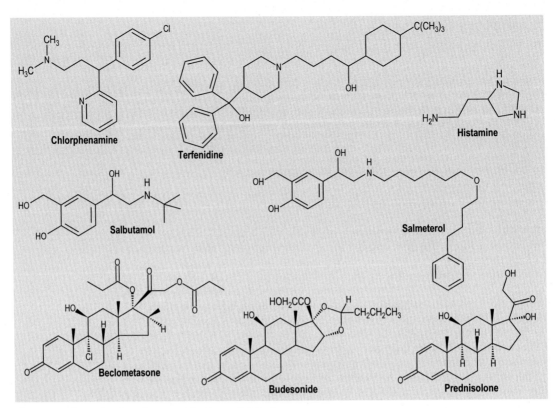

Figure 34.2 Examples of respiratory medication and histamine.

Chronic Asthma

Inflammation of the mucosa occurs in chronic asthma.

Corticosteroids can be used in chronic asthma. The actions of corticosteroids on the bronchi are not properly understood, but they might be effective due to the reduction of the inflammation of the mucosal oedema. They are no use for acute episodes, as they do not work fast enough. The dose is given via an inhaler, which is effective at limiting the dose because the liver clears corticosteroids administered in this way very quickly. So there is a good local effect that should not spread systemically.

Drugs such as **beclometasone** and **budesonide** can be used. In chronic asthma that is deteriorating, a short course of an oral glucocorticoid can be given, e.g. **prednisolone**.

• Adverse Effects

Local

- Candidiasis of the pharynx and larynx.
- Laxity of the vocal cords causing hoarseness.

Systemic

- Adrenal suppression leading to suppression of the immune system and poor response to infection or injury.
- The patients' ability to synthesize their own corticosteroids can be impaired because the adrenal glands have had their function taken over by drugs.
- Osteoporosis.
- Cushing syndrome.

- ## Contraindications for Orthodox Medication
  - Asthmatic patients should only take non-steroidal anti-inflammatories under medical supervision.
  - Beta-blockers are contraindicated in individuals with asthma because they are beta-antagonists (see Chapter 31 'The nervous system', p. 244).

Chronic Obstructive Pulmonary Disease (COPD)

Obstruction of the airflow is progressive and generally not reversible because of the tissue changes that have taken place. The two diseases associated with COPD are:

- bronchitis
- emphysema.

The two very often coexist.

Chronic Bronchitis

Signs and Symptoms

- Cough and sputum for 3 months a year for 2 years.
- Thickened mucosa, enlargement or increase in the number of mucous glands: results in secretion of large amounts of mucus and loss of cilia.
- Finger clubbing.
- Emphysema.
- Enlargement of alveolar air spaces with destruction of elastin in the alveolar wall.
- One-third of the lungs is usually destroyed before clinical symptoms appear.

Treatment

Treatment is given on clinical findings of frequent attacks of bronchitis, dyspnoea, productive cough, wheeze and cyanosis.

Emphysema

Signs and Symptoms

- Loss of elasticity of the lung tissue, leading to an enlarging of the alveoli and therefore surface area available for gas exchange.
- Shortness of breath on exertion and, as disease progresses, at rest.
- Finger clubbing

Treatment

- Anticholinergics
- Bronchodilators.
- Steroids.
- Oxygen if necessary.

As smoking is an important cause of COPD (see p. 267 for the effects of smoke on respiratory tract tissue) the patient is advised to stop smoking and is given adjunctive help.

Lung Cancer

Most common causes due to:

- smoking
- occupational exposure to carcinogens.

271

- ## Signs and Symptoms

  - Cough.
  - Dyspnoea.
  - Chest infections: these are often hard to resolve.
  - Chest pain.
  - Haemoptysis.
  - Finger clubbing.
  - Weight loss.

- ## Treatment

  - Radiotherapy.
  - Chemotherapy.
  - Surgery.
  - Palliative care.

Gastrointestinal disorders

35

Anatomy of the Gastrointestinal Tract

There are five layers in the gastrointestinal wall (Figure 35.1):

- Serosa.
- Longitudinal muscle layer: the outer layer of muscle. Combined with the inner circular muscle layer, its coordinated contraction creates peristalsis, which propels food through the gut.
- Circular muscle layer.

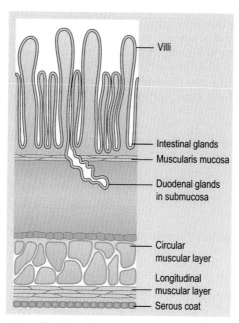

Figure 35.1 Cross-section of small intestine.

- Submucosa: a layer of dense irregular connective tissue with large blood vessels, an extensive lymph system and nerves branching into the external muscle and mucosal layer. This supply and drainage system becomes an important factor in the spread of secondary cancers.
- Mucosa: the innermost layer, which is in direct exposure to the lumen (i.e. the space within the tube of the tract). The composition of the mucosa varies depending on the area of the gastrointestinal tract. For example, in the stomach it has qualities that make it resistant to the effects of a low pH; in the small intestine it contains villi, which maximize absorption.

The blood flow from the small intestine is significant because it passes directly to the liver via the hepatic portal vein. Most of the water-soluble nutrients absorbed from the gut are transported to the liver in this way. Fat-soluble substances are absorbed by the intestinal lymphatic system and distributed to the blood by the thoracic duct, thus bypassing the liver.

The stomach mucosa contains many mucus-secreting cells; the mucus creates a protective layer over the lining of the stomach wall. The lining of the stomach is highly glandular and consists of four types of gland:

- Parietal cells: secrete hydrochloric acid (HCl) and intrinsic factor (see Chapter 13 'Vitamins and minerals', p. 105).
- Mucous cells: secrete an alkaline mucus that protects the epithelium against damage due to shearing of the membranes and the acid environment of the stomach.
- Chief cells: secrete pepsin, a proteolytic enzyme. Its activity is low at a low pH (see Chapter 8 'Acids and bases', p. 54) and the enzyme is therefore not fully active until it reaches the more basic medium of the small intestine (pH approximately 7.8).
- G cells: secrete the hormone gastrin.

Different areas of the stomach vary in their secretions.

Microflora of the Gastrointestinal Tract

The gastrointestinal tract is a complex and self-contained ecosystem of over 400 bacterial species. Anaerobic bacteria (bacteria that live in an environment where there is little or no oxygen) outnumber aerobic bacteria (those that require the presence of oxygen to function). Fungi are also present but, due to the population of the normal **commensals**, tend not exceed limits, except for a problem such as that caused by an overgrowth of, for example, *Candida albicans*.

Due to the existence of the commensals, a situation exists where host, bacteria and fungi live together without any adverse effects on one another. In many cases in the gastrointestinal tract, bacteria provide a very useful service, producing vitamins that are vital for health or taking part in chemical reactions necessary to activate compounds (see Chapter 13 'Vitamins and minerals', p. 108). These bacteria are usually non-pathogenic. Most of the gut flora is found in the colon and lives in the lumen of the bowel; it does not normally penetrate the gut wall.

Ingestion of certain substances, e.g. antibiotics, can disturb the normal balance of these commensals, which is why carefully consideration of gut health after a course of antibiotics is important.

Gastrointestinal Disorders

Dyspepsia
This is a general term for a group of signs and symptoms:

- heartburn
- pain or discomfort in the upper abdomen

- bloating and feeling 'full' after eating
- belching
- nausea or vomiting.

All these symptoms are intermittent.

Causes of Dyspepsia

- Acid reflux, oesophagitis or gastro-oesophageal reflux disease (GORD).
- Hiatus hernia.
- Functional dyspepsia: does not involve ulcer formation.
- Duodenitis: can be a precursor to an ulcer; a possible cause is NSAIDs.
- Gastritis: can be a precursor to an ulcer; a possible cause is NSAIDs.
- Duodenal and gastric ulcers.

Conservative Treatment

- Check patient's medication: patients who are taking NSAIDs or some other medications (e.g. some antibiotics, steroids) are required to stop medication.
- Patients must try to abstain from foods and drinks such as chocolate, coffee, alcohol, spicy foods and peppermint.
- Patients should try to stop smoking: chemicals inhaled from cigarettes are thought to relax the oesophageal sphincter.
- Patients might have to change posture if they habitually bend over during the day, and might have to avoid sleeping horizontally.
- At night, patients are discouraged from drinking or eating at least 2 hours before bedtime.
- Patients who are overweight should be encouraged to lose weight: the extra pressure on the stomach encourages reflux.

Orthodox Medication

Antacids

- Attempt to neutralize the available stomach acid: they are weak alkalis.
- Are thought to stimulate the mucosal repair mechanisms around ulcers: possibly by stimulating local prostaglandin release.
- **Medications include: magnesium hydroxide, magnesium trisilicate, aluminium hydroxide gel.**
- Magnesium is a more effective antacid than aluminium but has a tendency to create diarrhoea.
- As small amounts of magnesium can be absorbed, any antacid preparation containing magnesium should be used with caution.

H2-Receptor Antagonists

These compete with histamine at the H2-receptor level. They are more effective when the stomach is empty, e.g. at night or when fasting, and less effective when food is present.

Adverse Reactions

- Diarrhoea and other digestive disturbances.
- Headache.
- Dizziness.
- Fatigue.
- Ranitidine (Figure 35.2): can be associated with darkening of the tongue and black stools.
- Cimetidine: has been associated with hair loss.

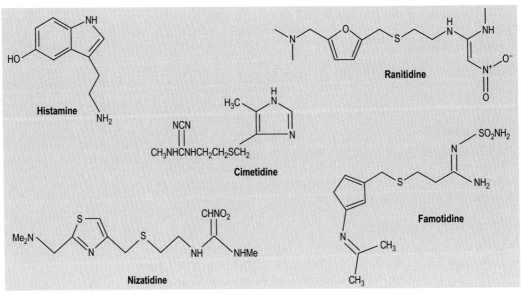

Figure 35.2 Chemical structure of histamine and various H2-receptor antagonists for comparison.

Drug Interactions

Cimetidine affects one of the liver detoxification pathways and thus can increase the time of metabolism of drugs removed by this pathway, leading to a build-up that can be toxic in some cases. **Theophylline** (a bronchodilator) and **warfarin** are two drugs that can be affected.

Proton Pump Inhibitors

These bind irreversibly to the proton pump mechanism on the parietal cell membranes. The proton pump is really an enzyme that actively secretes hydrogen ions into the gastric cavity. The medication is enteric coated to allow it to reach the small intestine, where it can be properly absorbed.

Omeprazole (Figure 35.3) interferes with the liver detoxification system and prolongs the presence of diazepam, phenytoin (an anticonvulsant; see Chapter 33 'Neurological disease', p. 256) and possibly warfarin.

Proton pump inhibitors are used only in the short-term management of duodenal and gastric ulcers, particularly those caused by NSAIDs. They can also be used in combination with antibiotics when treating for *Helicobacter pylori*.

Adverse Effects

- Diarrhoea.
- Skin rash.
- Headaches.

Treatment of Helicobacter pylori

The patient is given a non-radioactive isotope of carbon to drink. *Helicobacter pylori* breaks this down to ammonia and carbon dioxide. The labelled carbon dioxide is then tested. *H. pylori* is treated with antibiotics such as **clarithromycin, tetracycline, amoxicillin** and **metronidazole** (see Chapter 29 'Antimicrobials', p. 218) and a proton pump inhibitor for 2 weeks.

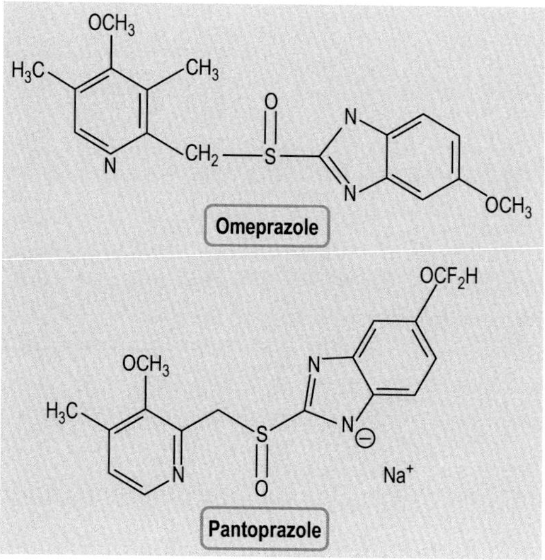

Figure 35.3 Chemical structures of proton pump inhibitors.

Peptic Ulcer

● Aetiology

- NSAIDs can damage the lining of the gut. NSAIDs work by blocking the cyclo-oxygenase (COX) enzymes involved in producing prostaglandins (see Chapter 30 'Inflammation and the immune system', p. 229). COX-1 helps to maintain the gut lining; COX-2 is less involved in this process. COX-2 inhibitors are supposed to help gastrointestinal effects because they allow the COX-1 pathway to carry on working while blocking the COX-2 pathway. The overall result is an anti-inflammatory effect and less gastrointestinal disturbance.
- *Helicobacter pylori*.
- Stress: originally thought to have an effect on the blood flow to the stomach; the damage by NSAIDs and *H. pylori* are now accepted as prime causal factors but stress might exacerbate the condition in some way.
- Diet: poor nutrition creates changes in the function of the gastrointestinal tract and secretions.

The entire gastrointestinal tract is covered by a protective mucus layer. Any reduction in the effectiveness of this layer renders the lining accessible and prone to attack by acid and enzymes, eventually creating an ulcer.

● Treatment

As above for dyspepsia.

Irritable Bowel

Reasons for this should be investigated if the condition does not quickly resolve with conservative treatment or other signs are present, such as blood in stools.

Constipation

● Contributing Factors

- Poor diet.
- Age.
- Metabolic conditions such as hypothyroidism.

- Medication.
- Cancer.

Reasons for chronic or painful constipation are usually investigated.

● Treatment for Functional Constipation

- Fibre: addition of fibre to the diet is encouraged.
- Bulk-forming laxatives: swell with the addition of water to create a mechanical pressure against the gut wall, thus encouraging peristalsis, e.g. methylcellulose.
- Stool softeners: can be given as pessaries or enemas.
- Stimulant laxatives: usually contain anthraquinones (see Chapter 21 'Phenols', p. 153), e.g. senna.
- Osmotic laxatives: work by drawing more water into the bowel, e.g. lactulose.

● Treatment for More Complex Causes of Constipation

- Treatment of underlying problem.

Coeliac Disease

Inherited condition in which exposure to gluten atrophies the gastrointestinal villi in the small intestine.

● Investigations

- IgA anti-tissue transglutaminase (tTG): now favoured.
- Endoscopy.

● Treatment

Patients refrain from eating foods containing gluten.

Crohn's Disease

A chronic, inflammatory bowel disease that can affect any part of the gut, but in particular the distal end of the ileum and the proximal colon.

● Signs and Symptoms

The following might or might not occur:

- possible diarrhoea for more than 6 weeks
- abdominal pain
- weight loss
- anorexia
- general feeling of being unwell
- fever.

These can well occur in a fairly young patient.

● Investigations

- Blood tests: erythrocyte sedimentation rate (ESR) and C-reactive protein (see Chapter 41 'Scientific tests', p. 331).
- Biopsy of relevant tissue.

- ## Treatment

Depends on particular pattern of condition. Will include:

- Aminosalicylates.
- Sulfasalazine: this drug combines sulfapyridine and an aminosalicylate. Both are poorly absorbed as systemic anti-inflammatories but as this combination is being used to reduce the inflammation of the gut lining the treatment can be very effective.
- Corticosteroids: see Chapter 30 'Inflammation and the immune system' (p. 230).
- Immunomodulators: see Chapter 30 'Inflammation and the immune system' (p. 232).

- ## Chronic Crohn's Disease

If the pharmacological intervention is unsuccessful then surgery is necessary.

Ulcerative Colitis

Signs and symptoms are very similar to Crohn's, for example, diarrhoea and general malaise. There might also be bloody stools.

- ## Investigations

- Blood tests: possible anaemia due to blood loss, raised white cell count, raised ESR.
- Stool sample: to ensure no infection is present.
- Biopsy.

- ## Treatment

Nicotine derivates currently being investigated.

- ## Active Ulcerative Colitis

As for Crohn's disease.

- ## Active Distal Colitis

Suppositories can be used as a topical application.

- ## Chronic Ulcerative Colitis

If pharmacological intervention is not successful then colectomy might be necessary to prevent colon cancer.

Colorectal (Bowel) Cancer

There might be a history of abnormalities, such as polyps or bowel disease, for example, ulcerative colitis. Signs and symptoms can include:

- weight loss
- anaemia
- diarrhoea or constipation
- occult bleeding: hidden blood in the stool that can be detected only using laboratory tests.

- ## Examination

- Full blood count and liver function tests (see Chapter 41 'Scientific tests,' p. 331).
- Barium enema.
- Colonoscopy or sigmoidoscopy.

- **Treatment**
  - Surgery: a colostomy can be permanent (if the rectum and anus need to be removed) or temporary (to allow the joined ends to heal). The patient will need to wear a colostomy bag.
  - Chemotherapy: necessary to assess the patient for the type of chemotherapy being used.
  - Radiotherapy.

Urinary tract infection

36

Lower Urinary Tract

Infections include:

- Cystitis.
- Urethritis.

More common in females. Common pathogens are *Escherichia coli*, *Pseudomonas* spp., *Streptococcus* spp., *Staphylococcus* spp.

Signs and Symptoms

- Urinary frequency.
- Dysuria.
- Suprapubic pain and tenderness.
- Haematuria.
- Smelly, cloudy urine.

These conditions are the ones most commonly seen by complementary healthcare practitioners. More serious upper urinary tract conditions, such as glomerulonephritis or pyelonephritis, are more likely to refer themselves directly to orthodox medical care. It is worth noting, however, that a relatively straightforward cystitis or urethritis can develop into an upper urinary tract condition if not treated appropriately.

Investigations

- Midstream urine sample is cultured.

Very often, a broad-spectrum antibiotic is given without a sample being taken, but if the infection does not clear then a culture needs to be grown to identify the type of bacteria and the most effective antibiotic for that strain.

Treatment

- A short course of antibiotics (see Chapter 29 'Antimicrobials', p. 219).
- Plenty of water.
- Paracetamol or ibuprofen to ease symptoms.

Benign Prostatic Hyperplasia (BPH)

- Common in men over 50 years old.
- Urinary frequency and urgency with decreased urinary flow.
- Nocturia.
- Complications: infection due to the incomplete emptying of the bladder.

Laboratory Tests

The prostate-specific antigen (PSA) is elevated with a large benign prostate. Whether this level indicates a more pathological condition, i.e. malignant prostate, depends on the age group.

PSA Levels

- Under 50 years of age: below 2.5 ng/mL.
- Under 60 years of age: below 3.5 ng/mL.
- Under 70 years of age: below 4.5 ng/mL.
- Under 80 years of age: below 6.5 ng/mL.

Treatment

Alpha-Adrenoceptor Antagonists

- Can create partial reversal of smooth muscle contraction in the enlarged prostate and bladder base.
- Alpha-adrenoceptor antagonists are also helpful in patients with hypertension if they are not too specific (see Chapter 31 'The nervous system', p. 244).

5-Alpha-Reductase Drugs

- Prevent the synthesis the production of the androgen dihydrotestosterone from testosterone.
- Can take several months before they work.

Adverse Effects

Both reduce sexual performance.

Serenoa repens (Saw Palmetto)

Experimentally appears to inhibit 5-alpha-reductase but no well-constructed clinical studies have yet be run to say definitively whether this herb is effective with BPH. However, the possibilities are there (Fagelman & Lowe 2001).

Adverse Effects

There are no serious side effects.

Prostate Cancer

By 80 years of age, 80% men have some degree of malignancy.

Signs and Symptoms

Initially not dissimilar to benign prostatic hyperplasia (BPH), or there might be a history of BPH. Plus:

- blood in the urine or semen
- painful ejaculation
- lower back pain extending into hips and upper thighs.

Laboratory Tests

PSA; see above.

Treatment

- Patient might be in an age group that dies of old age first, so observation is used.
- Zinc supplementation.
- Removal of prostate (prostatectomy).
- Radiotherapy.
- Hormonal treatments: Chapter 39 'Chemotherapy' (p. 310).

Prostatitis

- Acute or chronic inflammation of prostate.
- Common pathogens: *Gonococcus, E. coli, Staphylococcus, Streptococcus.*
- Some chronic prostatitis can be non-bacterial.

Signs and Symptoms

- Frequency.
- Dysuria.
- Nocturia.
- Urgency.
- Urethral discharge.
- Low back pain.

Treatment

Antibiotics. However, chronic prostatitis does not always respond to antibiotics and can prove difficult to treat.

Urinary Stones

- Most kidney stones are composed of calcium phosphate or calcium oxalate.
- Their cause is usually unknown.
- Abnormally high urinary calcium (**hypercalciuria**) increases the risk of developing kidney stones.
- High doses of calcium will not cause **hypercalcaemia** (abnormally high calcium in the blood).

Causes

- Gout.
- Hypercalcaemia.
- Dehydration.
- Infection.
- Renal disease.
- Some drugs, e.g. diuretics can create dehydration. Tetracyclines bind readily to calcium.

Signs and Symptoms

- Can be asymptomatic.
- Kidney: loin pain, haematuria, possible proteinuria.
- Ureter: severe colic, tenderness over course of ureter, enlarged kidney.
- Bladder: frequency, haematuria, gravel in urine.
- The presence of stones will increase the chance of urinary tract infection.

Treatment

- Wait for stones to pass.
- Removal of stones: surgically or by lithotripsy (breaking up stones using shock waves).
- Antibiotics.
- Painkillers.
- Treatment of underlying problems.

Renal Cancer

Signs and symptoms

- Painless haematuria.
- Low-grade fever.
- Anaemia.
- Weight loss.
- Abdominal mass.
- Loin pain.
- Hypercalcaemia.

Treatment

- Surgical removal.
- Radiotherapy.

Bladder Cancer

- Uncommon below the age of 40.
- More common in men.

Signs and Symptoms

- Painless haematuria.
- Nocturia.

- Frequency, urgency, and hesitancy.
- Pain and weight loss: late features.

Therefore many features are similar to prostate conditions.

Treatment

- Surgery: the degree of this will depend on how far the cancer has progressed.
- Radiotherapy.
- Chemotherapy.

Reference

Fagelman E, Lowe FC. Saw Palmetto berry as a treatment for BPH. Reviews in Urology; 2001; 3(3):134–138.

Metabolic disorders

37

Pineal Gland

Synthesizes melatonin, which – because of its position in the third ventricle – is secreted directly into the cerebrospinal fluid (CSF), from where it finally ends up in the blood. Melatonin affects reproductive development and daily physiology.

Pituitary Gland

The 'master gland' of the body; possesses two lobes:

- Anterior (adenohypophysis): is attached but not directly connected to the hypothalamus.
- Posterior (neurohypophysis): directly connected to the hypothalamus via neural tissue. Does not produce its own hormones but stores and releases hormones when they are required.

Anterior Pituitary Gland

The anterior pituitary gland secretes:

- Growth hormone (GH): stimulates growth of bones, muscles, etc. by stimulating protein synthesis.
- Follicle-stimulating hormone (FSH).
- Prolactin (PL): stimulates the development of female breast glandular tissue during pregnancy and milk production after birth.
- Luteinizing hormone (LH).
- Thyroid-stimulating hormone (TSH): stimulates secretion of thyroid gland.

- Adrenocorticotrophic hormone (ACTH): stimulates secretion of adrenal glands.
- Endorphins.

The anterior pituitary gland responds to:

- Growth-hormone-releasing hormone (GHRH): causes the release of growth hormone (GH), which controls growth.
- Thyrotropin-releasing hormone (TRH): causes the release of thyroid-stimulating hormone (TSH) and prolactin (PL).
- Corticotrophin-releasing hormone (CRH): causes the release of adrenocorticotrophic hormone (ACTH), which controls blood pressure.
- Dopamine (DA): inhibits release of prolactin under normal conditions.
- Gonadotrophin-releasing hormone (GnRH): causes release of FSH and LH, which control pregnancy.

Posterior Pituitary Gland

The posterior pituitary gland secretes:

- Oxytocin: involved in childbirth.
- Antidiuretic hormone (ADH): affects blood pressure, water and concentration of salts in the nephron (see Chapter 26 'Cardiovascular disorders', p. 193).

Treatment of Pituitary Disorders

It is evident from the above that any patient with a pituitary condition of any kind will probably be under orthodox medical care. This can be complex and the patient is carefully monitored. However, it is worth being aware of the condition of **diabetes insipidus**, which is caused by a reduction in ADH. The patient will urinate excessively. The difference between this and **diabetes mellitus** is the normal blood sugar levels.

A careful case history should enable a practitioner to identify the medication the patient is on and consult a formulary for the actions of the drug and any side effects. Note that severe trauma to the head can be responsible for pituitary dysfunction.

Thyroid Gland (see Chapter 41 'Scientific tests' Table 41.1, p. 340, Table 41.2, p. 341)

Dysfunction of this gland is commonly encountered in clinical practice.

The thyroid is a double-lobed endocrine gland situated in the neck. It produces the hormones thyroxine (T4) and triiodothyronine (T3). These hormones are responsible for:

- regulating metabolic rate generally
- affecting growth.

Iodine is necessary for the production of both hormones. Disorders of the thyroid include:

- Hyperthyroidism: overactive thyroid
- Hypothyroidism: underactive thyroid.

Thyroid-releasing hormone is released by the hypothalamus, via the pituitary gland (see above); occasionally the pituitary is at fault.

Hyperthyroidsm

• Symptoms

- Palpitations, tachycardia.

- Agitation.
- Insomnia.
- Weight loss.

• Symptomatic Relief

Non-selective beta-blockers, 235 because tremor usually responds to beta-2 and not beta-1-blockers (see Chapter 31 'The nervous system', p. 235).

• Side Effects

See Chapter 31 'The nervous system' (p. 235).

• Treatment

- Radioactive iodine is used to destroy some of the thyroid cell, thus reducing production. Very often, however, this causes permanent hypothyroidism and the appropriate medication has to be given.
- Drugs that interfere with the synthesis of thyroid hormone, e.g. methimazole (US), carbimazole (UK).

Hypothyroidism

• Symptoms

- Fatigue.
- Weakness.
- Weight gain.
- Coarse dry hair, hair loss and dry rough pale skin.
- Muscle cramps.
- Depression and irritability.
- Abnormal menstrual cycles.
- Decreased libido.

Only severe cases have goitre.

• Treatment

- Thyroid replacement therapy: thyroxine (T4) is normally converted to triiodothyronine (T3). It is thyroxine that is normally used in treatment.

Adverse Effects

- Symptoms of hyperthyroidism.
- Disease related to calcium metabolism.

Parathyroid Gland

Calcium Regulation in the Body

- The amount of calcium in the blood and fluid has to be tightly controlled. There is always some loss of calcium from the body, (100–240 mg in the urine and between 45 and 100 mg in the faeces) but this is not a problem if it is being replaced.
- The parathyroid glands detect when the calcium concentration in the blood decreases and secrete **parathyroid hormone (PTH)**. PTH stimulates the conversion of **inactive vitamin D** to **active calcitriol**.
- Calcitriol increases the absorption of calcium from the small intestine.
- The **PTH** and **calcitriol** stimulate the release of calcium from bone by activating osteoclasts (responsible for bone resorption) and increase the absorption of calcium in the kidneys.

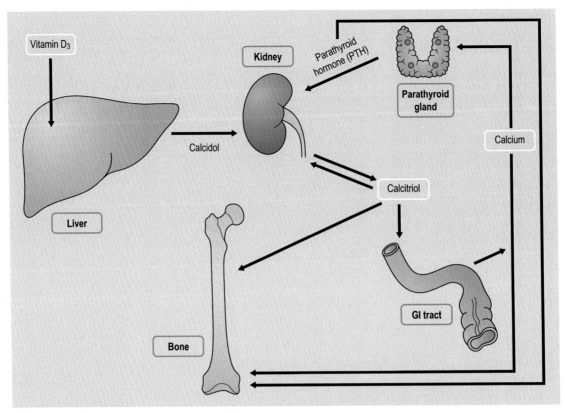

Figure 37.1 Demonstrating the interrelationship between calcium and vitamin D and calcium metabolism.

- An increase in the concentration of the calcium in the blood above normal levels will switch off the production of PTH. The kidneys will then begin to excrete excess calcium in the urine.

Although this system maintains good control of calcium in the body, it does so at the expense of the calcium in the bone.

Interestingly, the efficiency of absorption of calcium from a supplement is inversely proportional to the total amount of calcium ingested. The cells of the gut wall have a maximum capacity for how much calcium they can pass across from the lumen to the capillaries.

Vitamin D is required for optimal calcium absorption.

Interaction of Food Substances with Calcium

See Chapter 13 'Vitamins and minerals' (p. 96).

Osteoporosis

Bone continually remodels itself. This occurs due to action of the **osteoclasts**, which dissolve and reabsorb bone, and the **osteoblasts**, which synthesize new bone to replace that reabsorbed.

Osteoporosis can occur when the rate of bone resorption is greater than its formation. Although osteoporosis is thought to be a postmenopausal problem it is possible even in children. Osteoporosis is caused by more than one factor. Risk factors are:

- Female sex.
- Oestrogen deficiency.
- Smoking.

- Metabolic disease such as hyperthyroidism.
- Certain medication such as corticosteroids and anticonvulsants.

There is also an element of genetic and lifestyle factors.

Assessment of Osteoporosis or Osteopaenia

- Full blood counts and hormone levels are checked for underlying causes.
- Alkaline phophatase levels (see Chapter 41 'Scientific tests', p. 335) are usually raised.
- Single and dual X-ray absorptiometry (DXA) and digital X-ray radiogrammetry (DXR): these procedures assess the mineral content of the entire skeleton. DXA is considered to be the gold standard for diagnosis of bone density reduction, particularly in the hip area. DXR is a newer and simpler technique using a standard radiograph of the hand.

Treatment

Conservative Treatment

- Weight-bearing exercise has been showed to help osteoporotic patients but the exercise has to be high-impact based.
- Vitamin D and calcium supplementation (see Chapter 13 'Vitamins and minerals', pp. 95 and 107) have been shown to be beneficial.

Orthodox Medication

Bisphosphonates

These attach to bone tissue and are ingested by and kill the osteoclasts (the bones cell that break down bone tissue). This slows bone resorption but not bone forming. So, over a period of time, the bone density should increase.

Bisphosphonates have to be taken on an empty stomach and with at least 8 fluid ounces of water. The patient then needs to remain upright for at least 1 hour to be sure that the bisphosphonate has passed out of the oesophagus.

Hormone Replacement Treatment (HRT)

This is no longer considered a primary means of treating osteoporosis as it has been shown to increase the risk of breast cancer.

Selective Oestrogen (Estrogen) Receptor Modulator (SERM)

- Reduces bone loss and vertebral fracture but might increase the risk of blood clots and can exacerbate hot flushes.
- Does appear to be linked with a decrease in the risk of breast cancer.

291

Adrenal Glands

Responsible for the 'fight or flight response'. The adrenals secrete:

- corticosteroids (see Chapter 30 'Inflammation and immune system', p. 230).
- catecholamines (see Chapter 31 'The nervous system', p. 240).

Cushing Syndrome

Although this can be caused by a tumour in the pituitary or adrenal glands, the more common reason seen in complementary practice is the long-term usage of steroids, e.g. prednisolone, to reduce inflammation in arthritic conditions, or asthma.

Thymus Gland

- Involved in the immune system.
- Produces T lymphocytes.

Reproductive Hormones

See Chapter 38 'Reproductive hormones' (p. 299).

Pancreas

Diabetes

There are two types of diabetes:

1. Insulin-dependent diabetes mellitus (IDDM; type 1 diabetes):
   - the result of autoimmune destruction of pancreatic islet cells
   - the beta cells in the Islets of Langerhans are no longer able to secrete insulin.
2. Non-insulin dependent diabetes mellitus (NIDDM; type 2 diabetes).
   - a disorder of middle-aged and elderly patients, with a familial tendency
   - the cells in the body become insulin resistant.

Treatment of Type 1 Diabetes

- The aim is to reduce blood sugar levels.
- Patients are treated with insulin, as they are no longer able to make insulin themselves.
- The gut destroys insulin, which has to be injected into the body.
- The insulin can be porcine or bovine in origin, but these days synthetic insulin is produced.

● Adverse Effects

- Build-up of fat or localized tissue loss around the injection site; the site needs to be changed regularly.
- Antibodies can develop to insulin: the antibody then acts in the same way as a plasma protein, taking free insulin out of circulation making its action less effective.
- Hypoglycaemia: if too much insulin is administered patients can become irrational and aggressive; at worst, they can lapse into a coma.

Treatment of Type 2 Diabetes

The pancreatic islet cells are still functioning.

● Conservative Treatment

- Dietary control: the intake of simple sugars is reduced and that of more complex carbohydrates is increased (see Chapter 9 'Carbohydrates', p. 68).

● Orthodox Medication

Biguanides: Metformin

- Mechanism of action uncertain but might be due to decreasing absorption of glucose from the gut and increasing the passage into cells, effectively removing glucose from the bloodstream.

- Can reduce levels of vitamin B_{12} and folic acid, which can lead to an increase in levels of homocysteine (hyperhomocysteinaemia; see below), thus increasing the risk of cardiovascular disease.
- Not suitable for use in pregnancy.

Adverse Effects

- Anorexia.
- Nausea.
- Diarrhoea: this can be avoided by introducing the dose slowly and increasing gradually.
- Abdominal pain.
- Decreased vitamin B_{12} absorption.

Sulphonylureas: Gliclazide

- Augments insulin secretion and therefore some beta cell activity is required.
- Has a short half-life (see Chapter 17 'Metabolism', p. 129) and therefore reduces the possibility of hypoglycaemia.
- Not suitable in pregnancy.

Adverse Effects

- Gastric disturbances.
- Nausea.
- Vomiting.
- Diarrhoea.
- Constipation.

Thiazolidinediones: Rosiglitazone

- Increases cell sensitivity to insulin.
- Usually given in combination with biguanides or sulphonylureas.

Adverse Effects

- Gastrointestinal disturbances.
- Headache.
- Anaemia.
- Fatigue.
- Weight gain.
- Oedema.
- Hypoglycaemia.
- Dizziness.

293

Polycystic Ovarian Syndrome

The cause is not properly understood.

• Signs and Symptoms

- There might be no symptoms and the condition is only discovered on ultrasound examination.
- Menstrual dysfunction: irregular or absent.
- Ovaries are larger than normal and have an abnormally large number of small follicles, which remain immature and do not develop to ovulation or egg production. As a result, ovulation is rare.

- Infertility.
- Signs of androgen excess, e.g. excess weight and body hair (hirsutism).
- Acne.
- Often insulin resistant with hyperinsulinaemia (blood insulin levels are abnormally high).
- May be general endocrine disturbance.

• Diagnostic Blood Tests

- LH elevated.
- LH : FSH ratio increased; FSH is normal.
- Raised levels of prolactin in the blood.
- Thyroid function tests.
- Fasting glucose and oral glucose tolerance test to reveal any insulin-resistant diabetes.
- Fasting lipid levels.
- Testosterone and oestriol may be elevated. Very high levels of testosterone might be due to a tumour.

• Treatment

Usually according to symptoms:

- Diet and exercise: weight loss may help general symptoms and insulin resistance.
- Type 2 diabetes medication: see above.
- Clomifen: to induce ovulation.
- Anti-androgens: to counter hirsutism.

Other Metabolic Conditions

Metabolic Syndrome X

- Central obesity: excessive fat tissue in the abdominal region.
- Insulin resistance.
- Dyslipidaemia: high levels of triglycerides and low levels of high-density lipoproteins.
- Hypertension.
- Abnormal levels of blood-clotting factors (high fibrinogen or plasminogen activator inhibitors in the blood).
- Low levels of high-density lipoprotein and high levels of low-density lipoprotein cholesterol and triglyceride, ultimately encouraging plaque formation in artery walls (see Chapter 41 'Scientific tests', p. 340).
- Proinflammatory state: elevated high-sensitivity C-reactive protein in blood (see Chapter 41 'Scientific tests', p. 334).

• Reasons for Predisposition to Metabolic Syndrome X

- May be genetic: members of the same family are more likely to develop the condition.

• Treatment

- Exercise and diet can reverse insulin resistance.

If exercise does not work:

- Lipid-lowering drugs: e.g. statins (see Chapter 27 'Problems with lipid metabolism', p. 207)
- Aspirin: to prevent blood clotting.

- Hypertensive drugs if blood pressure is high (see Chapter 26 'Cardiovascular disorders', p. 195).
- Diabetic medication: if blood sugar levels are high.

Gout

Purines are excreted by soluble uric acid, but uric acid and urates are only just water soluble. This becomes a problem when the urine becomes particularly acidic (high meat intake, particularly red meat full of purines and pyrimidines; see Chapter 18 'Drug excretion', p. 134). High levels of uric acid in the blood (uraemia) can result in uric acid crystals in the joints, most frequently the first metatarsophalangeal joint. The attacks are acute and very painful. Repeated attacks lead to tissue damage and arthritic malformations.

• Treatment

1) Reducing the immune response to uric acid deposits.
2) Reduce the inflammation.
3) Reduce uric acid synthesis.
4) Increase renal excretion of uric acid.

1) Reducing the immune response to uric acid deposits:

Glucocorticoids

Non-steroidal anti-inflammatories (NSAIDs; see Chapter 30 'Inflammation and the immune system', p. 231):

Indomethacin is commonly used.

Colchicine

Thought to inhibit cell division of neutrophils. How colchicine works is not yet properly understood. However, it is thought to: (1) reduce lactic acid production by leucocytes, which results in a decrease in uric acid deposition; (2) reduce phagocytosis. This combined effect reduces the body's response to inflammation, thus allowing the inflammation to subside.

Adverse Effects of Colchicine

- Nausea.
- Vomiting.
- Abdominal pain.
- Diarrhoea.

2) Reduce Inflammation

- Glucocorticoids.
- NSAIDs.
- Cherries: the flavonoids in cherries can act as an anti-inflammatory, and also increase the renal filtration of urate (fitting into the fourth category of gout treatment), while decreasing its reabsorption (Jacob et al 2003).

3) Reduce Uric Acid Synthesis

Allopurinol is a competitive inhibitor (see Chapter 19 'Pharmacodynamics: how drugs elicit a physiological effect', p. 138) and attaches so securely to the enzyme-binding site that the normal substrate cannot attach itself and take part in the necessary reaction. This reduces the production of uric acid, leaving more soluble products in the blood, which are likely to deposit as crystals in the joints. It is used between attacks. There are few adverse effects.

4) Increase Renal Excretion of Uric Acid

- **Probenecid**: increases the excretion of urate. Few side effects but on withdrawal of drug there might be fever, a general feeling of being unwell, muscle pain and skin rash.
- **Sulfinpyrazone**: more powerful than probenecid but has antiplatelet effects and so is used with caution in patients on antiplatelet or anticoagulation drugs. Gastrointestinal disturbances sometimes occur. Avoid in patients with peptic ulcers.
- **Cherries** (see above): reduce inflammation.

Hyperhomocysteinaemia

A high level of circulating total homocysteine (tHcy) is an independent risk factor for vascular diseases:

- Homocysteine is an amino acid, but not one that is part of the metabolism or structure of the body, as it is an intermediary product. It is synthesized from methionine.
- Homocysteine is effectively at the centre of two pathways, one that requires folate and vitamin B_{12}, the other that requires vitamin B_6. Deficiencies in these vitamins are therefore likely to leave a high level of homocysteine in the body.
- It is possible that homocysteine encourages the formation of superoxide radicals (see Chapter 7 'Free radicals', p. 44) in the blood. These damage the blood vessels wall and, once damaged, plaques can form (Chapter 27 'Problems with lipid metabolism', p. 204).
- Homocysteine has prothrombotic effects and enhances the activities of factor XII and factor V (see Figure 28.1, p. 212).

● Predisposing Factors

- Sex: men have a tendency for high levels of homocysteine.
- Genetic: there are also genetic differences, as can be see with race.

● Exacerbating Factors

- Heavy coffee consumption (approximately eight cups a day) combined with smoking has been associated with high levels of homocysteine.

● Treatment

Plasma homocysteine levels can be lowered by taking folic acid along with vitamin B_{12}, which works synergistically. The higher the level, the greater the drop with this type of supplementation.

Wilson's Disease

- Recessively inherited disorder of copper metabolism.
- Causes the body to retain copper: the liver of a person with Wilson's disease does not release copper into bile as it should.
- Copper is absorbed from food and builds up in the liver, damaging the liver tissue: this damage eventually releases the copper directly into the bloodstream, resulting in copper being carried throughout the body.
- The copper build-up leads to damage in the kidneys, brain and eyes.
- If not treated, Wilson's disease can cause severe brain damage, liver failure and death.
- Wilson's disease is hereditary: symptoms usually appear between the ages of 6 and 20 years, but can begin as late as age 40.

● Signs and Symptoms

- Presents as liver disease in children and adults.

- Kayser–Fleischer ring present as a greenish brown or gold ring on the cornea in 90% of symptomatic patients.
- Reduced serum copper and ceruloplasmin concentrations (see Chapter 41 'Scientific tests', p. 340).

Early Signs and Symptoms

Asymmetrical tremor at rest or with movement. In older patients, Wilson's disease can be mistaken for Parkinson's disease.

Later Signs and Symptoms

- Arthritis with osteopenia.
- Spasticity.
- Dystonia: extended muscle contraction in a group of muscles.
- A small percentage may have psychological problems.
- Nephrocalcinoisis: excessive deposition of calcium in kidneys.
- Cardiomyopathy: damage of heart muscle.
- Increased concentration of copper in the brain and viscera: therefore neurological (e.g. epileptic seizures) and hepatic symptoms (possible cirrhosis).

• Initial Diagnostic Screening Tests

Blood Test

- Ceruloplasmin (copper-containing protein) levels: low (less than 20 mg/dL).

Urine Test

- If ceruloplasmin levels are low then urine is collected over a period of 24 hours.
- Normal levels of urinary copper are between 10 to 30 mg/24 hours.

• Treatment

- Patients are advised to abstain from alcohol to avoid damaging the liver further.
- Potentially hepatotoxic drugs are avoided.
- Avoidance of foods high in copper: dietary copper is kept below 2 mg a day (see Chapter 13 'Vitamins and minerals', p. 98).
- Zinc supplementation to interfere with absorption of copper.
- Chelating agent – penicillamine – forms a complex with the copper, thereby removing it from the body's metabolism. Readily absorbed from the gastrointestinal tract and quickly excreted in urine. Other chelating agents are available if there is lack of tolerance to penicillamine, e.g. trientine. However, this drug creates problems in patients with an iron deficiency.
- Patient has to undergo frequent urinalysis and complete blood counts.

Adverse Effects of Penicillamine

- Nausea and vomiting.
- Nephrotic syndrome: large amounts of protein leak into urine.
- Arthropathy: swelling or dysfunction of joints.
- Optic neuropathy.
- Various blood disorders.

Reference

Jacob RA, Spinozzie GM, Simon VA et al. Consumption of cherries lowers plasma urate in healthy women. Journal of Nutrition 2003; 133(6):1826–1829.

Reproductive hormones

38

There are several major classes of steroid hormone:

- Female sex hormones: oestrogens and progesterones.
- Male sex hormones: androgens.
- Adrenocorticoids: glucocorticoids.

These are all derived from cholesterol. There is an interconversion between male and female hormones, as the structures are very similar (see Figure 38.3, p. 305). This occurs naturally in both males and females, although in females there is a predominance of female hormones and in males a predominance of male hormones.

Female Hormones

- Oestrogen: secreted by the adrenal cortex as well as the ovaries.
- Progesterone: prepares the uterus for implantation of a fertilized egg and maintains pregnancy. The ovaries of sexually mature females secrete a mixture of **oestrogens** and **progesterone**.
- Adrenocorticoids: maintain electrolyte balance (see Chapter 26 'Cardiovascular disorders', p. 198).

The Menstrual Cycle

Gonadotrophin-releasing hormone (GnRH) stimulates the pituitary gland, which secretes **follicle-stimulating hormone (FSH)** and is responsible for the synthesis and secretion of oestrogen in the ovaries. When oestrogen levels rise to a critical point, production is switched off by shutting off the **GnRH** release from the hypothalamus (Figure 38.1).

Progesterone production is stimulated by **luteinizing hormone (LH)**, which is produced by the pituitary as a result of stimulation by **GnRH**. Progesterone levels cannot rise too high, as they are controlled in the same way as oestrogen. A new follicle begins to form in one of the ovaries at this stage and, when menstruation ceases, the follicle continues to develop while at the same time secreting **oestrogen** (Figure 38.2). The rising **oestrogen** levels cause the endometrium to thicken and become richly supplied with blood vessels and glands.

Rising levels of LH create a change in the follicle until a sudden surge in LH levels at about 2 weeks triggers ovulation (**mid-cycle**). The unfertilized egg is then released

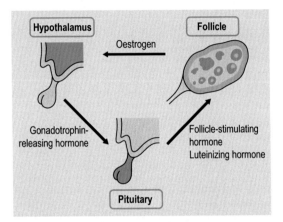

Figure 38.1 Hormonal feedback in the female reproductive system.

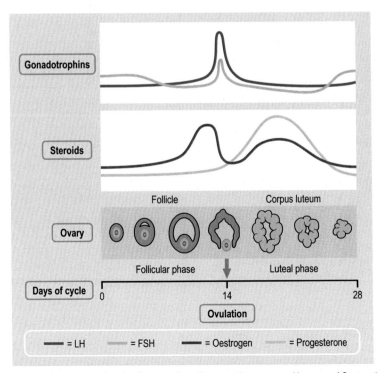

Figure 38.2 The menstrual cycle, showing the effects on the ovary and hormonal fluctuations.

into the fallopian tube. The presence of **LH** encourages the empty follicle to develop into a **corpus luteum**, which then starts to secrete **progesterone**. This:

- continues preparation of the endometrium for pregnancy
- inhibits the contraction of the uterus
- inhibits the development of a new follicle.

If fertilization does not occur then the elevated levels of **progesterone** inhibit the release of **GnRH**, which inhibits further production of **progesterone**. When the progesterone levels drops, the:

- corpus luteum and endometrium break down
- uterus is able to contract and menstruation begins.

Menstruation occurs every 28 days, when the lining of the uterus breaks down and is discharged.

Pregnancy

The menstrual cycle is arrested. The fertilized egg embeds itself in the wall of the uterus and forms a blastocyst, which has two parts:

- the inner cell mass, which becomes the fetus
- the trophoblast, which develops into amnion, placenta and umbilical cord. This part of the blastocyst starts to secrete **human chorionic gonadotrophin (hCG)**, which maintains the corpus luteum and stops it disintegrating. It is not inhibited by rising levels of progesterone.

The placenta then becomes a major source of progesterone, which is necessary to maintain the pregnancy.

Birth

- The placenta releases **corticotrophin-releasing hormone (CRH).**
- This stimulates the pituitary of the fetus to secrete **adrenocorticotrophic hormone (ACTH).**
- ACTH acts on the adrenal glands of the fetus.
- This releases an **oestrogen precursor**, which is converted to **oestrogen** by the placenta; the placental secretion of oestrogen rises.
- The rising level of oestrogen causes the muscle wall of the uterus to contract. This effect is increased by **oxytocin**, which is secreted by the posterior lobe of the pituitary as well at the uterine wall.
- Prostaglandins that encourage muscle contraction also appear in the mother's blood as well as in the amniotic fluid. The combination of the **oxytocin** and the **prostaglandins** start the labour.

Oral Contraceptives

The feedback inhibition of GnRH secretion by oestrogen and progesterone is utilized by most forms of contraceptive pill. The inhibition of GnRH prevents the mid-cycle surge of LH and therefore ovulation. With no egg to be fertilized there should, in theory, be no possibility of pregnancy.

Side Effects of Taking the Pill

There can be an increased tendency for blood clots to form, thereby increasing the risk of strokes and heart attacks, as oestrogen enhances the clotting of blood.

Infertility Treatment

Both the male and female partners are examined, although orthodox treatment in most cases is directed towards the female member of the partnership:

- Structural: to ensure that all the reproductive organs are normal and there are no obstructions.
- Viability: to ensure patients are capable of producing the appropriate amounts of viable eggs and sperm.
- Disease: sexually transmitted infections (STI) such as *Chlamydia trachomatis* can cause asymptomatic inflammation of the fallopian tubes.
- Metabolic disorders: systemic conditions, e.g. polycystic ovarian syndrome (see Chapter 37 'Metabolic disorders', p. 293).

Diagnostic Tests

- Laproscopy.
- Sperm count.

The Importance of Hormonal Levels in Infertility Blood Tests

- **Follicle-stimulating hormone (FSH)**: if levels are high, the woman might be low on eggs as this hormone triggers the follicle to release eggs. High levels indicate an overall imbalance of the hormone.
- **Luteinizing hormone (LH)**: high levels – usually in a surge – occur at around the time an egg is released. Blood tests are usually performed just before ovulation to look for these surges.
- **Prolactin**: high levels prevent the release of FSH and LH.
- **Progesterone**: has to maintain the luteal phase, which occurs 12–16 days after ovulation. The progesterone levels are expected to rise at this point.

Treatment

Infection

Any infection is identified and treated with antibiotics. Both parties can be treated in this case.

Improvement of General Health of the Patients

Diet and lifestyle should be addressed if this is an issue for both parties, including vitamin supplementation.

Infertility Drugs

Generally three classes of drug are used:

- selective oestrogen receptor modulators (SERM) – anti-oestrogens
- human menopausal gonadotrophin
- dopamine agonists (see Chapter 19 'Pharmacodynamics: how drugs elicit a physiological effect', p. 140 and Chapter 31 'The nervous system', p. 242).

Selective Oestrogen Receptor Modulator: Clomifene (Clomid)

- Taken orally on a daily basis.
- Stimulates the pituitary gland to produce FSH to trigger ovulation.

Adverse Effects

- Mood swings.
- Breast pain.

- Abdominal pain.
- Hot flushes.
- Menstrual disorders: menorrhagia, intermenstrual spotting.
- Endometriosis.
- Weight gain.
- Rashes.

Human Menopausal Gonadotrophin

- Purified FSH injected (subcutaneous or intramuscular injection) for 7–12 days to develop egg follicles. Then injected with:
- Human menopausal gonadotrophin (hMG) to stimulate the ovaries to release the egg (or eggs) that has developed.

This method is usually used in women with low oestrogen levels who have not responded to clomifene. This phase of the treatment is decided using a combination of blood tests and ultrasound.

Adverse Effects

- Nausea and vomiting.
- Bloating.
- Fluid retention.
- Weight gain.
- Joint pain.
- Fever.
- Overstimulation of ovaries: resulting in possible multiple pregnancy and miscarriage. It might also lead to a swelling of the ovaries to several times their normal size; the fluid in them might leak into the abdominal cavity.

Dopamine Agonists: Bromocriptene

- Usually offered to women with hyerprolactinaemia (high levels of prolactin in the blood).
- Hyperprolactinaemia can be due to a pituitary tumour, which is usually benign.
- Medication such as antidepressants, opiate drugs and painkillers can raise prolactin levels in the blood because they interfere with dopamine inhibition of prolactin response.

Adverse Effects

- Excessive sleepiness.
- Fibrotic reactions.

Menopause

This can start in the early forties and is due to the follicles becoming less responsive to FSH and LH. As the follicles secrete less oestrogen, ovulation and menstruation become irregular and finally cease. At this point, menopause occurs.

With the reduction of oestrogen, the hypothalamus is no longer inhibited and is able to stimulate the pituitary to secrete hormones at a much higher level. The high concentrations of FSH and LH can cause a variety of physical and emotional symptoms.

Hormone Replacement Therapy

This is a combination of oestrogens and progesterones. It is believed to be of benefit because:

- Unpleasant menopausal symptoms are reduced.
- Loss of calcium from the bones is reduced, decreasing the risk of osteoporosis.

This occurs only while HRT is being administered.

• Premarin

Adverse Effects

- Heavy menstrual bleeding, cramping.
- Breast tenderness.
- Fluid retention, oedema, weight gain, increased fat.
- Headache, migraine.
- Depression, anxiety.
- Glucose intolerance, insulin resistance.
- Oestrogen dominance.
- Stimulates growth of fibroids.
- Worsens endometriosis.
- Nausea, vomiting, cramping, bloating.
- Leg cramps.
- Eye problems.
- High blood pressure.
- Increased blood clotting.
- Venous thromboembolism.
- Increased risk of endometrial and breast cancer.
- Loss of scalp hair, growth of facial and body hair.
- Gall bladder disease.
- Pancreatitis.

• Progestins

Progestins are chemical or drug imitations of progesterone. Provera (medroxyprogesterone acetate) is the most common progestin. Most are made by taking natural progesterone and altering the chemical structure so it can be patented. Another type of progestin is made by altering a synthetic form of testosterone.

Adverse Effects

Because they suppress the production of natural progesterone in the body, they disrupt the steroidal hormone pathways as well, causing problems with adrenal and general gonadal function. This can lead to:

- depression
- anxiety
- fatigue
- fluid retention and breast tenderness, weight gain
- migraine
- angina, palpitations
- menstrual irregularities, spotting
- glucose intolerance (promotes insulin resistance)
- general oedema
- nausea

- insomnia
- skin rashes, acne
- hair loss on scalp, facial hair growth.

More serious effects are:

- coronary spasm
- stroke
- pulmonary embolism
- evidence suggesting increase in breast cancer with women taking this medication.

What are the Natural Alternatives?

Diadzein

Diadzein is naturally occurring isoflavone (Figure 38.3), which is classed as a phytoestrogen because it possesses oestrogen-like properties. It appears to have both weak oestrogenic and antioestrogenic effects and might also be an antioxidant, anticarcinogenic, antiatherogenic and provide some protection against osteoporosis. It is found as the glycoside **diadzein** in:

- Fabaceae: *Glycine max* (soy bean), *Psoraleae corylifolia* (*Bu Gu Zhi*), *Puerariae* spp. (*Ge Gen*), *Trifolium pratense* (red clover).

Dioscorea spp. (*Shan Yao*)

The plant sterol **diosgenin** (see Figure 38.3) comes from *Dioscorea* spp. (wild yam). It occurs as a glycoside. Diosgenin can be converted to progesterone via a chemical

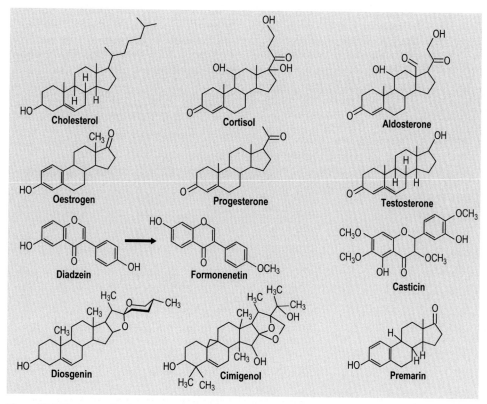

Figure 38.3 Structure of various reproductive hormones and related plant compounds.

process called 'Marker degradation', which gives access to many important steroids, e.g. testosterone and oestradiol.

Diosgenin has been shown to have some oestrogenic activity, but lacks progesterogenic activity. Neither can it be converted to progesterone in the body. This process can only occur in the laboratory.

Vitex Agnus Castus

This herb is used a great deal in Western herbal medicine. The decrease in oestrogen effects is thought to be mediated through the pituitary gland, by inhibition of anterior pituitary function. Vitex seems to be able to raise progesterone levels.

Casticin (Figure 38.3), a flavonoid, may be one of the active components, but its activity is far from clear.

Black Cohosh (*Cimicifuga racemosa*)

Pharmacological studies have shown that *Cimicifugia* can inhibit oestrogen-dependent breast cancer cells. The sudden release of LH during menopause leads to hot flushes. *Cimicifugia* prevents the release of LH and decreases the hormone's ability to bind with receptors in the hypothalamus.

The exact mechanism of the antioestrogenic activity of black cohosh is unknown, as extracts of black cohosh do not bind to the oestrogen receptors. However cimigenol (see Figure 38.3), which is found in *Cimicifugia*, has a steroidal configuration.

The Male Reproductive System

Testosterone

Testosterone, like progesterone and oestrogen, is derived from cholesterol. Testosterone is also secreted by the ovaries and placenta, as well as by the adrenal glands in women (although in very small amounts). Testosterone is significantly metabolized by the gastrointestinal tract. Approximately 44% is lost in the first-pass metabolism. Testosterone promotes protein synthesis and growth of tissues with androgen receptors, resulting in:

- muscle growth
- increased strength
- increased bone density
- maturation of the male reproductive organs
- a deepening of the voice: although this also occurs in females to a lesser degree due to a slight increase in testosterone
- increased body and facial hair.

Chemotherapy

39

Chemotherapy is used in treatment of cancer. There are two types of chemotherapy:

- antineoplastic: anticancer
- cytotoxic: kills the cells.

History

The treatment of cancer by chemotherapy started in the 1940s after military personnel were accidentally exposed to mustard gas. Examination of their blood showed abnormally low white cell counts and it was thought that this might have an effect on patients with cancer. It was tried out on patients with advanced lymphomas and given intravenously. Their improvement, although temporary, was enough to start research into chemotherapy.

Uses of Chemotherapy

Chemotherapy is a systemic treatment and is therefore used when the cancer has spread to various sites in the body. Radiation and surgery are used when the problem is localized.

The Cell Cycle

To understand how chemotherapy works it is necessary to understand the lifecycle of a cell (Figure 39.1):

- GO phase (resting stage): the cell is at rest and has not started to divide. This can last for a few hours to a few years, depending on the circumstances (reproductive cells have a very short resting phase whereas plant seeds have been known to germinate many years after they have been deposited). The cell becomes activated.

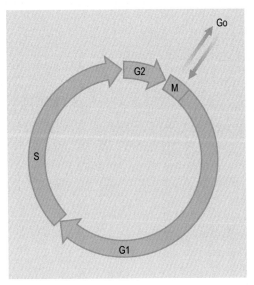

Figure 39.1 The phases of the cell cycle.

- G1 phase: the cell starts to make more proteins and is ready to divide. This usually lasts 18–30 hours.
- S phase: the deoxyribonucleic acid (DNA) chains are copied so that the new cell has the same DNA. This usually lasts 18–20 hours.
- G2 phase: this is just before the cell starts splitting into two cells. This phase usually lasts from 2–10 hours.
- M phase: the cell splits into two new cells. This phase usually lasts 30–60 minutes.

Chemotherapy works on actively reproducing cells. Different drugs act on different parts of the cycle. Oncologists use different groups of drugs to act on certain parts of the cycle. The problem with chemotherapy, however, is that it also acts on normal cells that are actively reproducing. The reproductive cells tend to be the ones that are most badly affected as they are multiplying relatively rapidly. The trick is to balance killing off too many good cells along with the bad cells.

The Aims of Chemotherapy Treatment

There are three aims.

- **Cure**: so the cancer does not return.
- **Control**: stopping the disease spreading and try to provide quality of life while the patient is alive.
- **Palliative**: if the cancer is in an advanced stage drugs are used to relieve the symptoms, even though they might not increase the patient's life span.

Terminology

- **Adjuvant therapy**: postsurgical treatment to prevent the growth of any remaining cells and metastasis around the body.
- **Benign tumour**: remains confined to original location. There is no invasion of surrounding material or general dispersal. Can be removed by surgery.

Generally not life threatening unless in an inoperable place, e.g. certain types of brain tumour.

- **Malignant**: tumour can invade surrounding material and generally disperse in the body. Often life threatening.
- **Metastasis or secondaries**: spreads from the main site of the tumour to a distant site, forming new centres of growth.
- **Neoadjuvant therapy**: can be used to shrink a large tumour so that it can be more easily removed by surgery.

Major Groups of Cancer

Carcinomas

- Solid tumours usually from epithelial cells.
- 90% of all human cancers.

Usually found in:

- Skin.
- Cells lining internal organs, e.g. lung and intestine.
- Glandular tissue e.g. breast and prostate.

Sarcomas

Tumours arising from connective tissue, for example bone primary tumours.

Leukaemia and Lymphomas

- From blood-forming cells and cells of the immune system.
- 8% of all human cancers.

Chemotherapeutic agents

The categories of drugs are based on:

- How the drugs affect specific chemical pathways within the cancer cells.
- How the drugs interfere with the cellular pathways.
- The specific cell phase.

This helps the oncologist to plan when to use a drug or which drugs are going to work best together. There are several forms of chemotherapy:

- alkylating agents
- cytotoxic antibiotics
- plant alkaloids: vinca alkaloids and taxanes
- antimetabolites
- hormones.

Alkylating Agents

Work in three ways:

- Attach to alkyl groups of DNA bases: DNA becomes fragmented by repair enzymes trying to replace the abnormal units.
- Causing mispairing of the nucleotides, which leads to mutations.
- Formation of cross-bridges so that DNA is unable to unzip.

Cyclophosphamide is metabolized in the liver to form several active metabolites. Its adverse effects are that prolonged use can lead to secondary cancers, particularly leukaemias.

• Cytotoxic Antibiotics

- Squeeze between the base pairs, creating problems with DNA and RNA synthesis.
- Inhibit the enzyme that 'unknots' the DNA so that it can unzip and form RNA.
- These work at all phases of the cycle.

• Plant Alkaloids

- Mitotic inhibitors.
- These work in the M phase of the cell cycle.

Vinca Alkaloids

Vincristine prevents cell division (mitosis) at a point where the cell pulls duplicated DNA chromosones to either side of the cell in special structures called spindles. Vincristine binds to tubulin which makes up the spindles thus preventing the formation of the spindles and cell division.

Taxanes

Work in the opposite way to the vinca alkaloids by forcing the spindles together, creating abnormal bundles of microtubules and thus disrupting mitosis.

• Antimetabolites (Figure 39.2)

- Compete with the essential components of metabolic processes and inhibit those processes.
- Interfere with DNA and RNA growth.
- Phase specific: work in the S phase.
- Used to treat leukaemias and tumours of the breast, ovary and gastrointestinal tract.

Methotrexate

Is an analogue of folic acid and interferes with folic acid metabolism. Folic acid is vital for normal cell function.

Azathioprine (AZA)

Becomes metabolized to **mercaptopurine** using glutathione. Although mercaptopurine can be used as a cytoxic agent in its own right, azathioprine has a longer duration of action than mercaptopurine.

• Hormones

- Alter the action or production of female or male hormones.
- Can be used to slow the growth of breast, prostate and endometrial cancers.
- Do not work in the same way as standard chemotherapy drugs.

Glucocorticoids

- Steroids are used to kill cancer cells or slow their growth.
- They are often combined with other types of chemotherapy drugs to increase their effectiveness.
- They are useful with brain tumours to reduce the swelling.
- **Prednisolone.**

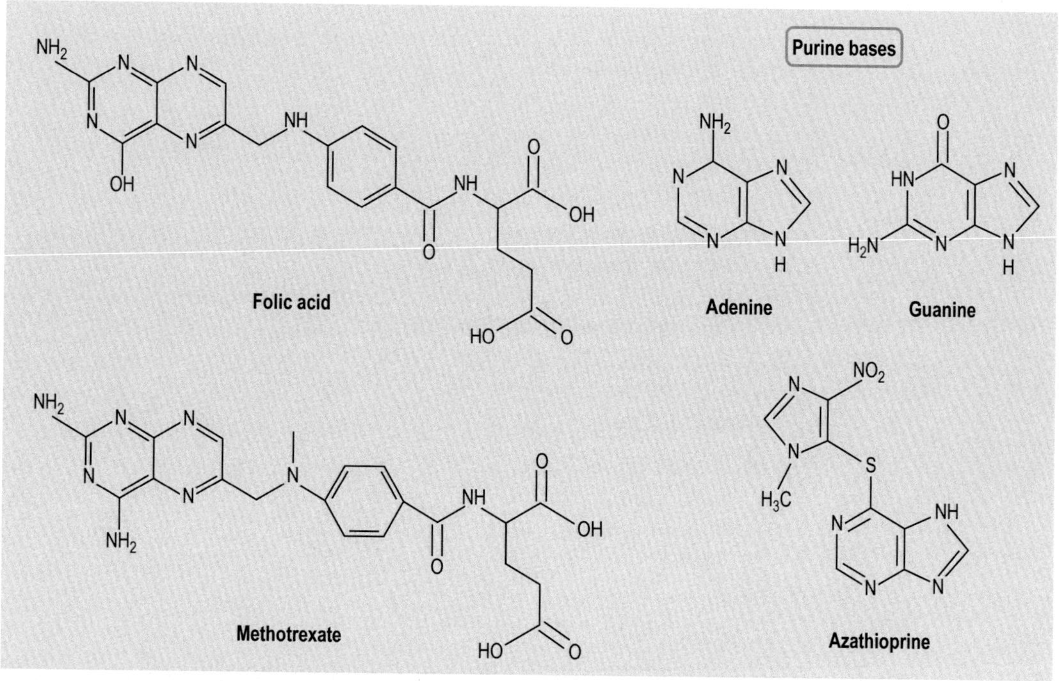

Figure 39.2 Antimetabolite drugs used in chemotherapy, showing the similarity in structure to normal metabolites. Methotrexate highlights the differences between the drug and the metabolite; azathioprine highlights the similarity.

Tamoxifen is an oestrogen receptor antagonist. It is the hormonal treatment of choice in women with oestrogen-receptor-positive breast cancer. **Buserelin** is used for prostate cancer.

Factors Considered in the Treatment of Chemotherapy

- Type of cancer.
- Stage of cancer (has it spread?).
- Age.
- General state of health.
- Any serious health problem (e.g. kidney or liver problems).
- Any anticancer treatments given in the past.

Cure requires complete eradication of tumour cells. By and large, the drugs kill a constant proportion of cells rather than a constant number. The fewer cells there are, the better the chance of recovery.

Why does Chemotherapy Fail?

- Anticancer drugs are still not specific enough for the cancer they are treating: the drugs rely on the biochemistry of the cancer cells being different to that of the biochemistry of the normal cells. In real life this is not really the case. *Note*: this principle is the same as antibiotics killing off the entire gut flora not just the bad bugs.
- Tumour cells can develop resistance to anticancer drugs: they divide rapidly and, like bacteria, a mutation of one cell, which develops resistance, will produce resistant progeny very quickly.

- Drugs might not be able to get to the site in high enough concentrations: a large mass means that the cells at the centre are not exposed to the blood supply that brings the drugs to the cells.

What Affects the Survival Rate of the Patient?

● Nature of the Cancer

- The stage it is at when diagnosed.
- How fast can it divide and multiply.
- If all the cells in the cancer are slightly different it makes it more difficult to choose the right chemical for chemotherapy.
- The phase in which the cell cycle is treated.

● Pharmacology

- How far on treatment is given.
- The gaps between treatments.
- The combination of drugs used.

● Patient

- The health of the patient.
- How efficiently the patient's blood supply is working. This is a double-edged sword. The tumour needs a good blood supply to deliver the drug, but this will also mean the tumour is well nourished.
- Whether the immune system of the patient is able to attack the tumour itself.

The Theory and Reality of Chemotherapy

● The Theory

- The drugs should vary in lethal toxicity around the cell cycle.
- If the drugs are specific enough to a specific point in the cycle then all those cells not at that point will not be affected immediately. Eventually, with enough therapy, all the cells will reach the same stage in the cycle at the same time to become synchronized. This makes killing more of them easier.
- Repeated chemotherapy in a consecutive treatment will maximize the effect of the treatment by eventually catching the cells it missed on the last round in the phase when they are most vulnerable.

● The Reality

- This is difficult to apply clinically: every person, and every cell, is unique.
- The tumour might regrow between treatments.
- Drug resistance.
- Not all the tumour sites might be exposed to a high enough level of chemical.

Adverse Effects

- Decrease of white blood cells, red blood cells and platelet counts: can lead to infections, anaemia and haemorrhage.
- Nausea and vomiting: due to stimulation of the vomiting centre in the CNS.

- Dysphagia, diarrhoea, pain and bleeding: due to the damage of proliferating mucosa of the gastrointestinal tract.
- Partial or complete alopecia: damage to hair follicles.
- Menstrual irregularities, premature menopause: fetal abnormalities. Oligospermia (decrease in sperm count) and infertility in males.
- Cancer patients might have an increase of second malignancies: the immune system might have been damaged by treatment, e.g. leukaemia.

Section 6

Toxicology

Toxicology

40

In the study of toxicology, a solid appreciation of pharmacokinetics and pharmacodynamics (see Chapters 14 to 19) is very important, as the mechanics of the two areas are very much a part of what makes a chemical harmful to a patient. Poisons or toxicants are chemicals that have harmful or adverse effects on living organisms. A chemical can be poisonous under one set of conditions and not under another. For example, potassium is a vital part of body metabolism, but too much will cause atrial fibrillation.

There are two different types of toxic reaction:

1. Irreversible: e.g. mutagenicity (mutation), carcinogenicity (cancer promoting), teratogenicity (congenital malformations) and death.
2. Reversible: providing the initial damage is not overwhelming, such as:
    - organ damage, e.g. liver, kidney or skin
    - functional damage, e.g. respiratory depression, loss of consciousness or convulsive effect.

When dealing with chemicals, the following must be kept in mind:

- The chemical must get to the effector site (such as a synapse or enzyme receptor site) in a biological system to produce a biological effect.
- Not all chemically induced biological effects are harmful, e.g. the therapeutic effects of herbs.
- The occurrence and intensity of chemical-induced biological effects are dose related.

- Interactions with other chemicals might potentiate the effect of one or more of the active compounds in the drugs, creating a toxic effect in the body.
- The chemical might be altered in the body and the metabolites might cause problems (see Chapter 7 'Free radicals', p. 41).

The Occurrence of Poisons

Virtually all chemicals can be considered toxic under certain conditions, e.g. pure water when inhaled is rapidly absorbed across the lung alveoli to cause lysis of red blood cells. Poisoning is either:

- **Acute**: this usually manifests as anaphylactic shock e.g. to nuts. Remember that some Chinese herbs are nuts, e.g. *Semen/Prunus persicae* (peach kernels, *Tao Ren*) so it might be worth asking patients if they have any known allergies to nuts; they will usually know.
- **Chronic**: the more usual type of poisoning encountered by herbalists. The chemical builds up over a period of time in the body, particularly anything fat soluble. The symptoms can be far less obvious than for acute poisoning, and in the long term might be lethal or sublethal (e.g. the patient might be ill and tired all the time).

Drug Absorption

The tissues that are most susceptible are those directly in contact with the environment, e.g. skin, mucous membranes of the lungs and gut.

Gut

This is a common route of entry. Different parts of the gut allow different rates of absorption:

- **Mouth**: rapid absorption. Chemicals in the mouth are in a fairly pure form, not having been diluted or transformed by enzymes or stomach acid. Chemicals entering the body via the mouth will not immediately enter the liver (which is the main detoxifying organ). If you are not sure whether a patient is likely to react to a decoction, ask him or her to take a small amount into their mouth, swill it around, then spit it out.
- **Stomach**: the change in pH alters the absorption of chemicals (see Chapter 8 'Acids and bases', p. 55). Decreasing pH leads to increased gastric clearance. Gastric movements mix the food material bringing it in close contact with gastric juices:
  - Gastric retention increases with decreased motility: the gastric retention will increase if the toxin favours gastric absorption.
  - Gastric retention decreases with increased motility: the toxin might be more of a problem in this case if it is better absorbed in the duodenum.
  - A fatty diet increases gastric retention time: this is why good movement around the gastrointestinal tract is important so that the normal toxins ingested do not hang around.
- **Small intestine**: the major site for absorption. The absorption area is large – approximately 250 m², which is the size of a tennis court.
- **Large intestine and rectum**: rectal absorption bypasses the liver and enters the bloodstream quickly. Thus suppositories can be used in cases where a drug is needed to act fast. However, because they initially bypass the liver, any reaction to the drug will be difficult to counteract.

Respiratory Tract

As much blood passes through the lungs as all the remaining parts of the body together. The lungs are therefore one of the most vascular and effective sites of absorption of the body. This is why it is possible for a patient to have an anaphylactic reaction from inhalation.

Skin

The total skin area of an average human is 2 m²; the skin is a relatively effective barrier to toxins. This is because the toxin has to reach the inner layer – the dermis – before it can diffuse into the bloodstream. The outer layer – the epidermis, through which the toxin must pass – is made up of dead, cornified cells and no active transport takes place. Only lipid-soluble substances will pass through the epidermis. This tends to occur at the sweat glands, sebaceous glands and hair follicles; however, these comprise only 1% of total skin's surface area.

• Factors Affecting Toxin Absorption through the Skin

- If a toxin is lipid soluble and is contained in a lipid then its absorption is enhanced. Ointments tend to keep the chemical in one area for absorption, so a local as well as a systemic reaction might occur.
- Strong detergents and lipid solvents can remove the surface lipid layer from the skin and make it more susceptible to toxins.
- Damage or injury to the skin, e.g. cut or graze, will cause problems, as the underlying tissue will come into direct contact with toxins present in the environment. This is why *Arnica* cream must only be applied to unbroken skin.

Distribution and Transport

The Role of Blood

- Only high-molecular-weight materials, e.g. proteins, will be prevented from passing through the blood vessel wall.
- Toxins can travel free in plasma (where they are more of a problem) or bound to plasma proteins or within red and white blood cells (Chapter 16 'How do drugs get into cells?', p. 123).
- The brain, cerebrospinal fluid and developing fetus are separated by a protective layer of cells from the blood (Chapter 16 'How do drugs get into cells?', p. 126). However, the placenta is not a very effective barrier to the entry of toxic chemicals. Many toxins enter the fetus by diffusion, e.g. thalidomide. Herbs containing volatile oils are thought not to be advisable for use during pregnancy as they can easily pass through to the fetus.

Enzymes

Chemicals can interfere with the enzymes that are vital as catalysts of metabolic processes in the body (see Chapter 19 'Pharmacodynamics: how drugs elicit a physiological effect', p. 137):

- Reversible and irreversible reactions: a toxin can attach itself to an enzyme, either reversibly or irreversibly. If the process is reversible then it might be a case of waiting until the toxin has been processed out of the body. If the process is irreversible then more enzymes have to be produced, which might take too long and result in the person's death.
- Competitive inhibition: if there is more toxin than normal substrate then the toxin, by sheer weight of numbers, attaches to the active site of the enzyme.

319

- Non-competitive inhibition: the toxin binds to another site on the enzyme, creating inhibition.
- Structural change: when a toxin has hooked up to an enzyme then it might force a change in the shape of the protein. This will mean that the normal substrate is not able to lock into the enzyme because it no longer fits.

The Importance of Correct Cell Structure

An intact cell membrane is crucial. Sometimes, however, the cell membrane might not be functioning properly:

- The membrane might break down and release the contents of the cell.
- The membrane structure might be altered more subtly, e.g. pore size or structures such as ion channels or the sodium pump might be affected, reducing movement or absorption of vital chemicals into cells.
- Organelles might be affected, e.g. mitochondria, endoplasmic reticulum, lysozymes. This can affect function, e.g. mitochondria are no longer able to produce energy, or lysozymes break down to release destructive enzymes.

Silicosis is well documented in miners and stonemasons, who work in conditions in which silica is converted to silicic acid. This ruptures the lung macrophages by destabilizing the lysozymes in the lung cells. Enzymes are released, which eventually break down the macrophages.

RNA and DNA synthesis can be affected and as a result growth, cell division and general metabolism are affected. This is most likely the metabolic system that is affected by **carcinogens** and **teratogens**.

Terminology

- **Carcinogen**: a toxin that induces the formation of tumours.
- **Teratogen**: a toxin that can cross the placenta during pregnancy and damage the developing fetus. The important stage of pregnancy is the critical period from the end of the first week up to the 9th or 10th week after conception.
- **Dose**: the quantity of a chemical involved or introduced into a biologic system in a unit period of time (g/kg single dose, repeated dose g/kg/day dose).

Route of administration or exposure is usually indicated.

Dose–Response Relationships

The LD_{50} is widely used: It is the best estimation of the dose of a compound that will produce death in 50% of the test animals (i.e. the lethal dose for 50%). But there are flaws with LD_{50}:

- It measures only mortality, and not toxicity that is non-lethal.
- There is a wide variation of LD_{50} between species so experimentation on animals cannot necessarily be extrapolated to humans. Rates also vary greatly with the age, health and sex of the patient.
- It measures only acute toxicity produced by a single dose, and not long-term toxicity.
- It cannot measure idiosyncratic reactions (abnormal sensitivity to toxins), which occur at low dosages in a small proportion of subjects.
- A great many animals are needed, which fuels the arguments against this type of experimentation.

Toxicity testing can be also dubious:

- The toxin is injected as a pure extract of an isolated chemical reputed to be an active ingredient (either as a toxin or with therapeutic qualities). Very high doses are administered to animals, whose size or metabolism might not necessarily match that of a human.
- It is important to remember that the usual way a herb or supplement is taken into the body is by ingestion as a whole product. The method of processing this chemical is likely to be very different, due to its exposure to the digestive system and processing in the liver.

Herbs can be tested on humans as standardized extracts, using a marker chemical, which is not necessarily the active ingredient. When reading research, it is necessary to discern the method that has been used in the study.

Degrees of Toxicity

- Extremely toxic: 1 mg/kg or less.
- Highly toxic: 1–50 mg/kg.
- Moderately toxic: 50–500 mg/kg.
- Slightly toxic: 0.5–5 g/kg.
- Practically non-toxic: 5–15 g/kg.
- Relatively harmless: more than 15 g/kg.

From this it is possible to see that the more toxic chemicals require a very low dosage.

Safety Versus Toxicity

All drugs, because of their ability to interfere with biological processes, are potentially harmful agents. This is particularly true if the action of the drug can also affect a normal life-preserving process, e.g. respiration. Once the therapeutic effect is exceeded then the vital process could be significantly affected to create harm to the patient, e.g. morphine produces analgesia but produces respiratory depression.

Potency

This is the relative dose of the drug required to produce an effect equal to that produced by a similarly acting drug. The margin of safety between the lethal effect and the desired effect is the therapeutic index. This must be large to be safe.

How is the Concentration of Chemicals in the Body Determined?

Blood is a handy sample material because it is the main method by which chemicals are carried to all parts of the body: movement of chemicals is largely via the blood and lymph systems. This is why blood tests are so commonly used for a range of diagnostic tests (see Chapter 41 'Scientific tests', p. 331).

Accumulation and Storage of Chemicals in the Body

- The shorter the half-life of a toxin, the more rapidly it is metabolized and removed from the body.
- Toxins deposited and metabolized in fat can diffuse back into the blood. The lipid-soluble pesticide DDT (dichlorodiphenyltrichloroethane) is easily stored in the fat and remains in the body for months, only to be released when the lipids are mobilized, for example if the person loses weight.
- Toxins can become incorporated into the body, for example into bone, and remain in the body for years.

Tolerance

Tolerance is the ability of an organism to have less of a reaction to a specific dose of a chemical than it did on a previous occasion with the same dose. For example, tolerance to a drug such as morphine can be acquired over a period of time, which means that patients on morphine for pain relief over a period of time will need gradually higher dosages to get an effect.

Tolerance to many of the drugs that affect the human brain is accompanied by a desperate desire to take the drug. If this is sufficiently strong, so that the drug is taken repeatedly, there is a progressive increase in tolerance. Sudden withdrawal of the drug can lead to serious illness or even death.

Detoxification

This term covers the range of biochemical processes in the body that help to maintain its health by converting toxic substances to non-toxic ones and excreting them through the liver, skin, lungs and intestinal mucosa. The liver is the main site of detoxification in the body (see Chapter 17 'Metabolism', p. 129).

Elimination of Toxins

• Skin

Many complementary practitioners believe that elimination of toxins thorough the skin is the reason for many skin reactions.

• Hair and Nails

The hair and nails are often used for detecting toxins. *Historical note*: it is possible that the emperor Napoleon was poisoned because arsenic was detected in his hair.

• Breast

The breast is an enlarged gland, and care should be taken when formulating herbs for a patient who is breast-feeding, as plant chemicals can come out in the breast milk.

• Lungs

Irritant substances can be removed from the respiratory tract by coughing and sneezing.

• Digestive Tract

Toxins are removed from the stomach by vomiting and from the gut by diarrhoea.

• The Liver

The liver is richly supplied by blood from the hepatic portal vein, which comes from the stomach and intestines. If the phase I and II pathways function properly then chemicals are rendered water soluble and pass out of the body via the kidneys.

An inefficient or impaired detoxification system can result in the accumulation and deposition of metabolic toxins and in increased free radical production and its ensuing pathology. Initially, the patient is usually unwell and lacks energy, but if this continues the effects may be lethal. It is also worth remembering the enterohepatic cycle (see Chapter 17 'Metabolism', p. 131).

Kidneys

The kidneys are a very important route for getting rid of water-soluble toxins. Good health of the kidneys is important, as is a reasonable amount of fluid consumption during the course of the day.

Genetic Factors

Some patients are more susceptible to allergens or toxins than others, for example hay fever and eczema run in families. As metabolic components such as enzymes are proteins, and as the information for producing proteins resides in the structure of the DNA, genetic input is now thought to be very relevant in this area as the whole of a patient's metabolism is likely to be affected.

The phase I and II pathways of the liver are thought to be influenced by genetic factors.

Factors that Alter Toxicity

Age

The Young

- The body is most susceptible to toxins before birth and when the growth rate is at a maximum and tissue and organ differentiation occurs.
- The toxins can cause **teratogenic effects**: e.g. thalidomide affects the limb buds.
- The **predifferentiation period** (the period before the cells differentiate into body tissues) occurs after 17 days; up to this point toxins can easily kill the fetus.
- From 17 to 55 days **organogenesis** occurs where the differentiation of the major body tissues occurs and organs are laid down. After this, limb-reduction deformities cannot occur because the limbs are fully formed.
- After birth, the enzyme system is not fully developed until 3 months of age.

The Elderly

- Altered pH in the stomach can affect the ability to handle toxins.
- **Renal clearance is reduced**: drugs excreted through the kidneys take longer to remove from the body.
- **Liver function might be reduced**: metabolism of the elderly is often impaired
- **Polypharmacy**: elderly people are usually on more than one drug, quite often for cardiovascular conditions.

Size

- The smaller a person is, the lower the dosage they will need for a drug to be toxic.

Pregnancy

- Very few drugs are safe during pregnancy.

Organ Damage

- Damage to the liver and kidneys has a dramatic effect on how efficiently a patient can clear toxins. Careful consideration has to be given when treating a patient with liver disease such as cirrhosis and hepatitis.

- Metabolic illnesses, e.g. Wilson's disease, can affect the function of the liver by damaging its cell structure; other inherited diseases might affect the function of the detoxification enzymes.

Stress

- Disease and nutritional deficiency lead to physiological stress.

Drug Interactions

This is a constantly changing field and a formulary will need to be consulted. Professional bodies should make practitioners aware of any particular changes in practice, but monitoring Medicines and Healthcare Products Regulatory Agency (MHRA) and Food and Drug Administration (FDA) sites should keep the practitioner aware of any developments. Reporting systems are in place throughout the world but as new drugs are developed the information will change.

Generally, care should be taken when treating a patient with herbs or supplements such as the following:

- Plants with alkaloid constituents: as alkaloids have the capability to interfere with metabolism at the genetic level (see Chapter 39 'Chemotherapy', p. 310) and at the receptor level (see Chapter 31 'The nervous system', p. 240), careful consideration has to be given to the potency of the alkaloid.
- Plants with constituents that are likely to upregulate cytochrome P450, e.g. *Hypericum* spp. (St John's wort).
- Drugs that are prone to interactions are those suppressing the immune system:
  - antiplatelet or anticoagulation
  - nervous or psychiatric disorders

Professional bodies send out regular newsletters commenting on possible interactions. The websites of national agencies for drug safety (see Chapter 41 'Scientific tests', p. 346) also have postings on the toxicology reports.

Plant Toxins

Correct preparation of herbs to prevent toxic reactions is vital. The use of an approved supplier should ensure that all herbs have been properly prepared. For example:

- *Pulsatilla* spp. have to be dried before a tincture is made.
- *Pinellia ternate* (*Ban Xia*) is treated with sulphur.
- *Da Huang* is a purgative if boiled for a short time; this quality is diminished if boiled for longer than 10 minutes.

Care must also be taken when using non-traditional preparations, e.g. a herb that has been extracted with alcohol when it is normally extracted using water.

Glycosides

Until the sugar is cleaved there is little risk of toxicity; as soon as the bacteria in the gastrointestinal tract remove the sugar the agent will work.

Oxalates

Generally, it is difficult to consume enough plant material for oxalates to cause problems. For example, it is found in high concentrations in rhubarb leaves, which are not normally eaten. Other examples include Polygonaceae: *Rheum* spp., which are varieties of rhubarb, including *Rheum palmatum* (Turkey rhubarb, *Da Huang*).

Lectins

Lectins are glycoproteins. They were discovered in the 1880s and found to be able to clump erythrocytes *in vitro*. They are now known to take part in several biological activities, including cell adhesion, the control of protein levels in the blood, glycoprotein synthesis (see Chapter 9 'Carbohydrates', p. 71) and cause mitosis in cells that are not actively dividing. Because of this, lectins have the potential to alter cell permeability and generally interfere with cell metabolism.

Of interest in toxicology is that lectins are found in the skins of uncooked beans (the red kidney bean is well known for being toxic if eaten uncooked). There have been problems with cooking raw beans in slow cookers or casseroles when the temperature of the mixture was not high enough to destroy the lectins (this usually requires 80°C). Soaking for at least 5 hours, followed by brisk boiling in fresh water for at least 10 minutes is required to break the lectin down.

Ricin, made from the castor oil bean, became a very well-known lectin following its use, in 1978, in the assassination of the Bulgarian dissident Georgi Markov, who was shot with a pellet coated with ricin from a modified umbrella on Waterloo Bridge in London.

Different lectins have different levels of toxicity and not all lectins are toxic.

Plants Absorbing Chemicals

Plants are very good at absorbing chemicals from the ground in which they are growing. It is therefore possible that, in an area where a high volume of fertilizer is used, excessive nitrate compounds will be incorporated into the plant. Selenium poisoning is well documented in areas where natural deposits are high. Heavy metals can also be absorbed by plants.

Reputable herbal companies will continually spot-check batches of herbs to assay for these compounds.

Arsenic

Arsenic is usually present in very small amounts in soil and water, but should not normally reach dangerous levels. It is found in:

- Fish: it is important to consider the quality of the source when giving fish oils.
- Cereal products.

• Toxicity

- Well known as a deadly poison.
- In low doses can be:
  - carcinogenic
  - teratogenic.

One of the best known signs of arsenic poisoning is Mee's lines or transverse lines across the nails.

Aluminium

Not an essential metal but is found in:

- Some medicinal products, e.g. antacids.
- Some antiperspirants.
- Some food additives, baking powder, cake mixes, self-raising flour, frozen dough and processed cheese.
- Many teas, although it is not easily absorbed.

Its interaction with the metabolism of the body is unknown.

• Toxic Effects

- • Osteomalacia.
- • Microcytic anaemia: the average size of the erythrocytes is smaller than normal.
- • Encephalopathy.

There is an ongoing debate as to whether aluminium might be a contributing factor to Alzheimer's disease.

Poorly Stored Herbs

• Mycotoxins

These are a potential problem with any food or herbal product.

Aspergillus flavus

This fungus produces aflatoxins, which are carcinogenic substances that have even been found in milk, linking the problem directly to grain contamination in cattle feed. It occurs mainly in contaminated cereals such as maize and legumes (e.g. peanuts), and most tree-based nuts. It is invisible to the naked eye but heat treatment and killing the fungus still leaves the aflatoxin behind. In the case of roasted peanuts, the fungus is not killed by roasting, so the longer they are left in storage, the worse the problem becomes.

Symptoms

There are is wide range, depending on the amount consumed:

- • Abdominal pain.
- • Vomiting.
- • Pulmonary oedema.
- • Liver cell damage: including fatty change.
- • Haemorrhage.
- • Loss of function of digestive tract.
- • Convulsions.
- • Cerebral oedema.
- • Death.

• *Claviceps purpurea* (*Ergot*)

This is a parasite of cereal grains. Baking bread kills the mould but leaves the harmful alkaloids behind. These contract the arterioles and smooth muscles of the digestive tract.

Symptoms

- • Gangrene in the extremities.
- • Vomiting.
- • Muscle twitching.
- • Staggering gait.
- • If consumption is continued, eventual death.

• *Ginkgo biloba* (Ginkgo, Maidenhair Tree, *Bai Guo*)

The ginkgo nut contains a neurotoxin that can result in convulsions and possibly death. This herb is traditionally prepared by boiling, which renders it safe.

Bibliograpy

Golan DE, Tashjian AH, Armstrong EJ et al. Principles of pharmacology. The pathophysiologic basis of drug therapy. Baltimore, MD: Lippincott Williams and Wilkins; 2004.

Hardman JG, Limbird LE. Goodman and Gilman's the pharmacological basis of therapeutics. 11th edn. New York: McGraw-Hill; 2005.

Loomis TA, Wallace-Hayes. Loomis's essentials of toxicology. 4th edn. London: Taylor and Francis; 2001.

Rang HP, Dale MM, Ritter JM. Pharmacology. 6th edn. Edinburgh: Churchill Livingstone; 2007.

Reid JL, Rubin PC, Whiting B. Clinical pharmacology. 7th edn. Oxford: Blackwell; 2006.

Waller DG, Renwick AG, Hillier K. Medical pharmacology and therapeutics. 2nd rev. edn. Edinburgh: Elsevier Saunders; 2005.

Section 7

The final analysis

Scientific tests

41

Blood Tests (Table 41.1)

The initial batch of blood tests will be a full blood count and erythrocyte sedimentation rate (ESR) which indicates inflammation or disease. Blood tests are not conducted randomly and cost is often an issue, so more expensive tests will be run only when a more definitive diagnosis is required.

Blood test results are now being delivered directly to the doctor's surgery by computer and abnormalities are identified by the laboratory, although normal ranges are demonstrated by the side of each test.

Full Blood Count

This is performed if there is:

* suspected blood disease
* inflammation
* cancer
* infectious disease.

Babies under 1 year and pregnant women can also be screened this way.

White Blood Cell Count (WBC)

* The number of white blood cells in a volume of blood.

A clinical condition known as leukopenia can occur where the bone marrow produces very few white blood cells. This reduces the efficiency of the immune system, leaving the body open to infection. This can be the result of exposure to:

* Gamma radiation.
* Drugs (such as chloramphenicol on rare occasions).
* Carcinogenic chemicals: e.g. chemicals that contain benzene.

Automated White Cell Differential

This allows the practitioner to see a breakdown in percentage of the different types of white blood cells.

Red Cell Count (RBC)

- The number of red blood cells in a volume of blood.
- An increase in the RBC can occur for several reasons:
  - living at high altitudes
  - strenuous physical training
  - smoking.
- Certain drugs have been associated with an increased RBC, e.g. gentamicin and methyldopa.

Haemoglobin (Hb)

- The amount of haemoglobin in a volume of blood.
- A low value indicates anaemia.
- A low haemoglobin value should always be considered alongside the components of the full blood count.

Haematocrit (Hct)

- The ratio of the volume of red cells to the volume of whole blood.
- If raised, can indicate reduced plasma volume, possibly due to dehydration, e.g. drug (diuretic) or alcohol induced. Might also indicate increased red cell mass due to certain types of tumours.

$$\text{Hct} = \frac{\text{Volume of red cells}}{\text{Volume of whole blood}}$$

• Mean Cell (Corpuscular) Volume (MCV)

- The average volume of a red cell (how big is it?).
- Low in microcytic anaemia, found in iron-deficient anaemia (see Chapter 28 'Blood disorders', p. 209).
- High in macrocytic anaemia, found in pernicious anaemia (see Chapter 28 'Blood disorders', p. 210).

$$\text{MCV} = \frac{\text{Haematocrit (Hct)}}{\text{Red blood cell count (RBC)}}$$

• Mean Corpuscular Haemoglobin (MCH)

- This is the absolute amount of haemoglobin in the average red blood cell in a tested sample.
- Usually, however, a combination MCV and MCHC is more useful:

$$\text{MCH} = \frac{\text{Haemoglobin}}{\text{Red blood cell count}}$$

• Mean Corpuscular Cell Haemoglobin Concentration (MCHC)

- Calculated from the haemoglobin measurement and the haematocrit.
- The average amount of haemoglobin in the average red cell.

- Calculated from the measurement of haemoglobin and the red cell count.
- Low in microcytic (hypochromic) anaemias.
- Normal in macrocytic (normochromic) anaemias: this is because although the cell size is larger than normal the amount of haemoglobin is high therefore making the concentration normal:

$$MCHC = \frac{Haemoglobin}{Haematocrit}$$

Red Cell Distribution Width (RDW)

- Measures the variability of red cell size, therefore a high number indicates greater variation in size.
- A high RDW with a normal MCV can indicate iron, vitamin B_{12} or folate deficiency.
- Normal range is 11–15%.

Platelet Count

- The number of platelets in a specific volume of blood.
- Platelets are not complete cells: they do not contain a nucleus and are actually fragments of cytoplasm from a cell found in the bone marrow called a megakaryocyte.
- Platelets play a vital role in blood clotting.
- Patients with liver disease develop an enlarged spleen: platelets then become trapped in the small pathways of the spleen, as the spleen is so large. The platelet count then reduces.
- Thrombocytopenia might also be due to failed platelet production (leukaemia, aplastic anaemia), increased platelet destruction or use or dilution of platelets.

Ferritin

Ferritin is a protein in the body which binds to iron. Most of the iron in the body is bound to ferritin, which is found in the bone marrow, liver, spleen and skeletal muscle. There is not much ferritin in the blood.

Under normal circumstances, serum ferritin most closely **indicates the amount of iron** stored in the body. Serum ferritin is the most convenient way to estimate iron stores in the body.

If ferritin levels are too low, anaemia due to iron deficiency arises from the following causes:

- Excessive menstrual bleeding.
- Pregnancy.
- Low iron in the diet (vegetarians and vegans).
- Bleeding from the gastrointestinal tract: ulcers, colon cancer, haemorrhoids.

If ferritin levels are too high:

- The amount of iron in the body is too high: this indicates an iron overload disorder such as haemochromatosis or porphyria (see Chapter 28 'Blood disorders', p. 211).
- Iron might be in excess because the body is sequestering iron in the form of ferritin to deprive bacteria of it: a C-reactive protein (CRP) test is used to see whether the elevated ferritin is due to infection or other causes. Both the CRP and the ferritin are made in the liver in response to inflammation. They are known as **acute-phase reactants.**

• C-Reactive Protein

This is a plasma protein, levels of which increase due to inflammation. If found to be present, it is an indicator for:

- cardiovascular disease
- hypertension
- diabetes
- rheumatoid arthritis
- infectious diseases

- autoimmune conditions: e.g. systemic lupus erythematosus.

• Glucose

This test usually occurs first thing in the morning, with the patient having fasted since the night before. An abn s above 7 mmol/L. However, it is possible for a patient with a normal glucose metabolism to have a 'false positive' due to the following.

Oral Glucose Tolerance Test (OGTT)

This is run when both a urine sample and a blood test indicates a problem with metabolizing glucose. It differentiates between a patient who might have had false positives and a normal pattern of glucose fluctuation and a diabetic pattern due to pancreas malfunction or insulin resistance.

- The patient fasts overnight before a sample of blood is taken.
- The patient then drinks 75 g of glucose dissolved in 250–350 mL of water.
- After 2 hours, another blood sample is taken.
- The levels of glucose in the two samples are compared.

The patient is considered to have a problem with glucose metabolism if the levels of glucose in the fasting blood sample are more than 7 mmol/L; if the OGTT is between 7.8 mmol/L and 11.1 mmol/L the patient is deemed to have impaired glucose tolerance; above 11.1 mmol/L and the patient is said to have diabetes.

In a patient able to process glucose normally, the glucose concentration approximately doubles in the first hour, returning to normal after 2 hours. The blood glucose in a diabetic patient will rise to a high level and takes more than 3 hours to return to normal.

The tests for glucose are normally combined and other aspects of the case history taken into account. False positives can occur particularly in women with gestational diabetes postpartum.

• Electrolytes

The electrolytes potassium, sodium and chloride are important for maintaining the:

- Correct amount of fluids in the body (see Chapter 26 'Cardiovascular disorders', p. 192).
- Proper function of the nervous system (see Chapter 31 'The nervous system', p. 235).

• Copper

See Wilson's disease (see Chapter 37 'Metabolic disorders', p. 297).

• Homocysteine

This is now considered a biomarker for inadequate folate, vitamin B_{12} and to a lesser extent vitamin B_6 status, as all these enzymes are involved in homocysteine metabolism (see Chapter 37 'Metabolic disorders', p. 296). Blood for measuring serum homocysteine levels is taken after a 12-hour fast. Levels between 5 and 15 μmol/L indicate insufficiency.

• Liver Function Tests

The liver is responsible for a great variety of metabolic processes in the body. Liver function tests are never performed in isolation and are usually additional information to a case history, examination and other test results.

Alanine Aminotransferase or Alanine Transaminase (ALT)

This is also known as serum glutamic pyruvate transaminase (SGPT). ALT is produced in the cells of the liver. The level is abnormally raised when these cells have been inflamed or have died. The ALT leaks out of the cells into the bloodstream if there is cell damage. Any form of liver cell damage can cause raised ALT levels. The levels are not necessarily an indicator of the degree of damage. **This test is the most sensitive marker for liver cell damage.**

Aspartate Aminotransferase or Aspartate Transaminase (AST)

AST is also known as serum glutamic oxaloacetic transaminase (SGOT). This also indicates liver cell damage. It is not as specific for liver disease as ALT. It can become elevated in situations such as a myocardial infarction, where heart cells are damaged.

Alkaline Phosphatase (ALP)

* Is an enzyme that is produced by the bile ducts.
* Is also found in bone and the placenta.
* Renal or intestinal damage can also cause an increase and it is therefore not specific to the liver.
* A serological test, called ALP isoenzyme test, can be run to determine the origin of the alkaline phosphatase. If the gamma glutamyl transpeptidase (GGT) test and the other function tests such as bilirubin are abnormal then the liver is involved.

Gamma Glutamyl Transpeptidase (GGT)

* This enzyme is also associated with the bile ducts.
* It is largely used to confirm whether the alkaline phosphatase is from the liver.
* If the GGT is an isolated finding then there might be a rare form of liver disease.
* Medications can cause the GGT to be raised as can alcohol or other liver toxins.

• Bilirubin

* A major breakdown product of haemoglobin.
* Haemoglobin comes from the red cells that are about 120 days old and have become too fragile to function. Their cell membranes rupture and the released haemoglobin is phagocytosed by the tissue macrophages throughout the body.
* The bilirubin that eventually forms is released from the macrophages into the bloodstream and immediately binds with the albumin in the plasma and is transported around the body.
* This bound form of bilirubin is called **free bilirubin**.
* The free bilirubin eventually reaches the liver, where it is released from the plasma albumin.
* It then undergoes a process called **conjugation** to form conjugated bilirubin, which is excreted in the bile.
* Bilirubin is converted to **urobilinogen** in the small intestine. This highly soluble compound is reabsorbed by the small intestine wall back into the blood.
* The function of bile salts is to emulsify fat in the small intestine, thus giving the digestive enzymes a larger surface area to work on.

There are two reasons for an increase in **total bilirubin**:

- **Haemolysis of red blood cells**: with haemolytic jaundice there is no blockage of the bile ducts. The red blood cells are broken down faster than the end product can be excreted. The plasma concentration of free bilibrubin rises abnormally. There is no blockage of the bile ducts, so the concentration of **urobilinogen** in the blood also increases. In this case, the **bilirubin** is largely in the '**free**' form.
- **Obstructive jaundice**: this is caused by obstruction of the bile ducts or liver disease. The ducts can be blocked by gallstones, by cancer or by damage to the liver cells. The **free bilirubin** enters the liver and is conjugated as normal but cannot enter the small intestine due to the blockage of the duct. The only route for the **conjugated bilirubin** is back into the bloodstream. This may be due to a congested bile duct rupturing and directly emptying its contents into the lymph system. The **bilirubin** in the plasma in this case is of the **conjugated** kind and not the '**free**' form.

• Total Proteins (TP) or Total Serum Protein

Measures total amount of protein in the blood. There are two main types of protein in the blood: albumin and globulins.

Albumin

- This is the most common protein in the blood.
- It is synthesized by the liver.
- Can give an idea of how well the liver is synthesizing proteins and acts as a '**marker**' protein.
- The test is a reliable and inexpensive way of assessing the degree of liver cell damage.
- Other tests and information have to be taken into account as malnutrition can also cause low albumin.

Globulins

- There are alpha, beta and gamma globulins.
- Some are part of the immune system (see Chapter 30 'Inflammation and the immune system', p. 225) and so can be used to see if the patient is susceptible to infection.
- Others bind to iron (see Chapter 28 'Blood disorders', p. 211) and so can be used to see if the patient is likely to have a rare blood disorder.

• Prothrombin Time (PT)

This gives an indication of the total quantity of prothrombin in the blood. The blood sample is prepared in a particular way so that the coagulation time can be measured. The normal prothrombin time is 10–15 seconds. This time is prolonged in patients with liver disease. This is not a specific test for liver dysfunction and should be used in conjunction with other liver tests.

• Platelet Count

See above.

• Efficiency of Liver Detoxification

This liver function test investigates the efficiency with which the liver can detoxify compounds. It is not the same as the liver function tests described above, which ascertains whether there has been destruction of the liver cells, but is a test of the efficiency of the detoxification pathways of the liver. The information gathered from this test will indicate to a practitioner the nutritional input and patient management that is required to improve the patient's detoxification pathways.

The patient is loaded with small amounts of caffeine, aspirin and paracetamol. These are taken in the morning and the clearance rates are assessed from two saliva samples at a specified time. Urine samples are also taken over a specified period of time. The efficiency with which these substances are cleared from the system will dictate the efficiency of the liver's detoxification efficiency:

- Low caffeine clearance indicates that phase I liver metabolism is not functioning efficiently enough.
- The efficiency with which the aspirin and paracetamol are handled indicates the efficiency of the phase II pathway.

Blood Lipids

- Total cholesterol: high levels indicate a high risk of cardiovascular disease.
- High-density lipoproteins (HDL): high levels indicate a lower risk of cardiovascular disease.
- Low-density lipoproteins (LDL): high levels indicate a high risk of cardiovascular disease.
- Triglycerides: high levels are associated with cardiovascular disease or pancreatitis. Patients with syndrome X tend to have high triglyceride levels.

Endocrine Tests

Thyroid Function Tests (see Chapter 37 'Metabolic diseases', p. 288)

The initial test used is for thyroid-stimulating hormone (TSH), which is deemed to be reliable because it does not fluctuate much on a daily basis. TSH is secreted from the pituitary gland; its production is controlled by a feedback system, which depends on the amount of thyroxine (T4) in the system. So TSH levels give an idea of how the function of the thyroid gland is perceived by the pituitary gland, and not by the peripheral tissues it has an action on. Thus, if the patient is known to have a pituitary problem, this test only gives a rough measure of thyroid output:

337

- Increased levels TSH = an effort to stimulate the thyroid gland = hypothyroidism.
- Decreased levels TSH = an effort to shut off the thyroid gland from producing too much thyroxine = hyperthyroidism.

T4 contains four iodine atoms. One atom is removed to form tri-iodothyronine (T3); so-called because it has three iodine atoms. The amount of T4 is controlled by TSH secreted by the pituitary. T4 enters the blood in two forms:

- Protein-bound T4: prevents T4 entering target tissues (see Chapter 16 'How do drugs get into cells?', p. 125).
- Free T4: can enter target tissues. This is therefore the most important method of ascertaining how the thyroid is functioning.

By combining the results from the TSH and free T4 (FT4), it becomes possible to discern whether the thyroid problem is secondary to a pituitary problem or primary.

T3 is useful for hyperthyroidism tests but not used for hypothyroidism as this is the last test to become abnormal (Table 41.2).

Female Hormone Levels

These tend to be performed for infertility, menopause or as part of the examination of menstrual irregularity and include:

- Prolactin, luteinizing hormone (LH) and follicle-stimulating hormone (FSH) levels – also found in men but for the purposes of this book are ignored.
- Infertility tests: see Chapter 38 'Reproductive hormones' (p. 302).

- **Urinalysis (Dip-Stick Testing)**

  - **Urinalysis**: reagent strips (known as 'chemical stix') are dipped into a urine sample. A colour reference chart on the side of the container denotes the results of the various tests. Urine samples are usually taken on a midstream sample to reduce any normal sediment present. Any sediment that is found can then be analysed for the presence of red and white blood cells, crystals, bacteria, etc. It is important to remember that some food stuffs, such as beetroot, will dye the urine red and that vitamin B_2 (riboflavin) makes the urine turn bright yellow.
  - **pH**: measures the acidity of the urine.
  - **Specific gravity**: measures how concentrated the urine is, but there will be fluctuations depending on how hydrated the patient is.
  - **Glucose**: there should be no glucose in the urine under normal circumstances. Glucose in the urine will result in a retest and in a blood test for glucose if this proves positive.
  - **Protein**: no protein should be present in the urine normally. However, children or athletes under intensive training might have protein in their urine.
  - **Blood**: no blood should be present in the urine under normal circumstances; female patients who are menstruating will have to be retested at another time as their sample might be contaminated. Blood can indicate trauma, infection, kidney stones or cancer of the bladder or kidney.
  - **Bilirubin**: there should be no bilirubin in the urine, although this might be present if there is liver or gall bladder disease.
  - **Nitrates**: should be negative; the presence of nitrates indicates a urinary tract infection.

- **Stool Analysis**

  - **Occult blood**: if bleeding occurs high up enough in the intestine to be blended sufficiently with the stools, it will not be immediately noticeable. Can be used as a screen for colon cancer (see Chapter 35 'Gastrointestinal disorders', p. 279).
  - **Parasites**: the stool sample is examined for parasites, e.g. those found in tropical diseases, such as pinworm or giardiasis.
  - **Infection**: the sample can be examined for bacteria or fungi.

Qualitative Analysis In Brief

Goldbeater's Skin Test

A membrane prepared from the intestine of an ox behaves similarly to an untanned hide. The skin is soaked in 2% hydrochloric acid then rinsed with distilled water and put into the test solution for 5 minutes. The skin is then transferred to a 1% solution of ferrous sulphate. A brown or black colour occurs if tannins are present in the test solution.

Chromatography

This is used to separate compounds out of a mixture. The test compound is dissolved in a solvent and then passed through **a stationary phase** substance. This substance remains static and the dissolved compounds either move through or adhere to it. High-performance liquid chromatography is the most common type of chromatography used in the quality control of herbs. The groups of chemicals are forced through the stationary phase in a column at high pressure, to speed the process up. The points at which the various chemicals stop are analysed by computer. This enables manufacturers or scientists to quickly analyse plant chemicals and isolate them.

Spectrometry

An optical instrument is used to measure light of specific frequencies but varying intensity. This enables scientists to calculate the concentration of a particular compound in a test solution. The concentration of a particular compound in a chosen plant can then be determined.

Table 41.1 Normal adult ranges in common diagnostic tests.

Test	Normal Range	
	Males	Females
FULL BLOOD COUNT		
Red blood cells	4.5–6.5 10^{12}/L	3.8–5.0 10^{12}/L
Haemoglobin	13–18 g/100 mL	11.5–16.5 g/100 mL
Hct	45–52%	37–48%
MCV	80–96 femto L	80–96 femto L
MCH	27–32 pg	27–32 pg
MCHC	32–36 g/dL	32–36 g/dL
RDW	11–15%	11–15%
White blood cell count	4–11 10^9/L	4–11 10^9/L
Neutrophils	2.0–7.5 10^9/L	2.0–7.5 10^9/L
Lymphocytes	1.3–4.0 10^9/L	1.3–4.0 10^9/L
Monocytes	0.2–0.8 10^9/L	0.2–0.8 10^9/L
Eosinophils	0.04–0.44 10^9/L	0.04–0.44 10^9/L
Basophils	0.0–0.10^9/L	0.0–0.10^9/L
Platelets	150–440 10^9/L	150–440 10^9/L
AUTOMATED WHITE CELL DIFFERENTIAL		
Segmented neutrophils	34–75%	34–75%
Band neutrophils	8%	8%
Lymphocytes	12–50%	12–50%
Monocytes	3–15%	3–15%
Eosinophils	5%	5%
Basophils	3%	3%
Prothrombin time	10–15 s	10–15 s
LIVER FUNCTION TESTS		
Bilirubin	0–21 micromol/L	0–21 micromol/L
Serum alkaline phosphatase	20–125 IU/L	20–125 IU/L
ALT/SGPT	0–40 IU/L	0–40 IU/L

(Continued)

Table 41.1 (Continued)		
Test	**Normal Range**	
	Males	Females
ALT/SGOT	0–48 IU/L	0–48 IU/L
GGT	0–45 IU/L	0–45 IU/L
Total serum protein	59–82 g/L	59–82 g/L
Serum albumin	30–45 g/L	30–45 g/L
Serum globulin	25–42 g/L	25–42 g/L
BLOOD LIPIDS		
Total cholesterol	<200 mg/dL	<200 mg/dL
HDL	>37 mg/dL	>47 mg/dL
LDL	<130 mg/dL	<130 mg/dL
Triglycerides	<150 mg/dL	<150 mg/dL
Ferritin	18–270 ng/mL	18–160 ng/mL
Fasting glucose	60–109 mg/dL	60–109 mg/dL
UREA AND ELECTROLYTES		
Serum sodium	133–145 mmol/L	133–145 mmol/L
Serum potassium	3.5–5.3 mmol/L	3.5–5.3 mmol/L
Serum urea	2.5–6.6 mmol/L	2.5–6.6 mmol/L
Serum creatinine	45–110 μmol/L	45–110 μmol/L
Erythrocyte sedimentation rate (ESR)	<15 mm/h	<20 mm/h
C Reactive protein	<10 mg/L	<10 mg/L
Rheumatoid factor	0–35 IU/mL	0–35 IU/mL
HORMONAL LEVELS		
Serum TSH	0.3–3 mIU/L	0.3–3 mIU/L
Serum thyroxine T4 (protein bound)	4.6–12 μg/dL	4.6–12 μg/dL
Free T4 (FT4)	0.7–1.9 ng/dL	0.7–1.9 ng/dL
Serum triiodothyronine (protein bound)	80–180 ng/dL	80–180 ng/dL
Free T3 (FT3)	230–619 pg/d	230–619 pg/d
Serum prolactin	N/A	0 to 20 ng/mL
Serum LH	N/A	5–20 mIU/mL
Serum FSH	N/A	5–30 mIU/mL
Serum FSH after menopause	N/A	50–100 mIU/mL
KEY VITAMIN AND METABOLITES		
Serum B_{12}	150–600 pmol/L	150–600 pmol/L
Red cell folate	360–1400 nmol/L	360–1400 nmol/L
Homocysteine	5–15 μmol/L	5–15 μmol/L
METALS		
Copper	<20 mg/dL	<20 mg/dL
Urinary copper	<100 μg/24h	<100 μg/24h

Table 41.2 Possible results of thyroid function test (See also Chapter 37 'Metabolic diseases', p. 288).

Thyroid dysfunction	Levels of TSH	Levels of FT4	Levels of FT3
Normal	Normal	Normal	Normal
Primary hypothyroidism (due to thyroid only)	High	Low	Normal
Secondary hypothyroidism (due to pituitary)	Low	Low	Normal
Hyperthyroidism	Low	High	High

42

Information gathering and the final analysis

As first-hand experimental evidence is not likely to be generally available to the normal complementary healthcare professional, it is important to know where to go to find reliable information and how to use it.

Internet Portals and Gateways

These are websites, quite often run by governmental bodies, which allow access to the databases of reliable websites in specialist areas. Entering through these portals and gateways usually ensures you will be accessing relatively reliable information.

Professional Journals

Many of these are available online and in many instances, providing the embargo date has passed, there is free online access to articles. *Note*: just because a paper is published in a professional journal does not mean it is flawless.

Critical Analysis of Papers

This requires some practice and it is not possible, given the scope of this book, to enter into a detailed discussion on evidence-based medicine or to dissect a scientific paper. However, a brief summary of the important factors should give an appreciation of what might constitute a well-written paper.

How is it Possible to make Sense of the Information Available and Place it in a Clinical Setting?

As a clinician exploring the subject of pharmacology, you will probably come across two main types of paper:

- Evidence-based medicine: a way of bringing together clinical experience with the best available clinical evidence from systematic research.

- Scientific experiment: limited to work in the rigidly controlled environment of a laboratory.

• Evidence-Based Medicine

Evidence-based papers can be:

- Quantitative: involving numbers and statistics.
- Qualitative: more descriptive, giving background to a study such as the participants' personal feelings or experiences. These are more like reading a story and do not involve statistics.

General Questions to be Asked of an Evidence-Based Paper

- Does the title of the paper reflect the content?
- Is the quantitative or qualitative approach appropriate?
- Was the type of study used appropriate: e.g. if the researcher wanted to examine the relationship between a particular drug and its effects on a group of people over a period of time it is more appropriate to use a cohort study than a randomized controlled trial (see below).
- Have the authors thoroughly justified the methods they used?
- Bias: was the study biased by, for example, the selection of participants or the funding body?
- Was the data that was collected appropriate?
- Had ethical considerations been taken into account?
- Has the data been analysed properly: in the case of evidence-based medicine the statistics should be directly relevant to the clinical situation, e.g. numbers needed to treat (NNT).
- Are statements appropriately referenced?
- Is the research of clinical value?

Both the Critical Appraisal Skills Programme (CASP) and the Scottish Intercollegiate Guidelines Network (SIGN 50) have more detailed work sheets for critical appraisal (p. 347).

Evidence-Based Statistics

These are becoming more user friendly; for example, numbers needed to treat (NNT) gives an idea of how effective a treatment might be, as the fewer the number of patients needed for a response, the more effective the treatment. Details of the statistics associated with evidence-based medicine are available at the websites listed at the end of this chapter.

• Scientific Experiments

These are done in a laboratory environment, which is much easier to control than the conditions under which evidence-based medicine investigations are carried out. However, scientific experimentation is not without its problems. Most serious is that the results of scientific experiments, because of the way the experiments are conducted, are far removed from the conditions encountered in everyday life.

In many cases, at the start of an experiment an assumption is made regarding a drug or an active plant metabolite that might not apply to the normal consumption of that compound. The experiment then proceeds as follows:

- An observation: e.g. crude extracts of a particular species are found to have antibacterial properties.
- The hypothesis: the crude extracts contain several compounds, therefore one, several or all of them are responsible for the antibacterial properties.
- The question: what is the answer to the hypothesis?

343

- Conduct a literature search: to see what has been done before.
- Testing of the hypothesis: an experiment is constructed to test the hypothesis. All details of the experiment, e.g. material, preparation and process of the experiment, should be included in the experimental description. It is important that the methodology is reproducible; 'one-off' experiments are not scientifically valid.
- Presentation of results: quite often tabulated for quick reference.
- Discussion: what conclusions can be drawn e.g. certain groups of compounds in the plant in isolation have an antibacterial effect.

General Comments

The paper should state:

- Why there might be flaws in the research.
- If there is any particular bias: e.g. does the research have any affiliations with an interested group, or was funding derived from an interested party.
- Statistics: are these relevant? A full appreciation of a paper will obviously be enhanced by a proper understanding of statistics.

Types of Paper

• Systematic Reviews or Meta-Analyses

- Very useful for the busy clinician: someone else has taken the time to look through several related articles, commenting on their conclusions and the reliability of the evidence.
- The Cochrane database website (details below) is an example of this and some journals are published with this specific intent in mind.

Disadvantages

- The conclusions drawn by the reviewer might reflect that person's own opinions, so care does have to be taken when reading reviews to identify any particular bias.

• Randomized Controlled Trials (RCTs)

- Considered the 'gold standard' of research and are an intervention approach.
- Patients are randomly allocated into groups. Usually, one is a control group that receives no intervention, e.g. this group is not treated with an active drug.
- The two patient groups selected should be identical in character.

Disadvantages

- Trial subjects do not lead life in a vacuum and will introduce variables into the trial, e.g. dietary habits.

• Cohort Studies

- Prospective studies following a specific disease or characteristic over a period of time to see how a particular condition in a group of patients develops in comparison to a control group.
- This is how smoking was linked to lung cancer; a group of smoking doctors was followed over 50 years.

Disadvantages

- Time taken for study to be completed.
- Influence of lifestyle variables.

- **Case-Control Studies**
  - Retrospective studies looking at what might cause a disease compared with a control group.
  - Show associations, e.g. linking thalidomide to limb-bud malformation.

Disadvantages

- Rely on good record keeping or patient's memory.
- Control groups are difficult to select.

- **Cross-Sectional Studies**
  - Measure of frequency of a disease or risk factor in a carefully selected part of the population.
  - Data is collected at a single point in time.
  - Data might be retrospective.
  - Cross-sectional studies suggested linkages between vitamin A deficiency and cataracts.

Disadvantages

- Cannot establish the cause of a disease.

Websites

UK Portals

- National Electronic Library for Health: http://www.nelh.nhs.uk (This is a virtual library for the NHS.)
- Healthsites: http://www.healthsites.co.uk/index.php (Gives extensive list of medical gateways and portals.)
- Institute of Health and Life and Sciences: http://www.intute.ac.uk/healthandlifesciences (Has replaced Organising Medical Network Information, OMNI. It is a database that enables you to be confident of accessing high-quality internet sites covering health and medicine because they have been assessed by specialists in the topics covered. It is possible to use the database to search for a subject or as a gateway to other reliable sites.)
- PubMed: http://www.ncbi.nlm.nih.gov/entrez/PubMed (A service provided by the US National Library of Medicine that includes millions of citations from journals back to the 1950s. There may be abstracts or links to full text articles denoted by an icon. This service is the database most used by scientists and health professionals.)
- The Cochrane Library: http://www.interscience.wiley.com/cgi-bin/mrwhome/106568753/HOME?SRETRY=0 (A collection of databases that contain high-quality information related to healthcare. The residents of the following countries have full access to the Cochrane database through a 'national provision': Australia, Denmark, England, Finland, Ireland, New Zealand, Norway, Scotland, Sweden and Wales.)

Reviews of Healthcare Papers

- University of York NHS Centre for Reviews and Dissemination: http://www.york.ac.uk/inst/crd/index.htm (Provides research-based information about the effects of interventions used in health and social care.)

Online Formularies

- MIMS: only available on subscription.
- Australia: Australian Medicines Handbook: subscription only.
- UK: BNF online: http://www.bnf.org/bnf (UK medication: free registration.)
- USA: http://www.ashp.org/ahfs (American hospital formulary service online; see Chapter 5 'Nomenclature', p. 33.)

US Portals

- US Government Science and Technology gateway and portal websites: http://www.science.gov (Sites that pull together information from across government agencies.)

Gateways

- BUBL: http://www.bubl.ac.uk/link/h/healthlinks.htm (A UK-based gateway enabling access to a wide range of websites on a variety of subjects.)
- United States National Library of Medicine: http://www.nlm.nih.gov

Many databases provide an online tutorial for new users to guide you through the process of excluding information you might not want and refining your search.

Evidence-Based Medicine

• Australia

- National Institute of Clinical Studies: http://www.nhmrc.gov.au/nics/asp/index.asp/(Australia's official body for marrying evidence-based medicine with clinical practice. As with UK NICE, this is a useful site to keep abreast of new medical guidelines.)

• Canada

- Public Health Agency of Canada: http://www.phac-aspc.gc.ca/dpg_e.html (medical guidelines.)
- Faculty of Medicine and Dentistry of the University of Alberta's evidence-based medicine website: http://www.med.ualberta.ca/ebm/ebm.htm (Provides toolkits to aid the practice of evidence-based medicine.)

• New Zealand

- New Zealand Guidelines group: http://www.nzgg.org.nz (Attempts to link evidence-based medicine with clinical practice. Good links to health issues sites.)

• UK

- Institute for Health and Life Sciences: http://www.intute.ac.uk/useful-websites/evidence-based (See p. 344)
- Centre for Evidence-Based Medicine: http://www.cebm.net (A brief run-down of what evidence-based medicine is, providing links to evidence-based websites.)

• USA

- National Guideline Clearing House: http://www.guideline.gov (Database of evidence-based practice guidelines.)
- Agency for healthcare research and quality: http://www.ahrq.gov

Tools for Performing Analysis on Evidence-Based Medicine

- National Health Service Critical Appraisal Skills Programme (CASP) website: http://www.phru.nhs.uk/Pages/PHD/CASP.htm
- Scottish Intercollegiate Guidelines Network (SIGN 50). Critical Appraisal. Notes and Checklists: http://www.sign.ac.uk/methodology/checklists.html
- National Institute for Health and Clinical Excellence: http://www.nice.org.uk (Provides guidance in the UK for promoting good health and preventing and treating ill health. For orthodox health professions with tools to implement guidelines given by NICE, so a useful site to see changes that are occurring in current thought on the use of orthodox medication.)

Regulatory Agencies for Healthcare Products

These bodies work to ensure the safety of the general public who are taking drugs, herbs or supplements or using medical devices. Although your respective associations should be keeping you informed of changes in the law or guidelines, these website will keep you abreast of any changes.

Quality Control

• Australia

- Therapeutic goods administration of the Australian government: http://www.tga.gov.au/index.htm (Covers orthodox and complementary medicines.)

• Canada

- Canadian government website on drugs and health products: http://www.hc-sc.gc.ca/dhp-mps/index_e.html

• New Zealand

- Medsafe: http://www.medsafe.govt.nz/ (New Zealand's medicines and medical devices safety authority.)

• UK

- Medicines and Healthcare Products Regulatory Agency: http://www.mhra.gov.uk

• USA

- Food and Drug Agency: http://www.fda.gov

Bibliography on Evidence-Based Medicine

Greenhalgh T. How to read a paper: getting your bearings (deciding what a paper is about). British Medical Journal 1997; 315:243–246. Online. Available: http://www.bmj.com/cgi/content/full/315/7102/243

Greenhalgh T. How to read a paper: assessing the methodological quality of published papers. British Medical Journal 1997; 315:305–308. Online. Available: http://www.bmj.com/cgi/content/full/315/7103/305

Greenhalgh T. How to read a paper: papers that summarise other papers (systematic reviews and meta-analyses). British Medical Journal 1997; 315:672–675. Online. Available: http://www.bmj.com/cgi/content/full/315/7109/672

Greenhalgh T. How to read a paper: statistics for the non-statistician. I: different types of data need different statistical tests. British Medical Journal 1997; 315:364–366. Online. Available: http://www.bmj.com/cgi/content/full/315/7104/364

Greenhalgh T. How to read a paper: statistics for the non-statistician. II: 'Significant' relations and their pitfalls. British Medical Journal 1997; 315:422–425. Online. Available: http://www.bmj.com/cgi/content/full/315/7105/422

Index

Page numbers in **bold** refer to figures or tables.

A

abbreviations
  long-chain compounds 32
  sugars 66
abridged phenylpropanoids 150
absorption (into body) 123–125, 126
  calcium 96
  drugs 318–319
    commensal bacteria on 119,
      130–131
    gastrointestinal tract 115–117,
      119–120, 123–124, 143, 318
  iron 97
  lipids 203
  nutrients 274
  pH and pK 55–57
  polarity of substances 24–25
  vitamin K 109
  zinc 99
absorption (into cells) 123–125
accumulation of drugs 321
acetaminophen *see* paracetamol
N-acetyl-*p*-benzoquinone imine
  (NAPQI) 49
acetylcholine 125, **242, 259**
  muscle contraction 237
  receptors 241, 245–246
    myasthenia gravis 259
N-acetylcysteine 49
acid–base reactions 53, **54**
acids 53–59
  amino acids as 86
  excretion 135
actin 237
action potentials 124, 235–237
  heart muscle 194
activated oxygen 43
active transport 125
  renal tubules 192
acute phase reactants 333
adenohypophysis 287–288
adenosine triphosphate (ATP) **91**
adequate intakes, dietary 93
adjuvant chemotherapy 308
administration *see* routes of administration
adrenal gland 291
adrenaline (epinephrine) 240, 244–245

adrenocorticotrophic hormone
  (ACTH) 288
adrenoreceptors 244
  beta-adrenoreceptors 198–199
aflatoxins 326
agar 69
agarose 69
aglycones 181, **184**
agonists 140
alanine aminotransferase (ALT) 335, **339**
albumin 336, **340**
alcohol
  abuse, on gastrointestinal tract 120
  on iron absorption 97
  on liver 45
  warfarin and 214
alcohol functional group **30**
aldehyde functional group **30**
aldosterone **196**, 198, 200
alginates 69
alkaline phosphatase 335, **339**
alkaloids 175, 176–180
  for chemotherapy 310
  isomerism 39
  monoamine oxidase inhibitors and 263
  muscarinic receptor binders 240
alkylating agents
  chemotherapy 309–310
  for immunosuppression 232, 233
allergic rhinitis 268
allergies 225, 267–268
  nuts 317
allopurinol 295
aloe emodin **184**
alpha-adrenoceptor antagonists 282
alpha 1-antitrypsin, cigarette smoke on 45
alpha helix 83, **84**
alpha linolenic acid 75, **76**, 78
5-alpha-reductase drugs 282
alpha sugars 66
alpha tocopherol (vitamin E) 49–50,
  107–108
  ascorbic acid with 47
aluminium 325–326
  antacids 275
Alzheimer's disease
  glutamate 241
  muscarinic receptors 246

amine(s) 175
  epilepsy 255
amine alkaloids 177
  monoamine oxidase inhibitors and 263
amine functional group **30**
  amino acids 86
amino acids 81–82, 86–87
  alkaloids from 177
  dipole moments 16
  hydrolysis **26**
  sulphur-containing, free radicals on 45
aminoglycosides 219–220
aminosalicylates 279
amitriptyline 263
amlodipine 199
amphetamines **242**, 243, 244, 245
amphipathic substances 25
amygdalin 184
anaemias 209–211
  copper deficiency 98
  iron deficiency 209–210, 333
  pernicious anaemia 105, 210
analgesics 247–254
  alkaloids, examples 180
  NSAIs as 231
angina 200–202
angiotensin II 192
  see also renin–angiotensin system
angiotensin-converting enzyme
    inhibitors 200
  captopril **196**
  on renin–angiotensin system 197
animal tests 320–321
antacids 275
antagonists 140
  adrenoceptors 282
    see also beta-blockers
  histamine receptors 106, 268,
    275–276
  opioid receptors 252–253
anthocyanidins 161, 163
anthocyanins 161
anthraquinones 153–154, 182, **184**
anthrones 154, 182
anti-inflammatory agents 230–232
  flavonoids as 158
  see also corticosteroids; non-steroidal
    anti-inflammatories

Printed in the United States
By Bookmasters